ANIMAL BREEDING AND INFERTILITY

ANIMAL BREEDING AND INFERTILITY

Edited by
Michael J Meredith

Blackwell
Science

© 1995 by
Blackwell Science Ltd
Editorial Offices:
Osney Mead, Oxford OX2 0EL
25 John Street, London WC1N 2BL
23 Ainslie Place, Edinburgh EH3 6AJ
238 Main Street, Cambridge
  Massachusetts 02142, USA
54 University Street, Carlton,
  Victoria 3053, Australia

Other Editorial Offices:
Arnette Blackwell SA
  1, rue de Lille, 75007 Paris
  France

Blackwell Wissenschafts-Verlag GmbH
  Kurfürstendamm 57
  10707 Berlin, Germany

  Feldgasse 13, A-1238 Wien
  Austria

First published 1995

Set in 10.5/12.5pt Plantin
by Land & Unwin (Data Sciences) Ltd
Bugbrooke, Northamptonshire
Printed and bound in Great Britain by
Hartnolls Ltd, Bodmin, Cornwall

DISTRIBUTORS

Marston Book Services Ltd
PO Box 87
Oxford OX2 0DT
(*Orders:* Tel: 01865 791155
          Fax: 01865 791927
          Telex: 837515)

USA
  Blackwell Science, Inc.
  238 Main Street
  Cambridge, MA 02142
  (*Orders:* Tel: 800 215-1000
             617 876-7000
      Fax: 617 492-5263)

Canada
  Oxford University Press
  70 Wynford Drive
  Don Mills
  Ontario M3C 1J9
  (*Orders:* Tel: 416 441-2941)

Australia
  Blackwell Science Pty Ltd
  54 University Street
  Carlton, Victoria 3053
  (*Orders:* Tel: 03 347-5552)

A catalogue record for this book is
available from the British Library

ISBN 0–632–04038–6

Library of Congress
Cataloging-in-Publication Data
  is available

CONTENTS

Contents

Contents

PREFACE

Another book on breeding management and infertility?

While teaching and speaking on these subjects, both at home and abroad, I am constantly asked to recommend a suitable textbook and reference source for farm animal and/or equine reproduction. I have had to respond with an unduly long reading list, some of which is rather out of date for this fast-moving subject area. Now at last I can recommend a single, comprehensive, up to date and authoritative learning and reference source!

Locating information quickly

Busy professionals often need to access information quickly, so this book has been particularly designed to give a choice of two strategies for doing this:

a) searching the (very extensive!) index for relevant keywords
b) locating the appropriate chapter, then browsing the headings and/or the boxed checklists of information.

Conventions used

For simplicity, the individual gender terms 'he' or 'she' are used non-specifically in the text; these are intended to be interchangeable.

Dating of the oestrous cycle or pregacy, unless otherwise specified, is based on *the first day of detected oestrus*, or *the first day of mating*, being day 0. This difference in dating the reproductive stage of mated and unmated animals can be quite significant, particularly in the mare. For post-parturient animals, day 0 is the day of parturition.

The spelling of *oestrus* follows the usual convention of have a *-us* ending when it is a noun and a *-ous* ending when it is an adjective. The corresponding US English terms are *estrus* and *estrous*.

References

The book is not intended to be a comprehensive literature review, but provides details of key publications which are intended to provide a route into the relevant specialist literature. The references are aggregated at the end of the book.

Errors and Suggestions

If you should locate any errors, or have any suggestions for improvement of the content of this book, I will be happy to acknowledge your help when an update of this material becomes necessary. Please communicate suggestions to Dr MJ Meredith, Department of Clinical Veterinary Medicine, University of Cambridge, Madingley Road, Cambridge, CB3 0ES, UK. [Electronic Mail:mjm10@hermes.cam.ac.uk].

Sources of further information (including current legislation, training and codes of practice)

American College of Theriogenologists, Dr Dickson Varner, Texas Veterinary Medical Centre, Texas A & M University, College Station, TX 77843, USA.

Ibero American Association for Animal Reproduction, Prof. Felix Perez y Perez, Facultad de Veterinaria, Universidad Complutense, 28004 Madrid, Spain.

International Congress on Animal Reproduction, Dept. of Obstetrics and Gynaecology, Box 7039, Swedish University of Agricultural Sciences, S-750 07 Uppsala, Sweden.

International Embryo Transfer Society, Carl Johnson, Business Manager, 309 W. Clark Street, Champaign, IL 61820, USA.

Ministries of Agriculture and State Veterinary Services of individual countries.

Society for the Study of Animal Breeding (and European AI Vets Organization), c/o British Veterinary Association, 7 Mansfield Street, London, W1M OAT.

Unit for Veterinary Legislation and Zootechnics, European Commission, Rue de la Loi 200, Brussels, Belgium.

Disclaimer

The information contained herein has been obtained or is based upon sources believed by us to be reliable but is not guaranteed as to accuracy or completeness. The information is supplied without obligation and on the understanding that any person who acts upon it or otherwise changes his/her position in reliance thereon does so entirely at his/her risk. It is recommended that breeders obtain on-site advice from a veterinarian or other animal breeding specialist who can consider their individual situation.

Michael J. Meredith
February 1995

ACKNOWLEDGEMENTS

I would like to thank the following experts who contributed valuable comments on various sections of this book: Dr. Mike K. Curran, Wye College, University of London; Dr. Peter G.G. Jackson, University of Cambridge; Dr. Jane M. Morrell, National Institute for Medical Research, London; Simone Knudsen, University of Cambridge. Thanks also go to the following who contributed greatly to the production of the manuscript: Linda Notton, Dianne Styles, The Photographic Department of the Institute of Animal Physiology and Genetics Research. The Longman Higher Education editorial staff have been patient, persistent and indefatigable in guiding this book through its gestation period. I would particularly like to acknowledge the hard work of the Publisher, Alex Seabrook and the Senior Editor, Jo Whelan. Finally I would like to thank one of my graduate students, Allie D. Buckle, for her skilled and painstaking help with the indexing.

Michael Meredith

We are indebted to the following for permission to reproduce copyright material:

Oxford University Press for Figs. 1.1 (Nicholas 1987) and 9.6 (ND Allen et al., in Mammalian Development: a Practical Approach (M Monk, Ed.), IRL Press Ltd, by permission of Oxford Univerity Press); C Whittemore for Figs. 7.1 and 7.3 (Whittemore 1993); Blackwell Wissenschafts-Verlag for Fig. 7.2 (Anat. Histol. Embryol. 2, 29, 1973); Journal of Reproduction and Fertility for Fig. 7.5 (Love et al. 1993) and Fig. 8.5 (Wilmut et al. 1985); F.A. Eales and J. Small for Tables 8.22.

Whilst every effort has been made to trace the owners of copyright material, in a few cases this has proved impossible and we take this opportunity to offer our apologies to any copyright holders whose rights we may unwittingly have infringed.

LIST OF CONTRIBUTORS

Katherine Bretzlaff, DVM, PhD
The Texas Veterinary Medical Center, Texas A&M University, USA

Hilary Dobson, BSc, PhD
Department of Veterinary Clinical Science and Animal Husbandry, University of Liverpool, UK

Patrick J Hartigan, MA, BSc (Vet), MVM, PhD, MRCVS
Department of Physiology, Trinity College, Dublin, Ireland

Susan E Long, BVMS, PhD, MRCVS
Department of Clinical Veterinary Science, University of Bristol, UK

Michael J Meredith, MA, BSc, BVetMed, PhD, MRCVS
Department of Clinical Veterinary Medicine, University of Cambridge, UK

Heather G Pidduck, BSc, PhD
Department of Farm Animal and Equine Medicine and Surgery, The Royal Veterinary College, UK

Don Powell, PhD
Institute of Animal Physiology and Genetics Research, Cambridge, UK

Sarah J Stoneham, BVSc, CertESM, MRCVS
Beaufort Cottage Stables, Newmarket, UK

Huw Ll. Williams, PhD, FRAgS, Hon. Assoc. RCVS
Emeritus reader in Animal Husbandry, Department of
Farm Animal and Equine Medicine and Surgery, The
Royal Veterinary College, UK

Ian Wilmut, PhD
The Roslin Institute, UK

Bird, beast and fish, the female and the male,
In flocks, in herds, in shoals and schools relating,
Hunters and hunted, – eating, sleeping, mating,
Something they lack!
By wood, hill, stream, and dale,
The Dark Blue Buddha shows an open book,
Jewel-charactered on leaves of burnished gold.
Behold the treasure of communication,
Treasure of knowledge, ne'er to be forsook:
Deeds of great heroes, thoughts of sages old,
Bequeathed to man's remotest generation!

From *The Realms of Existence*, by Sangharakshita

1 GENETIC CONSIDERATIONS IN ANIMAL BREEDING
H.G. PIDDUCK BSc, PhD

The aims of animal breeding
Methods of identification of the best breeding stock
Choice of breeding method
Chapter summary and future prospects in animal breeding

The aims of animal breeding

Introduction

Domesticated farm animals are bred with the aim of improving the quality and quantity of marketable products including replacement breeding stock, milk and its components and carcasses for the meat trade. Whatever the species, it is very important to have the breeding aims carefully set out. These aims must be formulated against a knowledge of economic circumstances, biological limitations and genetic theory.

Economic circumstances can and do change. For example, in the 1960s and 1970s dairy cattle breeders in the UK concentrated their efforts into maximizing the yield of milk from their herds through selective breeding and feeding for yield. The consequent over-production of milk was limited by quota in 1984. Since then breeding and management have been primarily for fat and protein yield reflecting the changed economic climate in the dairy industry.

Biological limitations are undefined for most characteristics in most species, although a slowing in response to the selection process may indicate an approaching biological limit. Limits to extremes of body size are known in some species because of associated reproductive difficulties. Classic examples are found in some breeds of poultry and miniature dogs. In the turkey, the ability of the male to mate sets an upper limit to its body size and weight. Beyond this limit artificial insemination must be used. In some miniature breeds of dog there appears to be a lower weight or size below which females cannot reproduce because oestrus is irregular or absent.

A thorough knowledge of genetic theory is essential before aims can be formulated. Characteristics differ in their mode and degree of genetic control and it is these and other considerations which determine the likely outcome of selective breeding.

Genetic theory

The characteristics in which the animal breeder is interested range, in terms of their genetic determination, from those controlled by single Mendelian genes to those under the control of many genes, polygenes.

All genes are composed of deoxyribonucleic acid (DNA). In almost all types of genetic determination these genes are chromosomal (mitochondrial DNA also controls inherited characteristics but this represents only a very small fraction of total DNA). The genetic code is essentially the same across all living organisms, with the same specific triplets of purine and pyrimidine bases coding for each particular amino acid. Different organisms differ in their chromosome number and in the particular gene assortment carried by each chromosome. Within a species the chromosome number is constant along with its gene array, but subtle variation in base sequences creates varied gene products, which in turn result in variation in metabolic processes and physiology and their quantifiable endpoints. The base sequence variation in genes means that they can exist in different allelic forms or alleles. An individual animal, being diploid, i.e. having each chromosome represented twice, can have identical alleles at a chromosomal location or locus, or can have two different alleles. If the alleles are identical, the individual's genotype is homozygous, if non-identical, heterozygous. When an animal breeds it produces haploid gametes each containing just one representative of each chromosome pair. Thus heterozygosity creates genetic variation between gametes and the opportunity for new allelic combinations at fertilization.

Characteristics controlled by single genes typically exhibit a limited number of manifestations or phenotypes. The presence or absence of horns in cattle provides a good example. The phenotype can be horned or polled (without horns). Two alternative allelic forms of the gene *P*, alleles *P* and *p*, are responsible for these phenotypes. Homozygous *PP* and heterozygous *Pp* individuals are polled and homozygous *pp* animals are horned. Polled is said to be dominant to horned, and horned is recessive to polled. Polled cattle therefore may or may not be true breeding whereas horned cattle always are. Not all single-gene controlled characteristics show this dominant/recessive behaviour; in some cases the heterozygote may be distinguishable from or intermediate between both homozygotes. In this case co-dominance or no dominance exists.

Single-gene controlled characteristics with clearly defined phenotypes are relatively easy for the animal breeder to manipulate. Many aspects of coat colour and coat type are inherited in this way and provide the raw material for selection. The tremendous variety of coat in the present-day domestic dog and cat demonstrates how successful selection has been. Many diseases and abnormalities are the result of rare recessive deleterious alleles that manifest their effect in the homozygous condition. Examples are susceptibility to K88-positive *Escherichia coli* infection in piglets and bovine leucocyte adhesion deficiency (BLAD).

Characteristics controlled by many genes are generally those of most importance and interest to the animal breeder. These characteristics tend to be quantitative in their expression and their control is environmental in addition to genetic. They may be called multifactorial traits. The quantitative nature of these traits means that animals cannot be grouped into discrete categories, such as low and high yielding dairy cows; most individuals have values around the mean with progressively fewer towards the two extremes of the distribution (Figure 1.1). Other characteristics in dairy cattle that show quantitative variation are milk protein and milk

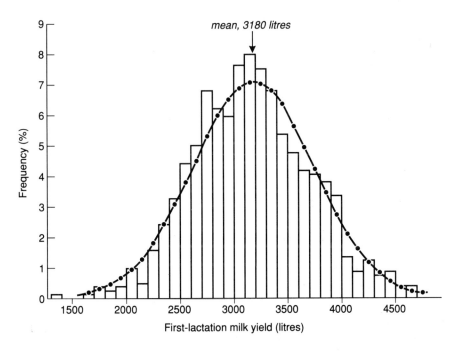

Figure 1.1 Frequency distribution of milk yield in Friesian cows. The histogram shows the first-lactation milk yield in a population of 840 Friesian cows. The mean yield is indicated, 3180 litres, and the variance is 315, 352 litres. A normal distribution with this mean and variance is superimposed in the figure (from Nicholas 1987).

butterfat, birth weight and weaning weight, and conformation traits such as the depth and support of the udder. Additionally, susceptibility of livestock to diseases, such as mastitis in dairy cattle and footrot in sheep, are examples of multifactorial traits. The phenotype that an individual animal displays is a result of its genotype plus the positive and negative effects of a variety of non-genetic influences. The variation in phenotype displayed by a population of animals arises from the combined effects of individual genotypes and non-genetic effects experienced by the animals. In other words the phenotypic variance (V_P) of a population for a quantitative trait has both genetic and non-genetic components. Taking milk yield of dairy cows as an example (see Figure 1.1), likely genetic effects include genes influencing body size, appetite, udder capacity and circulating levels of appropriate hormones. Allelic variation in these and other contributing genes collectively make up the genetic component (genetic variance, V_G) of the phenotypic variance. The sources of non-genetic variation might include differences between individuals in grazing, level of concentrates consumed, and bacterial infections of the udder. Collectively, these non-genetic sources of variation make up the environmental variance, V_E. The environmental variance can be subdivided into a general and a common component (V_{Eg} and V_{Ec}, respectively). V_{Eg} arises from aspects of the environment that are randomly distributed between individuals. V_{Ec} arises from environmental factors that are shared between specific pairs or groups of individuals, such as contemporary full siblings (e.g. piglet litter mates) sharing the same uterine and preweaning environment.

Thus, $V_P = V_G + V_{Eg} + V_{Ec}$
or, more simply, $V_P = V_G + V_E$

Quantitative traits differ in the relative proportions of V_G and V_E. The ratio V_G/V_P gives a parameter known as the degree of genetic determination, or broad sense heritability. A more useful statistic is narrow sense heritability (h^2), which is the proportion of the phenotypic variance that is amenable to selection and represents that fraction of V_G which is useful to the animal breeder. Thus, V_G has three main components distinguished by the effects of the contributing genes: V_A, additive variance; V_I, interaction (epistatic) variance; and V_D, dominance variance.

Additive variance arises from alleles whose contribution to the variance is additive and independent of other genes. In other words, an allele contributing to additive variance exerts its particular quantitative effect whatever its allelic partner at that locus and whatever alleles are present at other loci. Its effect is therefore repeatable from one generation to the next.

Interaction variance arises from alleles whose effects vary according to allelic combinations at other loci (epistasis). Therefore an allele contributing to V_I can change its quantitative effect from one generation to the next when it is likely to be recombined with a different assortment of genes.

Dominance variance arises from alleles whose effects depend upon the allele with which they are partnered at a locus. The contribution of such genes to genetic variance thus varies from one generation to the next as allelic pairings change.

In view of the above, the narrow sense heritability, which is the proportion of V_G that is predictable and amenable to selection, is based on V_A, i.e. $h^2 = V_A/V_P$. The difference between broad sense and narrow sense heritability should now be clear. Because broad sense heritability includes V_I and V_D in addition to V_A it gives an upper limit to narrow sense heritability, the difference reflecting the sum of V_I and V_D. In this text, in common with most others, the term heritability is used to mean narrow sense heritability unless indicated otherwise. By definition, heritability depends on variation. Thus, if all additive genes contributing to a characteristic become fixed, i.e. each gene becomes homozygous for a particular allelic form, and all animals in the population are genetically identical for these loci, there is no V_A left and the heritability becomes zero. This means that further selection will be ineffective as there is no useful variation left to exploit. It is important to note, therefore, that a very low or zero heritability does not mean that a characteristic is not under any genetic control. It simply means, as explained above, that there is no usable genetic variation (V_A) and, if improvement is sought, crossbreeding might be considered. A heritability estimate is a figure that relates to a specific trait at a specific time in a specific population of animals, such as a herd or a flock, because the variances upon which it is based are parameters derived from that population.

The estimation of heritability and typical values

Methods of estimating heritability are based on evaluating V_A as a proportion of V_P. Most methods depend upon analysing the phenotypic resemblance between relatives using regression, correlation or the analysis of variance. Interested readers are referred to Falconer (1989) and Becker (1984). Selection experiments can also be used to estimate heritability. Figure 1.2 illustrates the principles of this method. In the example shown, the selection is carried out by choosing the best 20% of the parental population as parents to breed the offspring generation. The response to selection is used to calculate the heritability, where $h^2 = R/S$. R is the response to selection; S is the selection differential, which is the difference between the selected parents and the mean of the population from which they are drawn. The relationship $h^2 = R/S$ can be rewritten as $R = h^2S$, thus providing a useful guide to expected response to planned selection for a

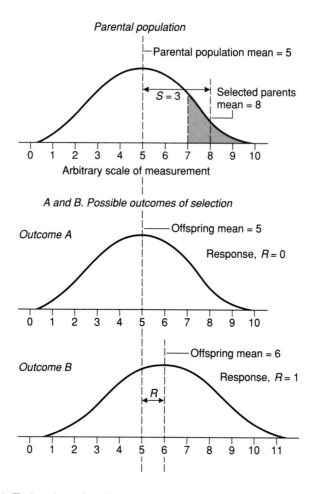

Figure 1.2 Estimation of realized heritability from the response to selection. The parental population mean is 5 units. The top 20% are chosen as parents of the next generation; their mean is 8 units, giving a selection differential, $S=8-5=3$. In Outcome A the offspring mean is 5, response is 0, i.e. $h^2 =R/S =0$. In Outcome B the offspring mean is 6, response is 1, i.e. $h^2= R/S=0.33$.

characteristic whose heritability is known. In general, the higher the heritability, the greater the response, and vice versa. Table 1.1 lists some important characteristics in livestock and some representative heritability values from various studies. Values below 0.2 might be referred to as low, 0.2–0.4 as medium, and greater than 0.4, high. In general it can be seen that production and growth traits of mature livestock have the highest heritabilities in contrast to biological fitness traits, such as reproductive performance and neonatal survival, with the lowest values. As a conse-

Table 1.1 Representative heritability values of various traits in cattle, sheep and pigs

Species, breed and traits	Heritability	Reference
Dairy cattle: Friesian/Holstein		
Milk yield	0.31, 0.47	MMB (1983), Brotherstone (1994)
Butterfat yield	0.31, 0.52	MMB (1983), Brotherstone (1994)
Protein yield	0.31, 0.45	MMB (1983), Brotherstone (1994)
Butterfat %	0.40, 0.72	MMB (1983), Brotherstone (1994)
Protein %	0.44, 0.64	MMB (1983), Brotherstone (1994)
Fore udder attachment	0.20, 0.29, 0.27	MMB (1986), Meyer *et al.* (1987), Brotherstone (1994)
Udder support	0.16, 0.16, 0.16	MMB (1986), Meyer *et al.* (1987), Brotherstone (1994)
Udder depth	0.29, 0.33, 0.39	MMB (1986), Meyer *et al.* (1987), Brotherstone (1994)
Beef cattle: various breeds		
Birth weight	0.42* (149)	Simm *et al.* (1986)
Growth rate	0.41* (354)	Simm *et al.* (1986)
Feed conversion efficiency	0.42* (45)	Simm *et al.* (1986)
Carcass lean proportion	0.39* (14)	Simm *et al.* (1986)
Days to slaughter	0.33	B. McGuirk (personal communication, 1993)
Killing out %	0.38	B. McGuirk (personal communication, 1993)
Eye muscle area	0.25	B. McGuirk (personal communication, 1993)
Sheep		
Scottish Blackface		
Fertility	0	Atkins (1986)
Lamb survival	0	Atkins (1986)
Litter size	0.12	Atkins (1986)
Various breeds		
Birth weight	0.28*	Parrat and Simm (1987)
Growth rate	0.20*	Parrat and Simm (1987)
Carcass lean proportion	0.35*	Parrat and Simm (1987)
Pigs: Large White and Landrace		
Litter size	0.05–0.13	Bichard and David (1985)
Ovulation rate	0.45	Johnson *et al.* (1985)
Daily gain	0.41, 0.41, 0.33	Smith and King (1962), Smith and Ross (1965), Gu *et al.* (1989)
Feed conversion efficiency	0.54, 0.48	Smith and King (1962), Smith and Ross (1965)
Fat depth (C)	0.65, 0.62, 0.41	Smith and King (1962), Smith and Ross (1965), Gu *et al.* (1989)

*Averages of many estimates. Figures in parentheses, where given, indicate the number of estimates contributing to the average.

quence, the former are generally amenable to change through classical selection procedures, whereas the latter require more elaborate strategies when attempting improvement.

Selection in practice

Selective breeding is carried out by mating together those animals whose superiority is most likely to be passed to their offspring. Essentially, this means mating the best males with the best females for the characteristic(s) one is trying to change. Depending on the species, the intensity of selection, which is related to the proportion of the population selected, may be very different in males and females. For example, in dairy cattle, a considerable proportion of adult females may be required for breeding herd replacements each generation, so there is little scope for selection. On the male side, very high intensities of selection can be achieved using artificial insemination. The choice of characteristics is influenced by their heritabilities and the practicalities of obtaining the necessary data. Some characteristics are more easily measured than others, e.g. feed conversion efficiency involves measuring an individual's daily feed intake as well as its weight gain, whereas a single weight such as weaning weight is intrinsically far simpler to obtain.

The number of traits under selection must also be considered. It is likely that improvement will be desired in more than one trait, and the most suitable approach must be chosen. Changing economic circumstances may encourage alternating periods of selection on different traits. For example, in intensively reared pigs, growth rate improvement might be pursued for some generations and then attention might be switched to feed conversion efficiency. Alternate selection for traits is known as tandem selection. As each trait is selected it responds, but when the selection pressure is relaxed on one trait in favour of the other(s) the response to the first trait changes. It may slow, stop or even reverse. This is because of genetic correlation, which results from quantitative traits sometimes sharing a proportion of their genetic determination. The degree of correlation reflects the extent of their shared genes. The correlation can be positive, when selection for one trait results in both responding in the same direction, or negative when the response of the two is in opposite directions. Table 1.2 gives some genetic correlations between traits in dairy cattle. Disadvantageous genetic correlations can sometimes be overcome by considering all traits of interest at the same time through one of two selection methods, independent culling levels or index selection. Independent culling levels can be set such that every animal chosen for breeding must reach a certain predetermined standard for each trait under consideration. Some exceptional individuals will therefore not be chosen for

Table 1.2 Estimates of genetic correlation in dairy cattle

	Milk (kg)	Fat (kg)	Protein (kg)	Fat (%)	Protein (%)	Reference
Milk (kg)		0.82	0.87	−0.27	−0.18	Gibson (1987)
Fat (kg)			0.86	0.26	−0.11	Gibson (1987)
Protein (kg)				0.04	0.22	Gibson (1987)
Fat (%)					0.55	Gibson (1987)
FUA	0.37	−0.14	−0.29	0.29	0.25	Meyer *et al.* (1987)
US	0.07	0.11	0.16	0.05	0.17	Meyer *et al.* (1987)
UD	−0.52	−0.23	−0.39	0.32	0.27	Meyer *et al.* (1987)

FUA (fore udder attachment), US (udder support) and UD (udder depth) are all linearly assessed from 1 to 9 as follows: FUA (weak, 1 to strong, 9); US (broken, 1 to strong, 9); UD (deep, 1 to shallow, 9). A positive correlation between one of the above udder conformational traits and a production trait is therefore favourable, but a negative correlation is unfavourable.

breeding even if they reach a very high standard in one trait but just fail to make the standard for another. Valuable genetic material may therefore be lost. A system that allows a degree of compensation between traits is index selection. In this method, animals are assessed for each trait and the measured value is weighted according to parameters such as the heritability and economic value of the trait. The figures are combined to give a total index score for each animal. Choice of breeding stock is then made according to scores achieved. Most commercial livestock breeding uses multitrait index selection.

There is a relationship between the number of traits and the effectiveness of selection: the greater the number of traits, the slower will be the individual response of the traits to selection. When considering which method to employ, index selection will give the greatest overall response to selection and tandem selection the least, but choice of method will also be influenced by practical management considerations. Any improvement is, of course, limited by generation time, so the earlier that measurements can be made, and breeding commence, the better.

Traits that are difficult to manipulate

Characteristics may be difficult to improve for a variety of reasons: heritability may be low (e.g. litter size), or the characteristic may only be expressed in one sex (e.g. litter size, milk yield) or only be measurable late in life (e.g. lifetime productivity, longevity) or only after slaughter (e.g. carcass traits). Various aids to selection are available in such cases. Low heritability traits concerned with reproductive performance, e.g. litter size in pigs and sheep, are notoriously difficult to manipulate. Not only is heritability low but the measurement is sex-limited to the female, and, in the case of sheep, whatever the underlying genetic control (see later) the phenotypic expression is limited to a narrow range of zero, one, two or exceptionally three or more lambs per ewe per season. Repeated measurements over the first two or three lambings are useful because the accuracy of assessing genetic capacity is improved with repeated assessment. This means, however, that choosing replacement breeders takes longer and consequently extends the generation time.

The measurement of component traits is another approach. Taking pigs as an example, the major components of 'the number of piglets reared per sow per year' are:

1. Mainly dam components:
    (a) rebreeding interval,
    (b) ovulation rate,
    (c) uterine capacity,
    (d) embryo/foetal loss,
    (e) mothering ability.
2. Mainly piglet components:
    (a) neonatal survival,
    (b) weaning weight.
3. Sire components:
    (a) sperm quality,
    (b) sperm quantity.

Most of the above are difficult to measure and of low or very low heritability. Attention has focused on ovulation rate because of its useful heritability (see Table 1.1) and relatively large phenotypic variance. Selection based on ovulation rate, measured at laparoscopy, is successful in increasing ovulation rate in pigs, but gestational losses rise to counteract the gain, so there is little net increase in the number of piglets born (Johnson et al. 1985). Unexpectedly, single genes seem to play a role in the reproductive performance of some species. A strain of Australian Merino sheep has been identified, the Booroola strain, in which a single fecundity gene can significantly augment ovulation rate. The normal 'wild type' variant is denoted +, and the fecundity variant, F. Homozygous FF ewes show a mean ovulation rate of over 4, compared with F+ at about 2.7 and ++ at 1.4. These differences are reflected in different mean litter sizes in the three genotypes of about 2.5, 2.2 and 1.4 respectively (Piper et al. 1985). Other sheep breeds have also been reported to have similar fecundity genes.

Another approach to female sex-limited characteristics with low heritability is the use of correlated or predictor traits. There is some evidence in sheep that future reproductive performance of ewe lambs is correlated with the testis size of their male siblings. However, results of selection based upon this association are confounded by a correlated response of decreasing body weight (Lee and Land 1985).

Characteristics that are only measurable late in life or after slaughter are most usually assessed on closely related animals. For late-in-life traits, often the only guide is information from the sire and dam, but this is of limited use. For characteristics assessed after slaughter, i.e. carcass traits, some information may be predicted from examination of the live animal, e.g. fat depth assessed with ultrasound. More detailed carcass assessment is obtained from slaughtered progeny or siblings.

Genotype–environment interaction

It is most important that selection is carried out in the environment appropriate to normal livestock rearing. This ensures that the selected genotype is adapted to that environment. A good example of how not to proceed is to develop an improved strain of livestock in a temperate climate and then transfer it to a tropical climate. Any improvement gained in production traits is likely to be offset by the animals' lack of adaptation to the climate.

Methods of identification of the best breeding stock

Introduction

The best breeding stock are those animals that are best able to transmit to their progeny the desired traits at the highest level. In other words, the best breeding stock are those animals with the highest breeding value (BV), which can be defined as the value of an animal judged by the mean value of its progeny. It is a property of an individual with reference to the population to which it belongs. It can be expressed in absolute units or, more usefully, as a deviation from the population mean. An example in dairy cattle is given by the following. Consider a population of dairy cows made up of daughters of a large number of sires. The population average for milk yield is 5000 kg. The daughters of two particular sires, sire A and sire B, within the population, average 5300 kg and 4950 kg respectively.

The deviation from the mean for sire A's daughters is therefore +300 kg and for sire B's daughters is −50 kg. The BV of a sire is given by twice the average deviation of its offspring from the population mean. Therefore BV of sire A = + 600 kg and BV of sire B = −100 kg.

The reason for multiplying the deviation by two is that a sire only transmits one-half of his genes to each offspring, so multiplying by two gives his entire genetic merit for that characteristic; it must be remembered, however, that only half his merit, i.e. ½ BV, is passed on.

True BV can only be obtained through assessing progeny merit, which is very time-consuming and expensive, so various indirect methods of estimating BV are employed. Estimated breeding value (EBV) is obtained from the individual's own merit or from records of its siblings or ancestors. Breeding value assessment (true or estimated) is more often made for males than females because of the far greater numbers of progeny left by individual males especially in species bred using artificial insemination (AI).

Methods of assessing real and estimated BV

Methods of assessing BV vary in suitability according to many factors including the heritabilities and ease of measurement of the characteristics. Assessment can be through progeny testing, sibling testing, individual performance testing and pedigree (ancestor) evaluation. Progeny testing is the most versatile and reliable method whereas estimating BV from ancestors is the least useful. Sibling and individual performance testing are intermediate in usefulness, the reliability of sibling testing increasing as sibling numbers rise. Whatever method is used, the primary aim should be to make assessment as early as possible in an animal's adult life, and, if feasible, to make repeated measurements of the characteristic (e.g. successive lactations) to increase accuracy, if this is compatible with the primary aim.

Statistical analysis of data for BV assessment is very complex as an individual animal's assessment arises from information from many related animals recorded in different environments, seasons and even years. Correction factors therefore need to be applied to take account of all these variables and their interactions. The statistical procedure used is the so-called best linear unbiased prediction (BLUP) and gives the BV or EBV of the animal from all the available and corrected data. Most recent developments of BLUP technology utilize computer-stored relationships of all recorded animals, thus providing genetic links that enable even more accurate BV assessments to be computed. This is known as individual animal model (IAM) methodology. IAM BLUP is applicable to any records of appropriate individuals provided correction factors and genetic relationships are known. It enables the valid comparison of BVs of sires born in different years taking into account all the measured environmental and genetic trends that occur.

An outline of the main methods of BV assessment follows.

Progeny testing

Progeny testing gives true BV. Potential sires are each mated (through AI) with a large number of unselected females and their progeny are reared in contemporary groups ensuring that any environmental differences are randomized. The characteristics of interest are measured at the appropriate stage of the animals' lives and each sire's BV is calculated. Progeny testing has particular application to assessment of BV for female sex-limited traits and carcass-limited traits in primarily monotocous livestock species. Progeny testing gives an increasingly accurate assessment of BV as the numbers of progeny and the heritabilities of the traits rise. It is this accuracy that is a major justification for the use of progeny testing in dairy and beef cattle, where each AI sire has the potential to leave a very large number of offspring. The major drawback to progeny testing in cattle is the time it takes coupled with the long generation interval. Consequently, proven (high BV) bulls are not in widespread use until they are over 6 years old, thus limiting the rate of genetic progress.

Individual performance testing

Individual performance testing is the evaluation of an individual (usually male) through its own performance to give its EBV. Characteristics most suitable for assessment through individual performance testing are those of medium to high heritability whose measurements can be completed by the time the animal reaches breeding age. Examples are rate of growth, feed conversion efficiency and weight at a specific age (e.g. 400-day weight in beef cattle). Characteristics that are sex-limited to the female or carcass-limited cannot be assessed by individual performance testing of the male. Breeding value estimated through individual performance testing is quick, relatively inexpensive and convenient. A comparison of individual performance testing and progeny testing (Table 1.3) shows that for low heritability traits, progeny testing with as few as 10 progeny gives a far more accurate result than performance testing, but for traits with heritability of 0.6 or more, performance testing gives comparable accuracy to progeny testing based on 10 progeny. At intermediate heritability values a performance test may suffice depending on the accuracy required. The accuracy of individual performance testing can be improved by back-up

Table 1.3 A comparison of the accuracy (0, minimum to 1, maximum) of individual performance testing and progeny testing in estimating breeding value (data from the Beef Improvement Federation, quoted by Lewis 1979)

Heritability	Performance test	Progeny test with			
		10 calves	20 calves	40 calves	80 calves
0.2	0.45	0.58	0.72	0.82	0.90
0.4	0.63	0.73	0.83	0.91	0.95
0.6	0.78	0.80	0.88	0.94	0.97

information from siblings or ancestors. Alternatively, animals with promising performance tests can then be progeny tested.

Sibling testing

Until the 1980s, sibling testing only found application in polytocous species such as pigs where individuals normally have a useful number of contemporary full siblings. The use of siblings for testing is well suited to medium to high heritability characteristics that are female sex-limited or carcass-limited. Thus EBV of boars for meat traits such as muscle area and lean percentage can be assessed through their male or female siblings. Sibling testing in cattle has become a practical proposition since the development of reliable multiple ovulation and embryo transfer (MOET) techniques. Matings can be made between selected superior females and proven sires to generate full sibling families. In order to do this, the breeding female is induced to superovulate and usually artificially inseminated and then the resulting conceptuses are removed and transferred to individual synchronized foster mothers. One superovulated cow may produce 10–20 embryos through a single treatment and the resulting mixed-sex full sibling group can be reared for testing and breeding as required. For dairy bull evaluation, the resulting female siblings can be assessed for lactational performance and dairy conformation; male siblings that are not intended for eventual breeding can be assessed for carcass traits and other beefing qualities.

A system of MOET assesses EBV of a bull far quicker than progeny testing. When MOET is used in cattle, the average generation interval is reduced to about 3.7 years compared with about 6.3 years for assessment through progeny testing. Despite the lower accuracy of sibling testing compared with progeny testing, a large-scale MOET scheme can achieve a rate of genetic improvement that is 30% greater than a large progeny testing scheme (Nicholas and Smith 1983). There are reservations regarding some forms of sibling testing because of the confounding effects of maternal environment. Siblings can be of three types:

1. Natural full-sibs, e.g. piglet litter mates, lamb twins/triplets, twin calves.
2. Natural half-sibs, e.g. piglets/lambs/calves of different dams but sharing a common sire.
3. MOET full- and half-sibs, e.g. full and half siblings of any species transferred as embryos from the genetic female parent to a foster mother.

The use of natural full siblings (type 1) for BV assessment is complicated by their common prenatal (uterine) and preweaning maternal environment (V_{Ec}, see p. 4). Accordingly the BV of an animal based on its own merit and the merit of its natural full siblings will reflect genotypic merit and the common environment, however good or bad, experienced by the whole sibling group. For example, a poor environment will give a misleadingly low estimate of BV. The problem does not arise with natural half-sibs (type 2) or embryo transfer full- or half-sibs (type 3), because it is likely that any differences in maternal environment are randomized.

Ancestor evaluation

Ancestor evaluation and pedigree selection are both terms used to describe the assessment of an individual's EBV from records on ancestors. This method finds limited application for various reasons: the number of close ancestors is limited to two parents and four grandparents, different generations experience different environments, and assessment depends on accurate past records being available. However, the evaluation of parents does provide a useful guide to an individual's subsequent BV but it needs additional evaluation through progeny or siblings. For late manifesting traits (e.g. longevity) and repeated measurements (e.g. successive lactations) parental records are the only indication of a young animal's subsequent performance.

Methods used in commercial livestock production

Dairy cattle

Income from dairy farming in the UK is derived from both milk and beef sales. The most important characteristics are protein and butterfat content of milk, dairy conformational traits related to production and health such as udder, teat and foot conformation, and beef quality. Most of the traits have useful heritabilities (see Table 1.1). Genetic correlations between traits (see Table 1.2) indicate that selection for some production traits will lead to correlated increases in other production traits (e.g. kg protein and kg fat, correlation coefficient $r = 0.86$). Selection for weight of either milk, fat or protein has a positive and favourable effect on both the other two variables. However it should be noted that some correlations between production and conformation mean that selection for weight of products does not always favour the desired shape or support of the udder for optimum function. Consequently if improvement is sought in these aspects of udder conformation, it must be selected for. Other conformational traits such as foot angle show no consistent or significant correlations with the production traits. Dairy cattle breeding is largely through AI so it is very important that every sire used has an accurately assessed BV. The method of BV assessment must also be suitable for female sex-limited traits of low to medium heritability. The method of choice in most countries including the UK has therefore been progeny testing, but the advent of MOET technology has made sibling testing also possible. Examples of each of these two methods will now be discussed in some detail.

Progeny testing has been used in the UK for many years, both nationally and on a smaller scale by cattle breeding clubs. Figure 1.3 outlines the Sire Improvement Programme (SIP), which is the scheme used by Genus. Potential dairy sires, primarily Friesian/Holstein (Friesians and Holsteins are considered to be strains of the same breed, because of the extensive gene exchange that has characterized their recent history), are procured as embryos from Canada, the USA and Europe or produced by contract mating of high genetic merit 'bull mothers' with high genetic merit sires. Bull calves thus obtained are reared and used to inseminate approximately 300 cows in recorded herds. Their daughters are recorded for at least 90 days of the first lactation for yields of protein, fat and milk and assessed for conformational traits. Daughters may also be assessed for beefing qualities. Progeny are reared in a range of herds, in each case alongside contemporaries, which are daughters of other 'on test' bulls. Each sire is evaluated for its predicted transmitting ability (PTA) for each of the production characteristics assessed, namely kg milk, kg fat, kg protein, fat% and protein%. Each figure, e.g. PTA +23 kg protein, predicts the merit of this sire in his offspring. For the example given, +23 kg protein, each daughter would be expected to produce 23 kg more protein in its first lactation than the daughter of a sire with a PTA for protein of 0 kg. Individual production PTA values can be combined into an index to indicate overall profitability or a profit index, abbreviated as PIN. A sire's production PIN is a valuation in monetary terms of his genetic potential for milk, protein and fat production taking account of feed, quota, milk transportation and processing costs. A sire with a PIN of £65, for instance,

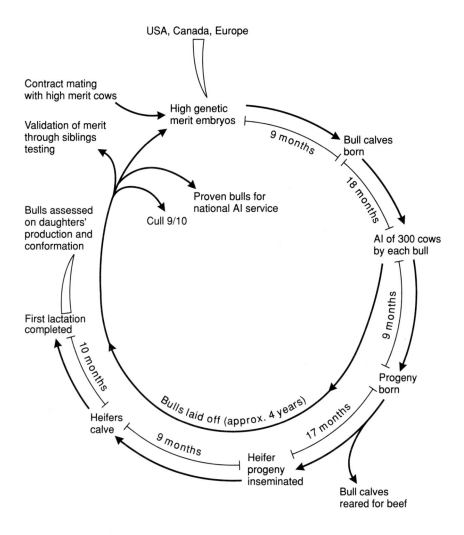

USA, Canada, Europe

Contract mating
with high merit cows

High genetic
merit embryos

Validation of merit
through siblings
testing

9 months

Bull calves
born

18 months

Proven bulls for
national AI service

Bulls assessed
on daughters'
production and
conformation

Cull 9/10

AI of 300 cows
by each bull

First lactation
completed

9 months

Progeny
born

10 months

Heifers
calve

Bulls laid off (approx. 4 years)

17 months

9 months

Heifer
progeny
inseminated

Bull calves
reared for beef

Figure 1.3 Outline of a progeny test for dairy bulls: Genus Sire Improvement Programme (GSIP). The Sire Improvement Programme was formerly known as the Dairy Progeny Testing Scheme (DPTS).

should produce daughters who outperform the daughters of an 'average' sire by a margin of £65 per lactation. The relationship between PTA, PIN and BV is that each PTA is equal to half the BV for that trait, and correspondingly the PIN value is equal to half the overall BV of the sire. PTA and PIN values can also be computed for cows and have equivalent predictive use.

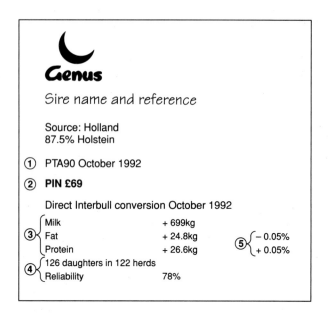

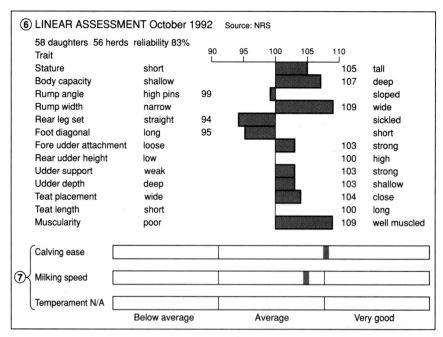

Figure 1.4 Extract from a dairy sire progeny test result (from Genus 1993).

Variables other than production can be incorporated into an index, such as assessments of longevity and health (particularly susceptibility to mastitis).

The number of female progeny providing data for each sire's BV assessment varies, greater numbers leading to higher reliability. Assessment of a sire's merit for conformational and behavioural traits is also carried out on its progeny and, again, predictive figures are computed.

All the computations for dairy sire and dam merit utilize information from the individual that is being assessed, corrected according to the merit of all recorded genetically related animals in the breed using IAM BLUP.

An extract of a dairy sire's progeny test assessment for production and conformation is given in Figure 1.4. Results of conformational assessment are tabulated as daughters' deviations from the breed average for each of the assessed traits. Table 1.4 lists four tested sires with PTA and PIN values to illustrate merit in different aspects of production.

Sibling testing using MOET is an alternative method for the assessment of genetic merit of dairy bulls. Figure 1.5 shows the MOET programme run by Genus (McGuirk 1990), which is an adaptation of the original proposal of Nicholas and Smith (1983). The scheme is based on an élite nucleus herd of 250 Friesian/Holstein cows of outstanding genetic merit bred from preselected parent stock. The nucleus herd was founded in the late 1980s. Each year the best females are chosen for superovulation,

Figure 1.4 *continued.*

1 Predicted Transmitting Ability and date of assessment. An estimate of the production merit of this bull compared with a fixed base (set at zero in January 1990).
2 Profit Index. This expresses the PTA 90 values for milk (kg), fat (kg) and protein (kg) in a single financial figure. PIN=$-0.039\times$PTA milk$+0.94\times$PTA fat$+2.75\times$PTA protein.
3 PTAs for milk, fat and protein. Predicts the daughter improvements for this bull compared with a bull with zero PTA values.
4 Distribution of progeny test daughters and the resulting reliability assessment of the PTA and PIN values.
5 PTAs for % of fat and protein. Predicts daughter improvements for fat and protein percentages compared with the zero base.
6 Linear assessment of conformation. Progeny of this bull have been graded for the listed traits. The bars represent, for each trait, the expected deviation of daughters compared with those of an average sire.
7 Other traits assessed and their results.

Note that in 1995, PIN 90 was updated to PIN 95 calculated as $-0.03\times$PTA milk$+0.60\times$PTA fat$+4.04\times$PTA protein. A new index of Total Economic Merit (ITEM) was introduced encompassing production and longevity.

Table 1.4 A selection of Friesian/Holstein sires and their breeding value assessments (from Genus 1993)

Sire	PTA90 (based on progeny testing unless otherwise stated					PIN (£)
	Milk (kg)	Fat (kg)	Protein (kg)	Fat (%)	Protein (%)	
Sunny Boy	1019	41.7	36.8	0.01	0.03	101
B757	391	32.3	23.8	0.27	0.15	81
MOET Masters III*	920	30.6	25.9	−0.07	−0.06	64
Lincoln	535	25.6	19.1	0.11	0.03	56

*Sibling tested.

inseminated with semen from high genetic merit sires, and the resulting embryos are transferred to recipient cows. It is aimed to generate 500 embryos each year to ensure the rearing of 130 female and 130 male calves. The females (comprising groups of full- and half-sibs) are reared, inseminated, calved and finally assessed for the economically important traits. These include milk yield and composition, individual feed intake, conformation, milking speed and temperament, fertility indicators and disease incidence. The merit of males is assessed according to the merit of their female full and half siblings using IAM BLUP analysis, each male being given a PTA equivalent. Those of sufficient merit to be used at stud are designated 'MOET masters'. The best females join the nucleus herd displacing those of lesser merit and the best males are used as sires for further rounds of MOET and for AI semen services. The breeding scheme is an 'open nucleus' with the continuing introduction of embryos and young females of appropriate genetic merit. The major advantage of sibling testing over progeny testing in dairy cattle is greater theoretical rate of genetic improvement in the former. This comes about through a substantial reduction in the generation interval (6–6.5 years in progeny testing, 3.7 years with sibling testing), which more than compensates for the inherently lower accuracy of sibling testing compared with progeny testing. Sibling testing, based on a nucleus breeding scheme, has the additional major advantage that the females are grouped into a single herd that can be effectively recorded for input (feed) as well as output (yield) and a far tighter control of management can be achieved than with a geographically diverse scheme such as the SIP. It is envisaged that sibling testing through MOET and the SIP will coexist for a number of years and that sires of high merit identified by the former will have their proof validated by the latter.

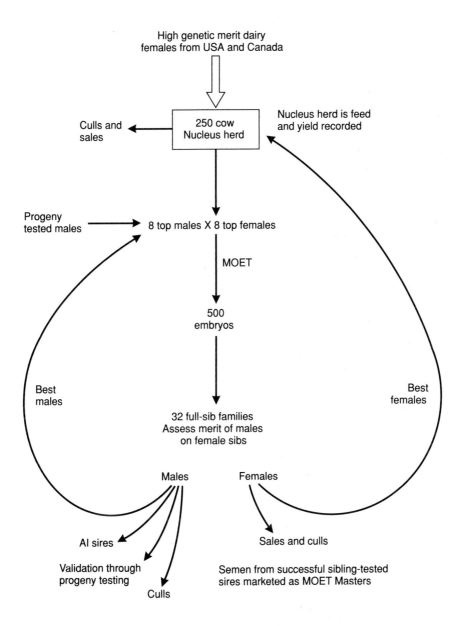

Figure 1.5 Outline of a sibling test for dairy bulls: Genus sibling testing scheme based on multiple ovulation and embryo transfer (MOET) technology.

Beef cattle

Improvement of beef cattle is sought for efficient production of saleable lean meat. Beef sires are used in pedigree beef breeding, in crossbreeding between beef breeds and, additionally, in dairy herds for beef cross calves. It is important that high merit sires are unequivocally identified, particularly in 'dairy-beef' breeding where AI is increasingly used. Some of the desirable characteristics such as growth rate, feed intake and fat depths can be assessed on the live animal, but other characteristics like carcass evaluation of sample joints can only be assessed after slaughter. The large numbers of different beef breeds and the relatively small average herd sizes in the UK (e.g. Charolais 16, Hereford 33, South Devon 11; MLC 1988) make a unified approach to BV assessment difficult. Most of the growth and carcass characteristics have useful heritabilities (see Table 1.1) but calving performance is less heritable. Characteristics that can be measured on the young animal are assessed through Meat and Livestock Commission (MLC) 'on-farm' performance testing of small groups of juvenile males. A test group may comprise animals from that farm alone, or animals from two or more cooperating farms. Each group is reared from weaning to 400 days of age under standard management and records are made of 200- and 400-day weight and daily feed intake, muscling score and (ultrasonic) fat thickness. Calving information is also collected for each male through test inseminations of up to 200 females, either heifers or cows depending on the breed of sire under test. In this way calving difficulty associated with the use of each sire is monitored and calf birth weights are recorded. All the above information is combined into the MLC Beef Index, which gives a measure related to BV. A financial assessment, the Beef Value can be derived from this index and is a predictor of profitability to be gained in using each particular sire. The Beef Index is designed 'to improve the financial margin between the value of saleable meat and the cost of feed, taking into account the cost of difficult calvings' (Allen 1990). The animals are assessed in groups, as explained above, and the average Beef Index score for each group is set at 100. This means that the Beef Index has a somewhat limited use as it only allows within-group comparisons. Progeny testing is therefore used to more accurately assess beef sires identified as promising on the Beef Index. The progeny are crossbred steer calves from dairy cows and are reared from a few days to 18 months of age. Rearing takes place at a testing station with standardized management. Liveweight gain is monitored and, after slaughter, progeny are assessed in detail for carcass quality. The results for each progeny-tested sire are presented as transmitting abilities for growth, lean, conformation and calving ease (the latter is assessed through the calving survey). An indication of calf quality for beef is also given. Valid comparisons can be made between sires within a breed because of use of the same IAM BLUP statistical methods used in dairy assessment. The results of two beef bull evaluations are shown in Figure 1.6.

MOET technology also finds application in beef improvement programmes. An élite nucleus herd of females can be formed by bringing together superior animals owned by co-operating members of a breed society. The best females can be superovulated and bred with progeny-tested sires to generate mixed sex full-sib families. These families can be used to assess both growth and carcass traits, retaining some female siblings from the best families for nucleus herd replacements and some male siblings for AI both in the nucleus herd and commercial herds. From a genetic point of view this scheme has great appeal, but in practical terms it is only suitable for the numerically largest beef breed societies such as Simmental, Aberdeen Angus and South Devon, which have all initiated their own schemes.

Pigs

In the UK, pig breeding is based on a pyramid structure as shown in Figure 1.7. At the top of the pyramid are the élite pure-bred herds where selection for improvement is carried out. The next layer consists of pure-bred multiplier herds and at the base of the pyramid are the commercial herds of hybrid females and their progeny. Very large pig companies may construct their own pyramids, but the UK national improvement scheme run by the MLC will be outlined here. In its current form this scheme evaluates the individual performance of élite herd boars and gilts based on weight for age, feed intake and fat depths. These traits are all of medium to high heritability (see Table 1.1), are not restricted to one or other sex, and can all be measured on the live animal. Individual performance testing is therefore a most appropriate method. The testing is carried out in the normal farm environment and each individual assessed is awarded a points score based on a multitrait index. Stock with the highest indices are used for breeding in the élite herds. In the multiplier herds, élite-bred males and females are used as foundation stock for lines of pure Landrace (L), Large White (LW) and other breeds. Hybrid gilts (usually L × LW) are also produced and then crossed with high indexing pure-line boars to generate the commercial pigs for pig meat production.

A criticism of this 'on-farm' performance test is the possible bias in the evaluation of individuals due to the varied farm environments. It could be countered that variation in feeding, housing and other aspects of pig husbandry is likely to be small. There is evidence in pigs that the genetically superior stock will outperform those of lesser genetic merit regardless of limited environmental differences.

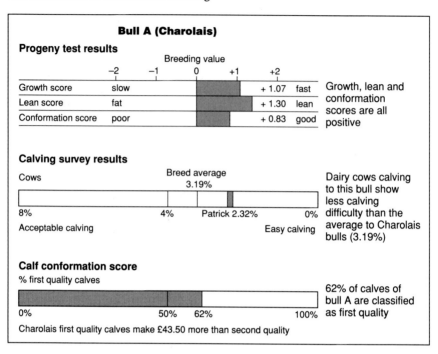

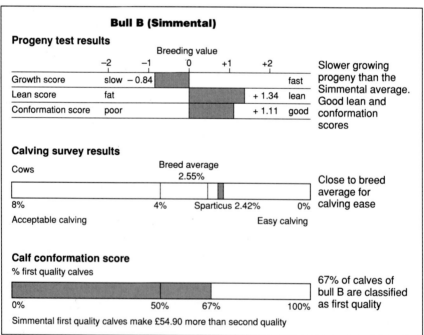

Figure 1.6 Beef bull assessment: progeny, calving and calf information (from Genus 1994). Progeny test breeding values are expressed as standard deviations.

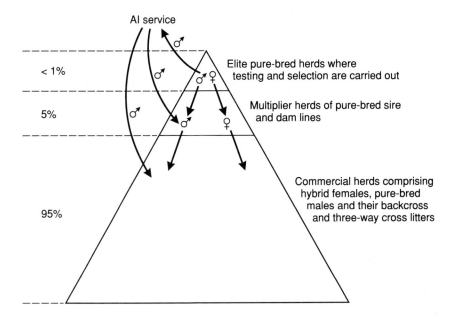

AI service

< 1%

5%

95%

Elite pure-bred herds where
testing and selection are carried out

Multiplier herds of pure-bred sire
and dam lines

Commercial herds comprising
hybrid females, pure-bred
males and their backcross
and three-way cross litters

Figure 1.7 Pyramid structure of pig improvement and production. Genetic improvement is carried out at the apex of the pyramid and the improvement is disseminated first to the multiplier layer and thereafter to commercial herds.

In the past in pigs, fairly intensive selection of breeding stock has been carried out based on progeny testing and sibling testing at test stations and 'on farm'. Very considerable improvements in leanness, growth, feed conversion and carcass quality have been achieved; the present limited 'on-farm' performance test maintains this improvement and keeps a degree of selection pressure on the most important traits.

The past success in pig growth and carcass improvement has been accompanied by an undesirable development in many breeds. The extreme leanness of pig carcasses means that the meat has a tendency to separate if sliced thinly, as it is for bacon. Of greater concern is the associated presence in very lean breeds of pigs of a single gene (N) with a recessive variant (n) at a significant frequency which when homozygous (nn) results in a combination of deleterious consequences. These consequences are halothane sensitivity (a short exposure to the anaesthetic gas, halothane, results in hyperthermia, rigidity, and death if not removed from the gas), an extreme sensitivity to stress (porcine stress syndrome, PSS) and pale soft exudative meat (PSE). The fact that this deleterious gene has reached very high levels in commercially important breeds is explained by its overall benefits in the heterozygous condition. Heterozygous pigs (Nn) have superior growth rate, carcass quality and carcass conformation compared with *NN* pigs, and do not suffer from stress-related deaths or poor meat quality typical of the *nn* genotype. The three genotypes can be distinguished by gene sequence analysis allowing breeders to manipulate genotype to best advantage.

Sheep

Sheep breeding in the UK is very traditional with no coherent single national improvement scheme. An enormous diversity of breeds is farmed in widely differing environments. AI is not routinely practised. Selection criteria in hill breeds are ill defined, the overall aims being hardiness, good mothering ability of ewes and survivability of their newborn lambs. Lowland breeds are generally managed in much more favourable environments, giving scope for easier recording and the opportunity to select for growth and carcass traits of lambs for market. Large flocks have the most scope for selection, but large flocks require more extensive recording. Despite the above limitations, classical selection programmes and other schemes for breed improvement can be established. Nevertheless remarkably few of the major breeds, particularly the hill breeds, have improvement schemes beyond a limited amount of 'importation' of genetic material from one breed to another by occasional crosses with chosen breeds (e.g. Swaledale genes into Scottish Blackface, North Country Cheviot into Cheviot). More organized methods for sheep improvement follow with specific examples where relevant.

Ram and ewe assessment

Both sexes can be readily assessed on their growth records for liveweight gain as well as accurate assessment by ultrasonic scanning of fat and muscle depths. A multitrait index derived from these measurements is particularly useful in selecting sires in terminal sire breeds such as the Suffolk and Texel. In the Suffolk breed, the use of a lean meat index over the first four generations of selection resulted in significant improvement (MLC 1990). Ewe and ram lamb gains in the 150-ewe selection flock compared with the 70-ewe control flock averaged 4.9% for 150-day liveweight, 6.4% for muscle depth, and −3.5% for fat depth. Detailed carcass classification can be carried out on slaughtered lambs using the MLC method of sheep carcass classification (MLC 1989). The prolificacy traits are more difficult to approach being low in heritability and sex-limited to the female. Repeated measurements on successive lambings gives improved response. Ewe prolificacy is usually recorded as lambs born per ewe lambing, but ovulation rate, measured at laparoscopy, may be a more promising selection criterion. Six years of selection for litter size in the UK Romney breed based on a group breeding scheme approach (see below) resulted in average figures of 1.78 (highline) and 1.54 (control line) (Anderson and Curran 1990).

Group breeding schemes

Group breeding schemes (GBSs) are a method of pooling the best genetic material (breeding stock) from a number of sources (cooperating flocks), and, after selective breeding, redistributing the improved stock to the members of the group. Group breeding schemes thus overcome the genetic isolation experienced by individual flocks by linking them through common breeding stock. Cooperating farmers initially contribute an agreed number of their best breeding females to the nucleus flock. This flock is subjected to detailed recording and selection for the required characteristics. Each year the best rams and ewes produced in the nucleus are used as nucleus breeding stock and high merit rams from the nucleus are distributed to the members. Occasionally, ewes from the nucleus herd may be displaced by superior recorded ewes drawn from the members' farms. This two-way flow of genetic material is an open nucleus scheme, which maximizes genetic gains and minimizes inbreeding but does increase the risk of disease in the nucleus flock. Nucleus flocks are likely to become closed after the first few generations because their animals' genetic merit will be higher than that of animals belonging to members' flocks. A particular feature of GBSs is the initial genetic lift that can be achieved if the élite nucleus foundation stock are correctly identified. This lift can be around 15% with annual gains in subsequent years of up to 2% (Land *et al.* 1983), making GBSs a very simple and rewarding approach. Group breeding schemes were first launched in New Zealand in the late 1960s and have had considerable success there. Australia followed with schemes for sheep and beef cattle. In the UK a small number of breeds have developed their own GBSs, mostly in association with agricultural colleges and universities. Breeds included are Welsh Mountain (initiated in 1976), Lleyn (1978), Romney (1979), Beulah Speckleface (1979) and Texel (1987) (MLC 1989).

Sire reference schemes

Sire reference schemes (SRSs) have some features in common with group breeding in that a number of participating members agree on their breeding objectives and share genetic material. However, the need for recording differs. In GBSs, only initial recording of members' flocks is required until the nucleus flock (itself fully recorded) is established. In sire referencing, full recording is needed in all members' flocks. Sire referencing is designed to allow valid between-flock comparisons as it provides 'genetic links' between flocks that are physically isolated from each other. The essential requirement for sire referencing is the use of the same rams, as the genetic links, in all participating flocks. Ideally this would be through the use of clones of animals across all flocks as the progeny of each clone would be a half-sib group. Comparison with progeny of other flock sires would lead to valid between-flock assessment of rams. Currently, until cloning is a practical possibility, SRSs take the following form. Member flocks, per-haps numbering 10, nominate a small team of reference sires (e.g. 4). Each sire is mated, ideally using AI, with a specific number of ewes (e.g. 15) within each flock. The other ewes are mated with homebred sires. The progeny of both the reference and homebred sires are evaluated, and, based on these results, a new team of reference sires is nominated. In theory these do not need to be of any particular standard, as they provide the genetic reference, but in practice it makes economic sense to use the highest merit sires available in all participating flocks. The Suffolk and Charollais breeds both embarked on sire referencing in 1989. Sire refer-encing has the advantage that a nucleus flock is not required and therefore the organization is less complex than for a GBS. However, AI and ram sharing are novelties to a rather traditional industry, which may need time to be more widely accepted.

Group breeding and sire referencing both require a high level of cooperation between members and agreed selection objectives, the latter generally in the form of a multitrait index. Both types of scheme benefit from breeding through AI, particularly SRSs where using the same sires in different flocks has practical difficulties if natural service is used. Whilst conception rates as high as 90% can be achieved with intrauterine AI, using laparoscopy and fresh semen, the same approach with thawed frozen semen only achieves conception rates of 56–58% (Findlater *et al.* 1991). As semen preservation techniques develop it seems likely that the figures for thawed frozen semen will rise.

Exploitation of prolificacy genes

Single genes with significant effects on ewe prolificacy were a surprising discovery in the 1980s. The most well documented of these is F, the fecundity gene of the Australian Booroola Merino (see p. 10), but genes with similar effects are also reported in other breeds, including the Ice-landic (Iceland), Javanese (Indonesia), Cambridge (UK), Belclare (Ireland), Romney (New Zealand) and Olkulska (Poland) (Elsen *et al.* 1991). Programmes designed to incorporate these prolificacy genes into other, less prolific breeds are in progress (e.g. F gene transfer to UK Romney). The consequences in terms of litter size will depend very much on how repeatable the gene's effect is when transferred to a different genetic background.

Choice of breeding method

Introduction

The breeding method has a marked effect on the profitability of any livestock breeding enterprise. The genetically superior stock, identified through their true or estimated BV, can be used in a system of pure breeding, crossbreeding or a combination of the two. The method chosen depends upon many factors including the species, the breeds available, the desired traits and the fate of the animals (breeding or slaughter). In this section the theory will be covered first followed by short sections on breeding methods in the main livestock species.

Theory

Figure 1.8 lists a range of breeding methods from the most intense form of inbreeding through to interspecific hybridization. Reading down the figure, the major consequences are an increase in heterozygosity and corresponding increase in scope for change through selective breeding. In general, the higher up the figure the more predictable is the outcome of a mating. At one extreme, full-sib matings generate and maintain inbred lines, where all individuals are identical, genetic variation is minimized and each mating produces further identical progeny. At the other extreme, breed crosses produce F_1 hybrids with maximum heterozygosity which, if interbred, generate maximum genetic variance in their progeny. Species crosses usually create sterile hybrids and feature very little in livestock breeding. Where they are performed it is to produce a tough working animal such as the mule, the hybrid offspring of a donkey (stallion) and a horse (mare). These hybrids are almost invariably sterile having in the case of the mule an unbalanced chromosome complement of $2n = 63$ derived from the donkey ($2n = 62$) and the horse ($2n = 64$) parents. This section will not deal with interspecific hybridization further.

Pure breeding

Pure breeding is breeding within a breed. It is carried out so that the characteristics of a breed may be maintained. Pure breeding can be classed

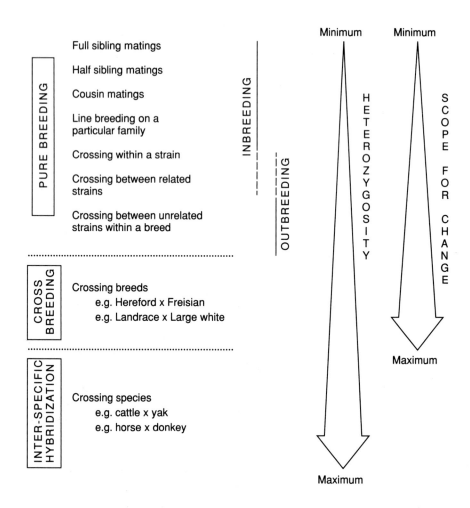

Figure 1.8 Range of breeding systems available to the animal breeder.

as inbreeding or outbreeding. Inbreeding is the breeding together of individuals that are more closely related than the average relationship within the breed. Outbreeding (or outcrossing) is the breeding together of individuals that are less closely related than the average relationship within the breed. The distinction between inbreeding and outbreeding therefore depends on the overall breed structure. A second cousin mating might be a relative outcross in a numerically small highly related pedigree dog breed but it would constitute inbreeding in an average-sized beef cattle breed. Inbreeding reduces genetic variance and leads to increased homozygosity. This is beneficial in some situations and detrimental in others. Inbred lines of rats and mice are bred that way to produce a defined product for a wide range of research uses. The reduction in genetic variance is brought about by many generations of inbreeding until, in theory, every genetic locus is homozygous and the inbreeding coefficient reaches 100%. The inbreeding coefficient, F, gives the chance that two allelic genes in an individual are identical by descent. The inbreeding coefficient can range from 0 to 1.0 (or 0 to 100%). The development of an inbred line begins by setting up a large number of individual full-sibling matings from desirable stock. Each generation some lines need to be culled for not meeting the required phenotypic standards, and others die out because recessive lethal genes become homozygous and are therefore manifest. Yet more lines are lost because of poor reproductive performance. After 20 generations of full-sibling mating, when essentially all genetic loci are homozygous or fixed and F approaches 100%, no further genetic change can take place except through mutation or introduction of different genetic material. Each surviving line thus becomes a separate inbred line, its genotype representing a selection of the genetic material present in the original sibling pair. An inbred line can be perpetuated by mating any individuals within that line (usually full-sibs). As many as 90% of inbred lines may die out during their development thus underlining the need for initially setting up very many lines. A general deterioration of quantitative traits usually accompanies inbreeding; this is inbreeding depression. Fitness traits are particularly susceptible to inbreeding depression. Fitness traits are traits associated with reproduction and neonatal survival, the fittest animals being those that contribute most genes to the next generation. Selection to maintain optimum levels of fitness traits must be carried out during the development of inbred lines. Typical losses due to inbreeding depression for a range of traits in pigs are shown in Table 1.5. It should be noted that inbreeding levels are assessed separately for dams and offspring. A dam's inbreeding affects her maternal performance in characteristics such as prenatal uterine environment and postnatal lactational performance,

Table 1.5 Effects of inbreeding on various performance traits in pigs (from Pirchner 1985)

Trait		Change per 1% inbreeding as a percentage of the mean
No. born alive	(O)	−0.28
No. born alive	(D)	−0.70
No. weaned	(O)	−0.73
No. weaned	(D)	−0.46
Daily gain on test		−0.42
Back fat thickness		−0.20

D, inbreeding of dam; O, inbreeding of offspring.

which in turn affect her offspring. The inbreeding level of the offspring affects their own performance for growth and survivability. Most investigations into inbreeding have shown a roughly linear relationship between increasing levels of F and decreasing levels of performance.

Crossbreeding

Crossbreeding means crossing different breeds, such as Hereford and Friesian breeds of cattle. The term is also rather more loosely (and incorrectly) used to describe crossing different strains of a breed or different inbred lines. The term outcrossing should be used for these situations. Traditional types of crossbreeding are shown in Figure 1.9. In contrast to the deleterious consequences of inbreeding, crossbreeding and outcrossing usually, but not invariably, generate hybrid vigour, the hybrid having superior performance to the mean of the two (or more) parental breeds. This hybrid vigour is measured as heterosis (H) and is exhibited to the greatest extent by those characteristics that are most susceptible to inbreeding depression. Furthermore, for these heterotic characteristics, the fitness lost on inbreeding tends to be restored on crossing. The concept of heterosis is illustrated in Figure 1.10. Heterosis can be positive or negative, and if the heterosis is positive, and the hybrid value exceeds that of the better parent, the heterosis can be said to be both positive and useful. Positive heterosis is measured on a scale of 0–100%. Like inbreeding

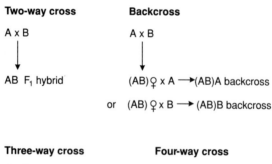

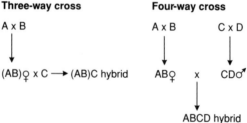

Figure 1.9 Traditional types of crossbreeding. A, B, C and D are pure breeds.

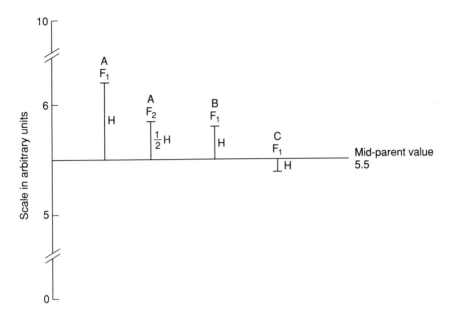

Figure 1.10 Diagrammatic representation of heterosis showing three possible outcomes of crossing two different parent breeds.
Parent breed 1 (P1) mean=5
Parent breed 2 (P2) mean=6

Possible outcomes, A, B and C.

A Positive useful heterosis, $F_1=6.2$, $H = \dfrac{6.2-5.5}{5.5} = 0.127$

    (note that in the F_2, the heterosis is halved)

B Positive heterosis, $F_1=5.8$, $H = \dfrac{5.8-5.5}{5.5} = 0.055$

C Negative heterosis $F_1=5.4$, $H = \dfrac{5.4-5.5}{5.5} = -0.02$

depression, heterosis can take effect at more than one level. Crossbred dams benefit from maternal heterosis and crossbred offspring benefit from their own individual heterosis. Offspring resulting from backcrosses, i.e. $(A \times B) \times A$, and three-way crosses, i.e. $(A \times B) \times C$, benefit from both maternal and individual heterosis.

How is it that inbreeding depresses and crossbreeding augments fitness traits? It seems likely that the decrease in heterozygosity with inbreeding and the increase in heterozygosity with crossbreeding are in some way responsible. It may be that high levels of generalized heterozygosity in the genotype are favoured by natural selection and lead to optimum expression of fitness traits. Another theory is that specific genetic loci, when heterozygous, have a beneficial effect on fitness. A third theory suggests that every genotype has a certain number of favourable dominant alleles. By combining (crossing) two different lines, the F_1 hybrid will contain a higher number of favourable dominants than either parental line, thus raising its level of the characteristics that are influenced by these dominant alleles. Whatever the mechanisms of inbreeding depression and hybrid vigour, breeding systems should be organized with due regard for the consequences of inbreeding and crossbreeding. Specific disorders of livestock that are inherited in a single-gene recessive or multifactorial manner are increased in incidence through inbreeding because related animals share a proportion of their variant alleles. This is of particular significance where extensive use of particular sires occurs in species largely bred through AI, such as dairy cattle. Known single-gene disorders in Friesian/Holstein cattle include BLAD and factor XI (plasma thromboplastin antecedent) deficiency. An individual heterozygous AI sire can transmit the gene to many hundreds or thousands of progeny. Where some of the dams are also carriers, the abnormality can be manifest. These defects should therefore be screened for in AI sires, and matings that result in inbreeding should be avoided.

Breeding methods: the main livestock species

Dairy and beef cattle

Cattle breeding includes examples of pure breeding and crossbreeding, the former more commonly in dairy cattle and the latter in beef cattle. Synthetic breeds have also been developed in some countries. In countries with widespread dairy industries, dairy cattle tend to be pure-bred Friesian/Holsteins for milk, or Channel Island breeds such as the Jersey for cream, butter and cheese production. The reasons for this are in part historical, dairy farming being a very traditional enterprise, and part biological. The biological reason is simply that suitable dairy breeds for crossing do not exist. The closest breed to the Friesian/Holstein for milk production is probably the Ayrshire, but hybrids between the two do not surpass the Friesian/Holstein parent breed. There is, however, interest in crossbreeding in countries with less productive indigenous dairy or dual-purpose cattle. For example, the Jersey has been used for crossing with native Criollo cattle in Costa Rica, Sahiwal in India and Sinhala in Sri Lanka. Lactational data from Jersey (J) × Criollo (C) crosses are shown in Figure 1.11. The F_1 hybrid, J × C (2052 kg milk), shows positive and useful heterosis in milk yield and most milk components, and retains the adaptive traits of the indigenous breed such as heat tolerance and tick resistance.

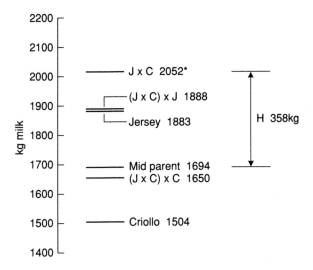

Figure 1.11 Jersey and Criollo milk yields in Costa Rica: parent breeds, F_1 and backcross data. J, Jersey; C, Criollo. *Unweighted mean of J♂ × C♀ (2022 kg) and C♂ × J♀ (2082 kg) (data from de Alba and Kennedy 1985).

There are organizational problems associated with crossbreeding schemes such as the Jersey × Criollo example. In practical terms there are two options: either both breeds need to be maintained, the exotic perhaps with difficulty, or the indigenous breed is maintained to supply females and AI is carried out using imported semen from the exotic breed. Both options are expensive and wasteful of stock. An alternative method of achieving a comparable endpoint is to create a synthetic or composite breed from an appropriate mix of the two. This takes many generations of crossing and selection, but has the major advantage that, once created, it can be 'pure bred' without need for further crossbreeding. It is, nevertheless, very important to conserve native breeds because of their unique gene pool and the unknown requirements of future livestock breeding. Examples of synthetic cattle breeds are the Belmont Red (Hereford/Africander/Shorthorn) in Africa and the Brangus (Brahman/Angus) in southern USA.

Another form of crossbreeding, crossing beef breed sires on dairy breed females, is carried out in the UK and overseas to produce calves for beef. The breeding females are those that are selected not to be replacement breeders for the dairy herd. Approximately 50% of UK beef comes in this way from the dairy herd. Typically, smaller beef breeds such as the Hereford are used on dairy heifers, and larger continental breeds such as Charolais, Simmental and Belgian Blue on dairy cows. Heterosis in the crossbred calf benefits neonatal survival and early growth rate, and beefing characteristics are much improved compared with a calf of a pure dairy breed.

Crossing between beef breeds is carried out in many countries using two-way, three-way and even four-way crosses. There is such a multitude of beef breeds even within a single country that very many crossing combinations are possible. In the UK the aim is often to combine the best characteristics of the slower growing later maturing British breeds with the faster growing earlier maturing qualities of the continental breeds. In genetic terms this advantage is known as complementarity. The cross benefits from an intermediate level of each of the traits in question; its overall merit is therefore higher when compared with any one of the parental breeds.

Pigs

In the UK pigs are either pure bred or crossbred depending on their role in pigmeat production. The slaughter generation is invariably crossbred, being derived from pure-bred boars and crossbred gilts. Two or three breeds may contribute to the scheme. A two-breed scheme is usually a backcross; typically a Large White (LW) × Landrace (L) hybrid gilt is backcrossed to a boar of either parental breed, i.e. LW × (L × LW) or L × (LW × L). The two levels of heterosis generated benefit both maternal reproductive performance and piglet survivability and early growth, all low heritability traits, which are particularly responsive to crossbreeding. Table 1.6 gives some Swedish data comparing reproductive performance of pure-bred, two-way cross and backcrossed litters. It can be seen that sow productivity, measured as piglet numbers between birth and weaning, is least good in pure litters, intermediate in F_1 crosses and best in back-crosses. Schemes involving three breeds such as a Hampshire sire on Large White × Landrace hybrid gilts do not appear to result in any significant further reproductive improvement. It is also found that sire fertility is not a limiting factor, therefore no heterotic advantage is gained by using a boar

Table 1.6 Comparison of pig litter sizes in pure, two-way cross and backcross systems (from Ral *et al.* 1978)

Breeds and crosses			Piglet numbers		
Boar	Sow	Litter	Born	Born alive	Alive at 6 weeks
LW	LW	LW	11.47	10.91	9.13
L	LW	L × LW	11.73	11.18	9.46
LW	L × LW	LW × (L × LW)	12.02	11.38	9.68

LW, Large White; L, Landrace.

that is crossbred rather than pure. Sire breeds other than Large White and Landrace can confer advantages in meat quality on their offspring. An example of this is the use of the Duroc as a terminal sire breed on Large White × Landrace hybrid gilts. However, reported gains in meat eating quality are somewhat subjective and are achieved at the expense of higher production costs for feed and higher carcass fat content (Walkland 1992). Another interesting crossing breed is the Chinese Mieshan. Mieshan pigs are highly prolific and early maturing but they are slow growing and their carcasses are rather fat. There may be overall benefits in using hybrid Mieshan × Large White gilts crossed with a lean sire line as a three-way cross to produce commercial pigs.

Sheep

Worldwide there are many hundreds of breeds of sheep, some predominantly specialized for wool production, some for sheep meat, and yet others for milk. Many breeds are self-contained, but a certain amount of crossbreeding is carried out, particularly between breeds specialized for different functions in order to achieve complementarity by combining the merits in the hybrid offspring. This crossbreeding may be repeated each generation, or synthetic breeds may be created. Well-known examples of synthetic sheep breeds are the Cambridge (UK) based mainly on the Finn, Lleyn, Llanwenog, Clun Forest and Kerry Hill breeds, and the Coopworth (New Zealand) derived from the Border Leicester and Romney breeds. A unique and highly organized scheme of crossbreeding operates in the UK between pure breeds utilizing the country's range of hill and lowland environments and exploiting hybrid vigour and complementarity. The scheme is illustrated in Figure 1.12. The hill breeds, such as the Scottish Blackface, have been subjected to generations of natural and artificial selection for hardiness and fleece quality and for the ewes' ability to rear a single lamb each spring. The Border Leicester and other longwool ram breeds are noted for their prolificacy, milking capacity and growth rate. The terminal sire breeds are typified by leanness, fast growth, and carcass quality. It is these sire breeds in which selection schemes based on group breeding and sire referencing are most applicable (see earlier). The stratified system illustrated in Figure 1.12 generates two-way cross females for breeding (half-bred ewes) and three-way cross slaughter lambs. The hybrid vigour and complementarity in the half-bred ewes augments their prolificacy and mothering abilities; the three-way cross lambs benefit from this maternal heterosis and their own individual heterosis for growth and carcass traits.

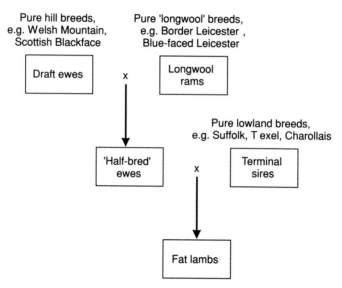

Figure 1.12 The stratified system of crossbreeding in the British sheep industry.

Chapter summary and future prospects in animal breeding

The aims of livestock breeding are well defined in most cases and the methods of selection of breeding stock are firmly based on established genetic theory. Breeding methods involve both pure breeding and cross-breeding and are organized to make the best use of the genetic resources in each species.

In the future it looks likely that animal breeders will achieve their aims with rising levels of technology. Breeding strategies will more and more make use of AI, embryo transfer and other methods of manipulating reproduction. Increasingly, molecular genetic advances will permit the identification of specific genes of interest for their deleterious or favourable properties. This will lead to major advances in selecting genotypes confer-ring productivity, fecundity and even disease resistance. The isolation of specific desirable genes will lead to their transfer between members of a species, and across species barriers.

The combination of traditional animal breeding skills with the new molecular technology promises a most exciting future.

2 CYTOGENETICS
S E Long BVMS, PhD, MRCVS

Methods of chromosome examination
Chromosome identification
Types of chromosome abnormalities
Chromosome abnormalities in domestic animals

Cytogenetics is the study of chromosomes. Chromosome anomalies can give rise to a number of fertility problems, which can be avoided if affected animals are identified and eliminated from the breeding stock. Whilst chromosome anomalies are not at the moment a major cause of fertility problems in domestic animals, as the infectious and management causes of reproductive failure are overcome genetic causes will become increasingly significant.

It is possible to examine the chromosome complement of an individual in a number of different ways. In the resting, or interphase, cell the chromatin is dispersed throughout the nucleus and individual chromosomes are not usually visible. Thus, chromosomes are most easily examined when they are dividing since during cell division they condense and separate (Figure 2.1).

Methods of chromosome examination

Mitotic chromosomes

Chromosomes are usually examined during mitotic metaphase. At this stage of cell division the chromatin has begun to divide to form two chromatids but they are held together at the centromere. Thus the chromosome morphology will vary depending upon where the centromere is located (Figure 2.2).

For the purposes of a clinical diagnosis it is desirable that results are obtained quickly but accurately. For this reason a 2–3 day, short-term blood culture is the method of choice because peripheral blood lymphocytes can be used as a convenient source of easily obtainable cells.

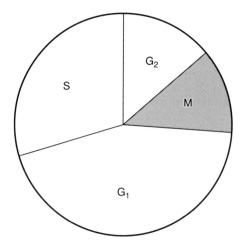

Figure 2.1 The cell cycle. DNA replication takes place during the S period. This is followed by a short period of growth and metabolic activity, the G_2 phase. Mitosis, the M phase, follows G_2 and the resultant cells enter another period of growth and metabolic activity, the G_1 phase. The stages of mitosis are prophase, when the chromatin contracts; metaphase, when the chromatids part and are only held together at the centromere; anaphase, when the chromosomes line up and pull apart on the spindle apparatus; and telophase, when the cytoplasm divides and the nuclear envelope reforms.

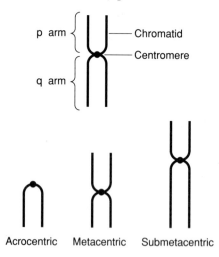

Figure 2.2 Diagrammatic representation of chromosomes at mitotic metaphase. The chromatin has divided to form two chromatids, which are held together at the centromere. If the centromere is at the end, the chromosome is acrocentric. If the centromere is in the body of the chromosome then it has two arms. The short arm is called p and the long arm is called q. If the length of the two arms is equal the chromosome is metacentric; when they are unequal the chromosome is submetacentric.

Terminology

Centromere: the region of each chromosome with which the spindle fibres associate during mitosis.

Chromatid: one of the two longitudinal subunits of the chromosome that separate at anaphase.

Chromatin: the material forming the chromosomes.

Heterochromatin: highly condensed areas of chromatin that stain darkly, replicate late in the cell cycle and are transcriptionally inactive.

Homologous chromosomes: chromosomes that are identical with regard to their genetic constituents.

Meiosis: two successive divisions of the nucleus preceding the formation of the gametes.

Mitosis: mode of nuclear division producing daughter nuclei that contain identical chromosome numbers and that are genetically identical to one another and to the parent nucleus.

Spindle apparatus: collection of fibres seen in the dividing cell that assist in chromosome movement and separation.

Telomere: the free end of the chromosome.

Blood cultures

Heparinized whole blood or buffy coat samples are placed into tissue culture medium supplemented with foetal calf serum, L-glutamine, antibiotics and a mitogen to stimulate the lymphocytes to divide. The two most commonly used mitogens are phytohaemagglutinin (PHA) and poke-weed mitogen (PWM). After 24 hours in culture at 37 °C the polymorphonucleocytes die and the lymphocytes begin to divide. The dividing cells can then be harvested after 48 or 72 hours in culture.

To harvest, a mitotic inhibitor, colchicine or its synthetic analogue, colcemid, is added for the last 30 minutes to 1 hour of the culture period. This inhibits the formation of the mitotic spindle and results in cells accumulating at metaphase. A hypotonic solution of potassium chloride is added that lyses the red blood cells and swells the lymphocytes. The cell suspension is then fixed with a 3:1 mixture of methanol and acetic acid. Multiple changes of the fixative are usually necessary. Slides are prepared by dropping a few drops of cell suspension on to a cold, wet slide. As the methanol and acetic acid evaporate the chromosomes spread out and stick to the slide (Basrur and Gilman 1964).

Fibroblast cultures

Dividing cells can also be obtained from other tissue by establishing fibroblast cultures. This method requires 2–3 weeks before a diagnosis can be made but it is necessary if it is suspected that the blood does not reflect the chromosome complement of all the tissue. To initiate *in vitro* division the cell suspension or small tissue block must be left undisturbed in tissue culture medium at 37 °C for a lag period during which time the fibroblasts adapt to the artificial conditions and attach to the surface of the culture flask. Once a primary culture has been established and cell division is quite rapid, the tissue should be subcultured. To do this the cells are lifted from the flask surface by a weak trypsin solution (0.15%), centrifuged, resuspended in fresh tissue culture medium and distributed to new tissue culture flasks. Two or more subcultures are derived from the primary culture which will also continue to grow. The subculture procedure can be repeated but the longer the tissue remains *in vitro* the greater the chance that the chromosome number and morphology will alter as the tissue adapts to the artificial conditions.

Peak mitotic activity occurs 18–24 hours after subculturing. To harvest, the flasks can be shaken vigorously and the dividing cells will detach and go into suspension in the tissue culture medium. This is then decanted and treated with hypotonic solution and fixative as for the blood cultures (Hyman and Poulding 1972).

Bone marrow cultures

Dividing cells can be obtained directly from the bone marrow but this is relatively difficult to obtain and is much more of an invasive procedure. Nevertheless, once bone marrow cells have been sampled, chromosome preparations can be made quite quickly. The cells are simply incubated at 37 °C in tissue culture medium with colchicine for a couple of hours and then treated with hypotonic and fixative solutions in the normal way (Tjio and Whang 1962).

Meiotic chromosomes

To identify small chromosome rearrangements it may be necessary to examine cells during meiosis. Any rearrangement will be revealed when the homologous chromosomes try to pair. Meiosis is much more easily studied in the male than the female since in males, after puberty, meiotic divisions normally take place throughout the animal's life. In the female, germ cells undergo the first stages of meiotic division during foetal development. They then remain dormant until just before ovulation when the meiotic division is completed. Therefore, examination of female meiosis requires either careful timing of oocyte collection or *in vitro* culture.

For male meiosis samples can be obtained at slaughter, castration or biopsy. Small samples of tissue are simply minced in a hypotonic solution and the disaggregated cells are fixed with a 3:1 mixture of methanol and acetic acid (Long 1978). For female meiosis, preovulatory oocytes obtained at slaughter can be cultured *in vitro* (Xu *et al.* 1986). For cattle, after approximately 12 hours in culture the oocytes will be at diplotene and after 24 hours they will have reached second metaphase.

Cells at diplotene and diakinesis provide information on pairing and chiasma formation. Cells at second metaphase allow calculation of the frequency of non-disjunction.

Submission of samples for chromosome analysis

Firstly, chromosome examination relies upon obtaining dividing cells. This means that samples must be submitted for analysis as soon as possible after collection so that the cells are still alive. Secondly, since the cells are grown in tissue culture medium that also supports bacterial growth, every effort should be made to obtain a sterile sample. Thirdly, because the different species have slightly different cultural characteristics it is important to label the sample clearly with the reference, species and type of analysis required so that the correct cultural procedures may be carried out.

Chromosome identification

With good techniques to produce well-spread metaphase chromosomes it is quite easy to establish the chromosome number and morphology for each of the domestic species (Table 2.1). However, with conventional Giemsa staining it is not always possible to identify each individual chromosome with confidence. This is particularly true for species such as cattle where all the autosomes are the same shape and only differ from each other in size (Figure 2.3). In some species, for example the pig, the chromosome complement can be subdivided on the basis of chromosome

Table 2.1 Chromosome number and morphology in domestic animals

Species	Diploid number	Autosomes	X	Y
Cattle	60	Acrocentric	Large, submetacentric	Small metacentric (*Bos taurus*) Small, acrocentric (*Bos indicus*)
Sheep	54	Three pairs of metacentrics, + acrocentrics	Largest, acrocentric	Small, metacentric
Goats	60	Acrocentric	Third largest, acrocentric	Small, metacentric
Pigs	38	Various	Large, metacentric	Small, metacentric
Horse	64	Various	Large, submetacentric	Small, acrocentric

morphology (Figure 2.4) but with conventional staining it is still impossible to detect minor chromosomal rearrangements. To do this a series of differential staining procedures have been developed that permit the accurate identification of homologous chromosomes in most species.

Differential staining techniques

For diagnostic purposes, C-banding and G-banding are the two most important differential staining techniques. R-banding is also used in some laboratories.

C-bands

These bands derive their name from the fact that it is usually the centromeric region that stains darkly whilst the rest of the chromosome remains rather pale. This can be achieved by treating the chromosomes first with an acid solution, then an alkali solution and then with a saline sodium citrate solution (SSC) before staining with Giemsa (Sumner 1972). This results in the double-stranded DNA first denaturing and then renaturing. The highly repetitive, constitutive heterochromatin at the centromere reassociates more quickly and so takes up the stain (Pardue and Gall 1970). The technique is particularly useful for identifying the X chromosome of the horse. In this species the X has a characteristic C-band on the long arm.

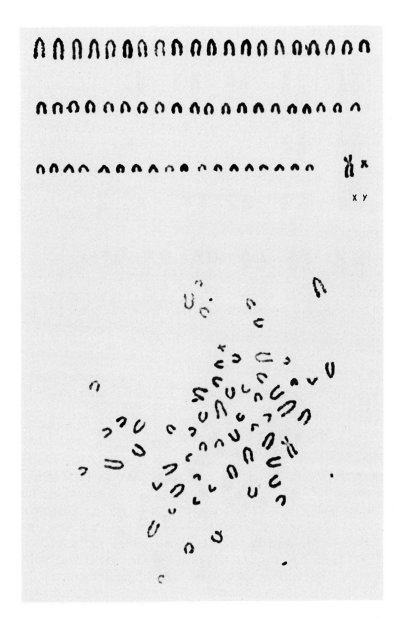

Figure 2.3 A karyotype and spread from a bull (*Bos taurus*). Conventional staining.

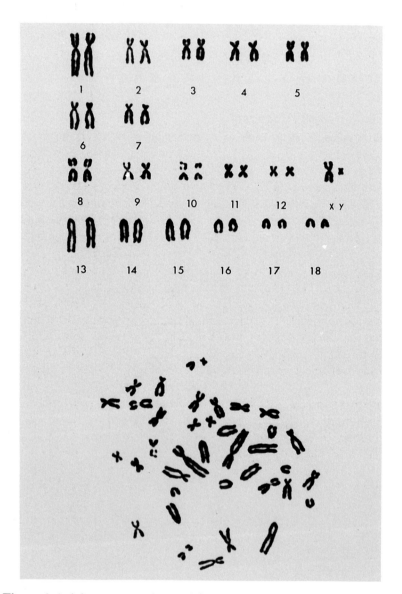

Figure 2.4 A karyotype and spread from a boar (*Sus scrofa*). Conventional staining.

G-bands

G-banding developed as a natural consequence of the C-band techniques, which occasionally produced a striped banding pattern along the whole length of the chromosome. The earlier techniques involved incubation with various salt solutions but the method now used almost universally consists of a partial digestion with trypsin and subsequent staining with Giemsa (Seabright 1972a, b). A standard nomenclature to describe the G-bands of domestic animals was agreed at an international conference at Reading in 1976 (Ford *et al.* 1980) and at Paris in 1989 (ISCNDA 1989, 1990).

R-bands

The banding pattern produced by R-band techniques is the reverse of the G-band pattern. R-bands can be produced either by incubating chromosome preparations in a phosphate buffer at 87 °C (Dutrillaux and Lejeune 1971) or by adding 5-bromodeoxyuridine (BrdU) to the culture for the last 6–10 hours of incubation. The latter procedure produces differential contraction along the chromosome and subsequent staining with acridine orange (a fluorochrome) results in distinct bands along the length of the chromosomes (Dutrillaux *et al.* 1973).

The major disadvantage to all the fluorescent techniques is that in order to visualize the band patterns the stained chromosomes have to be illuminated and the fluorescence fades under illumination. Thus, without immediate photographic recording the information is lost. To overcome this problem a fluorochrome (Hoechst 332258) plus Giemsa technique was developed that resulted in permanent bands which could be viewed with an ordinary light microscope (Perry and Wolff 1974).

Apart from these three main staining methods there are a number of others that can be used to provide even more detailed information on the chromosome structure or on chromosome rearrangements, e.g. Q-bands (Caspersson *et al.* 1968), T-bands (Dutrillaux 1973), centromeric staining (Eiberg 1974), NOR staining (Goodpasture and Bloom 1975; Bloom and Goodpasture 1976) and sister chromatid exchanges (Latt 1973). Since there is such a variety of different staining methods a code has been developed to describe each technique by means of a series of letters. The first letter denotes the type of banding, the second the general technique and the third letter the stain (ISCN 1978) (Table 2.2).

Table 2.2 Nomenclature for differential banding techniques

C	C-bands
CB	C-bands by barium hydroxide
CBG	C-bands by barium hydroxide using Giemsa
G	G-bands
GT	G-bands by trypsin
GTG	G-bands by trypsin using Giemsa
GAG	G-bands by acetic saline using Giemsa
R	R-bands
RF	R-bands by fluorescence
RFA	R-bands by fluorescence using acridine orange
RB	R-bands by BrdU
RBG	R-bands by BrdU using Giemsa

Types of chromosome abnormalities

Structural abnormalities (Figure 2.5)

During normal cell division the chromatin forming the chromosome may become damaged and break. If the breakage is not repaired, that portion of the chromosome that does not contain the centromere (i.e. the acentric fragment) is usually lost at the next cell division since it cannot attach to the mitotic spindle. This is a deletion. The deletion may be terminal, or interstitial, i.e. occurring in the body of the chromosome arm. If there is a deletion at the ends of both arms of a chromosome these may fuse to form a ring chromosome.

If there is a breakage followed by an incorrect reunion then a rearrangement occurs. When the rearrangement only involves one chromosome this is described as an intrachromosomal rearrangement. An example of this is an inversion. Inversions that do not involve the centromere are called paracentric inversions. Such inversions do not alter the gross chromosome morphology and cannot be detected without the use of one or more of the differential staining procedures. A single break and rotation will give rise to a terminal inversion whilst a double break and rotation will result in an interstitial inversion. Those inversions that do involve the centromere are called pericentric inversions. These will alter the shape of the chromosome if the break points either side of the centromere are not symmetrical. Shifts occur when there are two or four break points without rotation.

Figure 2.5 Diagrammatic representations of structural abnormalities in chromosomes.

Types of chromosome abnormalities

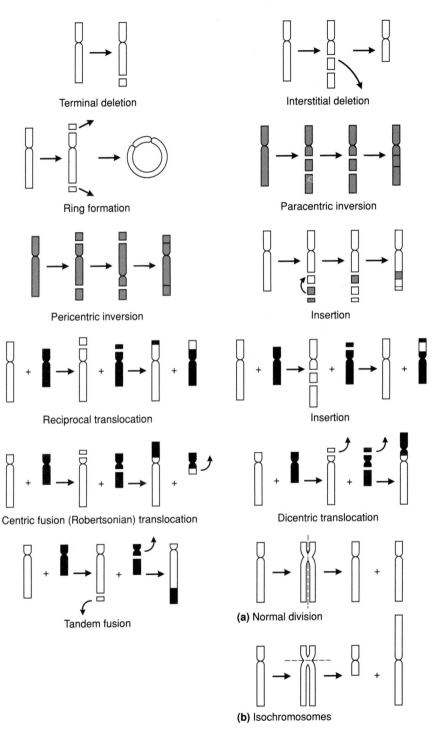

Terminal deletion

Interstitial deletion

Ring formation

Paracentric inversion

Pericentric inversion

Insertion

Reciprocal translocation

Insertion

Centric fusion (Robertsonian) translocation

Dicentric translocation

Tandem fusion

(a) Normal division

(b) Isochromosomes

When rearrangements involve more than one chromosome this is called a translocation. Reciprocal translocations occur when there is an exchange of material between two non-homologous chromosomes. If the size of the exchanged segments is different then there will be a change in the gross morphology of each participating chromosome. Insertions occur when there are two break points on one chromosome and only one break point in the other.

Centric fusion (Robertsonian) translocations occur between two acrocentric chromosomes. They are brought about by breaks in the minute short arm of one chromosome and the long arm of the other chromosome very close to the centromere. Fusion of the two large components results in a small centric fragment and a new submetacentric (or metacentric) translocation chromosome. After a number of cell divisions the centric fragment is often lost from the cell line. This is one of the easiest types of rearrangement to detect because not only is there a gross change in the chromosome morphology but also a reduction in the total chromosome number.

If the break point arises in the short arm of both acrocentric chromosomes then a dicentric chromosome is formed. Dicentric chromosomes are often less stable than normal because if the centromeres are sufficiently far apart each will try to act independently. However, if they are close together one centromere becomes suppressed and so the chromosome can sit on the spindle during cell division in the normal manner.

When there are breaks near the centromere of one chromosome and the telomere of another, with exchange of only the larger segment, then a tandem fusion is formed. Tandem fusions also result in the reduction of total chromosome number.

Sometimes there is abnormal division of the centromere during mitosis. Instead of dividing in the same plane as the chromatids, the centromere divides at right angles to this plane. The resulting two new chromosomes are called isochromosomes and each are metacentric with the two arms being genetically identical.

Rearrangements that do not result in any net loss or gain of genetic material are said to be balanced. Such abnormalities do not normally produce phenotypic changes in the affected animal. However, problems arise during meiosis. Meiotic pairing may be difficult or impossible and may result in non-disjunction. For example, with a centric fusion translocation a trivalent has to form during meiotic prophase and this leads to various degrees of non-disjunction at metaphase I, which can produce six different possible chromosome complements in the gamete (Figure 2.6). With reciprocal translocations a quadrivalent forms that may undergo adjacent 1, adjacent 2 or alternate segregation (Figure 2.7). This can result in 10 different possible gamete haplotypes (Ford and Clegg 1969) depending on where the chiasmata form.

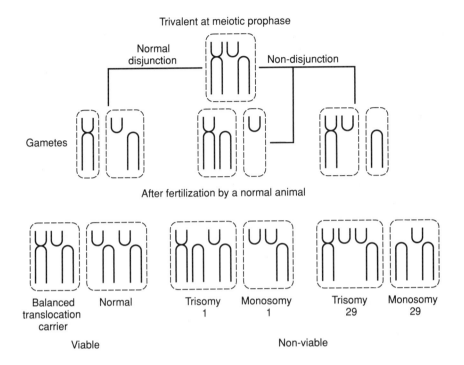

Figure 2.6 Diagrammatic representation of the effects of heterozygosity for a centric fusion such as the 1/29 translocation. The trivalent at meiosis can part in a balanced fashion to form gametes which, when fertilized, will form either normal offspring or balanced translocation carriers. However, if non-disjunction occurs, the gametes will be chromosomally unbalanced and any resulting offspring will also be unbalanced and non-viable.

If an abnormality is present in only one of a homologous pair of chromosomes the animal is said to be heterozygous for the abnormality. If the same abnormality is present in both homologous partners the animal is homozygous for the abnormality.

Numerical abnormalities

The normal somatic cell has the diploid number of chromosomes and is said to be euploid. Any deviation from the diploid number is known as heteroploidy. The gametes have only one of each homologous pair of chromosomes and so have half the diploid, i.e. the haploid, number of chromosomes. Somatic cells that have whole multiples of the haploid number above the diploid are called polyploid. For example, three times the haploid is triploidy, four times is tetraploidy, etc. Cells that have a few

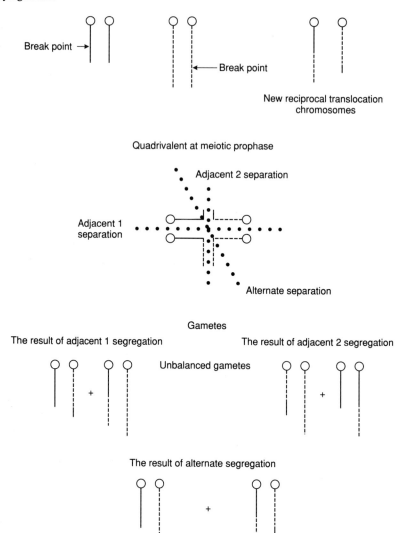

Figure 2.7 Diagrammatic representation of the effects of a reciprocal translocation. A quadrivalent develops at meiosis, formed from one copy of each of the normal homologues of the translocation chromosomes and the two new reciprocal translocation chromosomes. The chromosomes in the quadrivalent can part in one of three ways, adjacent 1, adjacent 2 and alternate segregation. Adjacent 1 and 2 separation results in gametes with an unbalanced amount of genetic material. These will result in non-viable embryos. Alternate segregation results in one gamete that contains both normal chromosomes and one gamete that has both translocation chromosomes and therefore has a balanced amount of genetic material. Offspring from these gametes are viable.

chromosomes more or less than the diploid number for the species are aneuploid. Where one of a homologous pair of chromosomes is missing this is called monosomy. When there is one extra chromosome with the homologous pair this is called trisomy.

Multiple cell lines

Animals with more than one cell line are said to be mixoploid, i.e. some cells with one chromosome complement and other cells with another chromosome complement. When the two or more cell lines derive from one original genotype the animal is a mosaic. However, when the two or more cell lines are derived from two or more cell lines this is a chimera. The different cell lines may be present in all the tissues of the animal, in which case it is referred to as a whole body chimera or whole body mosaic. Sometimes the multiple cell lines are only found in certain tissues, e.g. haemopoietic tissue.

Chromosome abnormalities in domestic animals

Most of the possible chromosomal abnormalities described above have been reported in the domestic species. Most are uncommon and many have been reported only as individual cases. However, certain anomalies are relatively common in some species and are important in the aetiology of fertility problems.

Freemartins

The commonest type of chromosomal abnormality encountered is sex chromosome chimerism, which is found in the freemartin condition. Freemartins have been diagnosed in cattle, sheep, goats and, rarely, pigs, but are most commonly seen in cattle (Marcum 1974).

Approximately 92% of the female calves born twin to a male are freemartins (Marcum 1974). The abnormalities of reproductive development seen in freemartins is due to the fact that the fusion of the placental blood vessels allows the anti-Müllerian substance (AMH) and testosterone, produced by the male, to circulate within the female (for review see Jost et al. 1973). However, the fused placental blood vessels also allow other material to transfer between the male and female foetuses.

During foetal development haemopoietic precursor cells migrate via the bloodstream to their final destination in the bone marrow (Winqvist 1954). When the placental blood vessels fuse the bone marrow precursor cells from each foetus become mixed and a common population of haemopoietic precursor cells is established in each animal. Thus, when the twins are of unlike sex, each will have bone marrow cells of male and female origin. That is, they are each blood cell chimeras. They have a mixed population of red cell antigens and chromosome examination of the peripheral blood lymphocytes reveals an XX/XY complement.

This chimerism was first demonstrated in cattle freemartins by Fechheimer et al. (1963) and it is a convenient way of diagnosing that placental anastomosis has occurred and thus that the female is likely to be a freemartin. It has to be stressed that the sex chromosome chimerism is in no way responsible for the freemartin condition and that its presence is merely used as a diagnostic tool.

In cattle the proportion of XX to XY cells is the same in each twin, i.e. there is not a reciprocal arrangement. However, the XX/XY ratio varies considerably between different sets of twins (Marcum et al. 1972). Therefore, for diagnostic purposes it is useful to be able to examine the bull twin at the same time as the female since some freemartins may have a very low percentage of XY cells. The bull will also have a low number of XY cells and so the fact of the placental anastomosis can be established through him and the inference made that the female will be a freemartin, despite having a preponderence of female cells. If the bull twin is not available, then sufficient cells have to be examined to reduce the probability that the XY cells are being missed because of their low incidence. For example, 90 cells must be examined to be 99% confident that there is not a second cell line with an incidence of 5% or more (Hook 1977).

The chromosome test for freemartinism is not 100% accurate. From the literature, 30 cows have been examined that were born twin to a bull and that have produced at least one calf (Eldridge and Blazak, 1977; Smith et al. 1977). Two of these (6.7%) were sex chromosome chimeras and would have been diagnosed as freemartins had they been examined as calves. On this basis the chromosome test for non-freemartins is only 93% accurate.

In sheep the incidence of freemartins is only about 4% of mixed sex twins. In addition, the clinical presentation is more varied in that animals may have an extreme male phenotype. However, a cytogenetic examination of a blood culture will reveal the sex chromosome chimerism.

The incidence of the freemartin condition in goats is not known although there are a number of reports in the literature, whilst the incidence in pigs is sufficiently low not to pose a practical problem.

Centric fusion (Robertsonian) translocations

In cattle the commonest structural chromosome abnormality is the centric fusion (Robertsonian) translocation: 28 different translocations have been identified although the 14/20 and the 14/21 may be the same (Table 2.3); both were found in the Simmental breed, the 14/20 in Scotland and the 14/21 in Hungary. Examination of the published photographs suggests that this may be the same translocation.

Most centric fusion translocations occur in only one breed of cattle. The notable exception to this is the 1/29 translocation, which has been found in numerous different breeds throughout the world and is seen in cattle of both *Bos taurus* and *Bos indicus* origin (Table 2.4). Most breeds of cattle carry only one centric fusion translocation and this is usually the 1/29. The Blonde d'Aquitaine breed appears to carry three different translocations (1/29, 9/23, and 21/27) and Simmentals have two or three (1/29, 14/20, and 14/21). The 5/18 that was reported in one Simmental bull appears to have arisen spontaneously in somatic tissue and was not in the germ line. One of the Italian rare breeds, the Podolian, also carries two different translocations (1/29 and 14/24).

Most of the British breeds do not carry translocations. The exceptions are the British White (1/29), Red Poll (1/29), Dexter (6/16) and the British Friesian (1/29). The Friesian breed was thought to be free of translocations (except for a few odd cases in central Europe) but recently some carriers of the 1/29 translocation have been found in pedigree British Friesian herds (Wilson 1990).

The incidence of the different translocations in each breed is, for the most part, unknown. Certain rare breeds of cattle have a very high incidence of 1/29 translocation carriers in the population. For example, the incidence is 67% in British White cattle (Long 1993), 22.5% in Romagnola and 18.9% in Marchigiana (Long 1985). This is presumably because the breed populations are small and there has been extensive inbreeding. However, some commercial breeds, with much larger populations, also have a high incidence, e.g. 14–22% in the Blonde d'Aquitaine (Gary *et al.* 1991) and 13.4% in the Swedish Red and White breeds (Long 1985).

With centric fusion translocations there is little or no loss of genetic material but the chromosome number is reduced. In general they cause problems in the heterozygous carrier animal because of the formation of a trivalent configuration at meiosis. The trivalent has a predisposition to undergo non-disjunction, the frequency of which varies with the different chromosomes involved in the translocation. The production of unbalanced gametes results in the formation of unbalanced zygotes, which die during early embryonic development. Animals heterozygous for the 1/29 translocation show a reduction in fertility of the order of 5–7% (for review

Table 2.3 Centric fusion translocations in cattle

Current name	Old name	Breed	Reference
1/4		?	Lojda et al. (1976)
1/23		?	Lojda et al. (1976)
1/25		Piebald	Stranzinger and Forster (1976)
1/28		?	Lojda et al. (1976)
1/29		Various	Gustavsson and Rockborn (1964)
2/8	(2/4)	British Friesian	Pollock and Bowman (1974), Eldridge (1985)
3/4		Limousin	Popescu (1977)
3/27		Friesian	Cited by Berland et al. (1988)
4/4		?	Cited by Berland et al. (1988)
5/18		Simmental	Papp and Kovacs (1980)
5/23		Brune Roumaine	Cited by Berland et al. (1988)
6/16	(5–6/15–16)	Dexter	Eldridge (1974), Logue (1978)
6/28		?	Lojda et al. (1976)
7/21	(5/21)	Japanese Black	Masuda et al. (1980), Hanada et al. (1981)
8/9		Brown Swiss	Tschudi et al. (1977)
9/23	(7/20)	Blonde d'Aquitaine	Darre et al. (1974), Cribiu et al. (1989)
11/21		Brune Roumaine	Cited by Berland et al. (1988)
11/22		?	Lojda et al. (1976)
12/15		Holstein	Roldan et al. (1984)
13/21		Holstein-Friesian	Kovacs et al. (1973)
14/20*	(11–12/15–16) (13/21)	Simmental	Bruere and Chapman (1973), Harvey (1976), Logue and Harvey (1978)
14/21*		Simmental	Papp and Kovacs (1978)
14/24		Podolian	di Beredino et al. (1979)
14/28		Holstein	Ellsworth et al. (1979)
15/25		Barrosa	Iannuzzi et al. (1991)
21/27		Blonde d'Aquitaine	Berland et al. (1988)
25/27		Alpine Grey	de Giovanni et al. (1979)
27/29		Guernsey	Bongso and Basrur (1976)

* May be the same translocation.

Table 2.4 Breeds of cattle in which the 1/29 translocation has been found

Alistana	Japanese Black
Asturiana Valles	Kuri
Bauole	Limousin
Blonde d'Aquitaine	Marchigana
British Friesian	Montebeliard
British White	Morucha
Brown Mountain	Norwegian Red
Brown Atlas	Nguni
Brown Swiss	Ottonese
Cachena	Pisa
Charollais	Podolian
Chianina	Red Poll
Czechoslovakian Red Poll	Retina
De Lidia	Rubia Gallega
Fleckvieh	Santa Gertrudis
Gascons	Sayaguesa
German Red Poll	Siamese
Grauviel	Simmental
Guernsey	Swiss Red and White
(Holstein Friesian)	Tudanca
Hungarian Grey	Vosgienne

see Gustavsson 1979). Other translocations have a much more severe effect. For example, the 25/27 translocation found in one bull of the Italian Alpine Grey breed had a non-disjunction rate of 46.7% (de Giovanni *et al.* 1980). This animal had poor semen quality (low volume and low density). However, the reduction in fertility in heterozygous females, daughters of this bull, was only of the order of 5% (Succi *et al.* 1982).

In Britain, bulls that are to be used for artificial insemination (AI) are screened for chromosomal abnormalities because of the reduction in fertility associated with centric fusion translocations. Those carrying the translocation are not used in the AI stud.

Five different centric fusion translocations have been found in sheep in New Zealand: 5/26, 8/11, 7/25, t_4 and t_5 (Bruere 1969; Bruere and Mills, 1971; Bruere *et al.* 1972; Pearce *et al.* 1990). Only the 5/26 occurs in Britain and that is in Romney Marsh sheep (Bruere *et al.* 1978a). However, contrary to the findings in cattle, there is no evidence that sheep which are heterozygous carriers of these translocations have any reduction in fertility. This is despite the fact that, as in cattle, there is an increase in the rate of non-disjunction at meiosis associated with the translocation chromosomes. However, in sheep, it is postulated that there is prezygotic selection against these abnormal gametes and abnormal zygotes are not formed (Bruere 1974, 1975; Long 1977).

Centric fusion translocations are rare in pigs. However, the one that has been reported, the 13/17, has been found in pigs in Japan (Miyake *et al.* 1977), Mexico (Alonso and Cantu 1982), Germany (Schwerin *et al.* 1986) and the USA (McFeely *et al.* 1988).

Reciprocal translocations

Reciprocal translocations are most commonly found in the pig. To date, 38 different reciprocal translocations have been identified (Table 2.5). The reduction in fertility, measured by litter size, varies between 5% and total sterility and probably depends upon which chromosomes are affected and also the size of the segments involved in the anomaly. Some chromosomes appear to be more commonly involved in these translocations than others, which suggests that there are specific 'weak' points on these chromosomes that are particularly vulnerable to damage. In France and Sweden national computer records are kept of the farrowing rates of sows. This enables sows and boars that produce low litters to be detected and monitored for chromosomal anomalies and this is how the majority of the translocations have been identified. In Denmark, a chromosome screening programme is being established for the pig industry (K M Hansen, personal communication).

Reciprocal translocations have also been reported in cattle (Mayr *et al.* 1979; Mayr and Schleger 1981; de Schepper *et al.* 1982; Mayr *et al.* 1983; Ansari *et al.* 1991) but they appear to be much less common than in pigs. Only two reciprocal translocations have been identified in sheep. The first was a 1p–; 20q + in Germany (Glahn-Luft and Wassmuth 1980) and the second a 13q–; 20q + in Iceland (Anamthawat-Jonsson *et al.* 1992).

Sex chromosome abnormalities

In the horse it is sex chromosome aneuploidy and sex reversal that are the chromosomal anomalies associated with infertility. Often, affected animals are mixoploids with multiple cell lines.

X chromosome monosomy (XO syndrome or Turner's syndrome) is fairly easy to diagnose. Clinically the mares are usually referred when they first go to stud because of a failure to show normal oestrous behaviour. Oestrus may be totally absent or the cycles be irregular and indefinite. The cervix is usually small, flaccid and open. There is an underdeveloped uterus and the ovaries are small and often difficult to palpate. Histologically the ovaries consist of undifferentiated ovarian stroma, although there

Table 2.5 Reciprocal translocations in the pig

Translocation	Reduction in litter size (%)	Reference
11p+; 15q–	56	Hageltorn et al. (1973)
		Akesson and Henricson (1972)
1q–;11q+	(malformed piglet)	Hansen-Melander and Melander
		(1970)
6p+;15q–	100	Bouters et al. (1974)
13q–;14q+	52	Hageltorn et al. (1976),
		King et al. (1981)
1p–;6q+	25	Locniskar et al. (1976)
6p+;14q–	(intersex)	Madan et al. (1978)
4q+;14q–	43	Popescu and Legault (1979),
		Popescu and Boscher (1982)
1p–;16p+	?	Forster et al. (1981)
9p+;11q–	50	Gustavsson et al. (1982)
7q–;11q+	50	Gustavsson et al. (1982),
		Gustavsson and Settergren
		(1984)
1p–;8q+	?	Gustavsson et al. (1982)
3p+;7q–	45	Popescu et al. (1983),
		Bahri et al. (1984)
1q–;17q+	40	Gustavsson (1984)
5p–;14q+	45	Popescu et al. (1984)
5q–;8q+	33	Gustavsson (1984)
1p+;14q–	34	Gustavsson (1984)
16q+;17q–	31	Popescu and Boscher (1986)
4q+;13q–	40	Makinen and Remes (1986)
7p+;13q–	?	Makinen and Remes (1986)
15q+;16q–	?	Makinen and Remes (1986)
1q+; 7q–	?	Makinen and Remes (1986)
7q–;12q+	40	Kuokkanen and Makinen (1987)
1q–;14q+	35	Tarocco et al.(1987)
2p;15q;4p	?	Makinen et al. (1987)
1p–;11q+	33	Kuokkanen and Makinen (1988)
1p+;15q–	43	Kuokkanen and Makinen (1988)
2p;4q	?	Gustavsson et al. quoted by
		Kuokkanen and Makinen (1988)
2p+;14q–	?	Gustavsson et al. (1989a)
Xq+;13q–	100 (males)	
	? (females)	Gustavsson et al. (1989b)
1p–;11q+	?	Tzocheva (1990)
1p:6p	?	Yang et al. (1991)
1q+;18q–	45	Villagomez et al. (1991a)
6q;8q	?	Bonneau et al. (1991)
6p;15q	?	Bonneau et al. (1991)
7q+;17q–	41	Villagomez et al. (1991a)
14q;15q	?	Gustavsson and Jonsson (1991)
Xp+;14q–	100 (male)	
	? (female)	Villagomez et al. (1991b)

may be small or degenerating follicles present. Many of these animals are said to have been abnormally small in stature.

Unfortunately, whilst such a clinical history is strongly indicative of a chromosomal abnormality it is not absolutely diagnostic since a number of mares with a similar history have been found to have a normal chromosome complement (Hughes and Trommershausen-Smith 1977; Bruere *et al.* 1978b; Long, unpublished data). A cytogenetic analysis is therefore necessary for a definite diagnosis. Examination of a heparinized blood sample will show a chromosome number of 63 in all cells and C or G banding will confirm that the missing chromosome is the X. The XO condition has been diagnosed in Arabs, Thoroughbreds, Quarter-horses, a Standardbred and a Welsh pony.

Most XY sex-reversed males present in a similar manner to XO mares. They arrive at stud as young 'mares' but fail to come into oestrus. Internally they usually have the same infantile development of the reproductive tract as the XO mares. However, the clinical picture in cases of XY sex reversal has shown some variations. There have been reports of XY 'mares' showing quite overt signs of oestrus and of having some follicular activity on the ovaries (Kent *et al.* 1986) There has even been one report of a fertile XY sex-reversed male but this animal may have had a normal XX cell line in the ovary (Sharp *et al.* 1980). All have the normal number of 64 chromosomes and C or G banding confirms the presence of the Y chromosome. Presumably the condition is caused by the deletion of a minute segment of the Y chromosome that carries the male determining genes. Alternatively, it could be due to a deletion of any one of the cascade of genes on the X and autosomes that are governed by the male determining genes on the Y. The condition was originally reported most commonly in the Arab breed but a number of cases have now been identified in Thoroughbreds in Britain and Ireland (Power 1986; Long 1988).

As well as XY sex reversal there have been a few cases of XY gonadal dysgenesis reported in the horse. These also present as infertile mares but have no gonadal tissue at all. Thus, they develop as phenotypic females but are, in fact, genetic males. There is some confusion in the literature between the terminology for XY sex reversal and XY gonadal dysgenesis and it may be that these are not two separate syndromes. XY gonadal dysgenesis may be an extreme form of XY sex reversal where there is so little gonadal tissue that it is not palpable *per rectum*.

The cases of XO/XX mixoploidy are more difficult to diagnose since they have presented no consistent clinical picture. Some XO/XX mares show irregular oestrous behaviour (Hughes *et al.* 1975) and some XO/XX mares are reported to have produced a foal when young (Halnan 1985). One mare with only 2% XO cells eventually produced a foal at the age of

9 years (Long, unpublished data). Thus it is often difficult to give a prognosis even when a diagnosis has been made. Furthermore, diagnosis can be difficult because mixoploidy cannot be positively excluded unless every cell is examined, so the probability of the existence of a second cell line has to be calculated from the number of cells examined. This is a situation where fibroblast cultures might establish whether the chromosome complement is consistent in other tissue.

X chromosome aneuploidy has been reported in cattle, sheep and pigs but only rarely and it does not seem to be of importance in these species.

3

REPRODUCTIVE ENDOCRINOLOGY AND PHARMACOLOGY

H DOBSON BSc, PhD, DSc

Introduction

In order to understand hormonal treatments, either for clinical or management purposes, it is necessary to appreciate (1) how an animal controls its own hormones and (2) in clinical cases, what defects have occurred in the system, and why.

The classical endocrine definition of a hormone (as a blood-borne chemical messenger between different organs within the body) requires modification, mainly because it is now known that some compounds can act within the endocrine gland that produced them, e.g. prostaglandins, endorphins. Suffice it to say, however, that most actions of endogenous hormones are mimicked by exogenous administration. Reproduction involves several complex interactions largely orchestrated by hormones. Hence reproductive pharmacology largely concentrates on endocrinology, although from a veterinary point of view antibiotic control of infections within reproductive organs and manipulation of uterine muscle action are also important.

The chemical nature of some exogenous hormones and biologically active compounds is exactly the same as those which occur naturally. However, analogues are often preferred either for commercial reasons (including patents, ease of manufacture, shelf-life) or therapeutic reasons (longer half-life, greater tissue penetration, more efficacious). The most important thing is to choose the right compound for the right condition, thus placing great emphasis on initial diagnosis! The collective name for compounds that have a similar action to progesterone is progestins; and similarly oestrogens for oestradiol-like compounds.

Hypothalamus–pituitary–gonad interactions

In both male and non-pregnant female animals the major endocrine glands involved in the control of reproduction are the hypothalamus, the anterior pituitary and the gonads (testes and ovaries, respectively) (Figure 3.1). The hypothalamus situated in the lower brain receives neuronal input from other parts of the brain and central nervous system and is linked to the

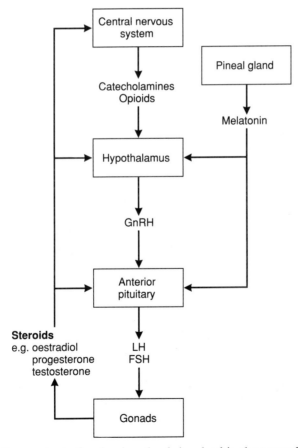

Figure 3.1 Interactions of endocrine glands involved in the control of reproduction.

anterior pituitary by a direct portal venous system. Gonadotrophin releasing hormone (GnRH) is produced by neurones within the hypothalamus and after release into the portal system acts on cells in the anterior pituitary to release luteinizing hormone (LH) and follicle stimulating hormone (FSH). Control of GnRH synthesis/release is of paramount importance in the correct functioning of the reproductive system. Neuronal input from higher parts of the brain is governed through catecholamine and opioid influences, which are in turn modulated by steroids produced by the gonads. Interaction with the pineal gland via production of melatonin is also thought to be largely exerted at this level. The feedback interactions between hypothalamus, pituitary and gonads are referred to as negative if production of a hormone is suppressed and positive if production is increased.

The behaviour of animals is also dependent on hypothalamus–pituitary–gonad interaction. It is well known that prolactin is essential for maternal behaviour during the postpartum period. Obviously oestrogens are closely implicated in symptoms of oestrus and evidence is accumulating for the involvement of opioids in both male and female reproductive behaviour.

The male

Testosterone is produced by the Leydig cells, which are situated between the spermatic tubules within the testis. Inhibin is produced by Sertoli cells and oestrogens are produced either by the Sertoli cells from steroid precursors synthesized in the Leydig cell or by the Leydig cell itself. The stallion and boar are remarkable for the amount of oestrone sulphate in the peripheral circulation, the reason for which remains obscure. The production of testosterone and oestrogen is enhanced by LH release from the pituitary; these steroids in turn feed back on the pituitary to control LH release. Peripheral plasma hormone profiles in most species reveal up to 4–10 peaks per day of testosterone, each being preceded by increases in LH concentration (Figure 3.2). Testosterone is thought to be converted to oestradiol both peripherally and within the behavioural centres of the brain, to control male reproductive behaviour. At present precise control mechanisms for the release of inhibin are unknown but it has a negative feedback effect on pituitary FSH secretion.

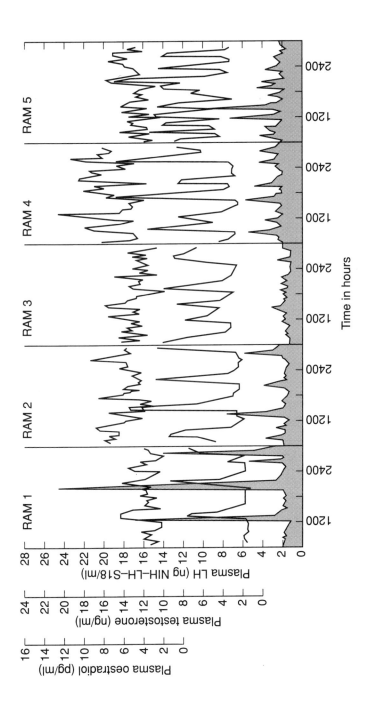

Figure 3.2 Plasma profiles of LH (lower, shaded area), testosterone (middle), and oestradiol (top) in crossbred rams sampled during the breeding season (from Schanbacher and Ford 1976).

Endocrine therapy of the male

As so little is known about endogenous endocrine regulatory mechanisms in males of all species it is not surprising that there is scant evidence for successful endocrine therapy. It has been suggested that any endocrine defects may be of a hereditary nature and hence treating and breeding from such males would be disadvantageous.

Attempts have been made to treat impotent males or those with low libido with testosterone or gonadotrophins, with no success. Indeed, experimental treatment of rams with testosterone resulted in a reduction in sperm output, and high endogenous plasma testosterone concentrations in bulls have been correlated with abnormalities in sperm morphology.

Nevertheless there are reports that gonadotrophins and testosterone plus possibly other intratubular factors are involved in regulating spermatogenesis. Only much more research in the future will lead to successful therapies.

While little progress has recently been made to enhance male fertility by endocrine therapy, success has been achieved in producing castrated males by immunological means—this involves immunizing males against natural GnRH. Once a high titre of antibody has been achieved, LH and testosterone concentrations diminish as does sperm output. Repeated booster immunizations maintain sterility. If necessary fertility can be restored by stimulation of gonadotrophin release with a GnRH analogue that is not neutralized by the antibody against natural GnRH (Keeling and Crighton 1984).

Tests for cryptorchidism

Another positive factor to emerge from research into male endocrinology has been the development of an endocrine test to confirm the presence or absence of retained testes (Cox *et al.* 1986). Owing to the great variation in testosterone concentrations throughout the day in normal males, it would be unreliable to depend on one peripheral plasma testosterone measurement to detect the presence of testicular material. Consequently the diagnostic test consists of taking two samples, one before and one approximately 90 minutes after an injection of human chorionic gonadotrophin (hCG) or GnRH. If both samples have low testosterone concentrations testicular material is assumed absent and explorative surgery can be avoided. However if the second sample has a higher testosterone concentration than the first, this provides evidence for the presence of retained testicular tissue.

The non-pregnant female

It takes about 4–6 months for follicles to grow from the primordial state to the point of forming antra to become Graafian follicles. The final 6–8 days of ovarian follicular growth are supported by pulsatile release of LH from the pituitary (Figure 3.3). During the mid-luteal phase the frequency of LH pulses is approximately six to eight pulses per day; early in the follicular phase this increases to 10–15 per day gradually becoming 1 pulse per hour by the late follicular phase (Goodman 1988). Each LH pulse is followed by an increase in oestradiol production by the growing follicle(s), which in turn stimulates further LH pulses in a self-perpetuating positive feedback system. Eventually, around the onset of behavioural oestrus a preovulatory surge of LH occurs, the ramifications of which are far reaching. As well as causing resumption of meiosis in the ovum of each mature follicle and further processes leading to ovulation, the LH surge switches off oestradiol production by each Graafian follicle and initiates the formation of a corpus luteum. After ovulation, for the first few days of the oestrous cycle there is nothing to suppress the resumption of frequent LH pulses and a second wave of follicles is encouraged to grow, resulting in considerable oestradiol production. However, usually before the LH surge and ovulation are achieved, progesterone production by the growing luteal tissue feeds back negatively on the hypothalamus–pituitary axis to suppress LH secretion. By the mid-luteal phase the regular frequency of LH pulsatility is again under progesterone domination.

It is now known that corpora lutea of many species produce oxytocin and progesterone in parallel. At the end of the luteal phase, possibly in response to luteal oxytocin, the uterus secretes prostaglandin $F_{2\alpha}$ ($PGF_{2\alpha}$) and this is thought to be the main luteolytic factor in some species such as the sheep, although in other species, such as the cow, additional factors (especially oestradiol) are thought to be involved.

Manipulation of ovarian cyclicity

Occasionally there are situations when negative suppression of ovarian cyclicity is required, e.g. in feedlot meat production systems. If ovarian cyclicity is suppressed, a 10–20% increase in weight gain will be achieved with an 8% greater feed conversion ratio. Similarly, animal handling is easier if cyclicity is suppressed in riding ponies or show horses.

Reasons for wishing to exert exogenous control of ovarian cyclicity upon animals are basically two-fold, clinical or managerial. Clinical reasons include either the need to counteract subfertility, for example during a

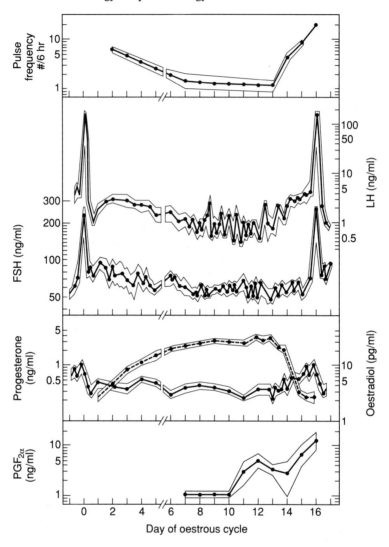

Figure 3.3 Changes in LH pulse frequency, mean peripheral concentrations of LH, FSH, progesterone and oestradiol, and uterine vein concentrations of prostaglandin $F_{2\alpha}$ ($PGF_{2\alpha}$) throughout the ovine oestrous cycle. Shaded areas depict ± SEM for each hormone (from Goodman 1988).

prolonged postpartum period, or when natural endocrine rhythms have become deranged. Managerial reasons include:

1. minimization of handling and heat detection procedures, especially for artificial insemination (AI) regimes;

2. to allow batch births and hence maximum perinatal supervision;
3. to realign the timing of births either for commercial reasons, e.g. in dairy cows to take maximum advantage of milk seasonality payments, or for agricultural reasons such as grass availability;
4. to control the length of the postpartum period;
5. to obtain more frequent births per dam per year, e.g. producing three lamb crops in 2 years.

For efficient successful manipulation of ovarian cyclicity certain requirements are necessary. All efforts will be wasted unless at least normal (or preferably increased) rates of fertility are obtained immediately following manipulation. Well-fed animals, not too thin nor too fat, should be used, and stress-free handling facilities should be available. Accurate animal identification is a necessity, as is good record-keeping. The application of hormones should be as trouble-free as possible. Obviously, adequate opportunities for insemination must be provided, either by artificial means, keeping in mind inseminator fatigue, or by natural means, not forgetting the need for a higher male:female ratio if many females are expected in oestrus in a very short time. Above all, especially in farming situations, the whole manipulation regime must be provided at reasonable cost, not only taking into account drugs but also the extra time and labour that are often involved.

Techniques in the absence of corpora lutea

The choice of method is very dependent on whether active corpora lutea are present or not. If there are no corpora lutea present progesterone is often administered, usually for a period of time similar to the animal's own luteal phase. The easiest way to do this is by orally active compounds that are fed daily, but this is only effective if the animals are fed individually (e.g. horses and pigs) to be certain each animal consumes an appropriate dose. Alternatively, for cows, sheep and goats, slow-release formulations such as intravaginal devices or subcutaneous implants are more desirable to overcome the need for frequent injections.

The theory behind progesterone administration relies partially on the ability of this hormone to initiate regular pulses of LH similar to those in the mid-luteal phase—very often in anoestrous situations LH, if secreted at all, is released in a random, disorganized pattern of pulses. Once appropriate pulses of LH are released, any Graafian follicles present will grow in the ovary and upon progesterone withdrawal a normal follicular phase will continue. However, sometimes in situations of deeper anoestrus, extra ovarian stimulation is required in which case pregnant mare's serum gonadotrophin (PMSG; now renamed equine chorionic gonadotrophin, eCG) or purified preparations of FSH are administered at the time of progesterone withdrawal to minimize handling procedures, although better results can be obtained if eCG (PMSG) is injected 1 or 2 days prior to the removal of progesterone.

As an alternative to progesterone therapy the use of repeated administration of low doses of GnRH to stimulate LH pulses has been suggested. In fact even continuous slow-release formulations of GnRH have been successful in inducing ovulations, but the quality of subsequent corpora lutea has only been adequate after pretreating the animals with progesterone (McLeod et al. 1982). Future research may result in the production of a successful combination treatment.

Other effective ways of increasing LH pulsatility include exposing females to males, especially in situations such as very late seasonal anoestrus. In this case an increase in LH concentration will occur within 5 minutes of exposure, probably via a pheromonal effect. Similarly, a substantial sudden increase in the plane of nutrition, i.e. flushing, or removal of sucking young, i.e. weaning, or altering hours of day length will initiate ovarian activity within 2–4 weeks, possibly via an influence on LH pulsatility or by a direct action on the ovary. (In breeds or species very sensitive to day length it has also been shown that male reproductive activity can be altered by changing lighting regimes.)

An awareness of the influence of light and its interaction with the pineal gland has led to the development of melatonin formulations that can be used to initiate early ovarian cyclicity in seasonal breeders, e.g. sheep and goats (Symons et al. 1988). Melatonin is endogenously secreted from the pineal gland during hours of darkness. At present it is not clear whether melatonin acts mainly at the hypothalamus, pituitary or ovary. Continuous application of melatonin means that if an animal does not conceive at the first induced oestrus, cyclicity will continue to allow a second chance of conception (unlike an application of progesterone too early before the onset of the breeding season).

Techniques in the presence of corpora lutea

In order to synchronize oestrus in the presence of corpora lutea decisions must be made whether to prolong the luteal phase or shorten it. Prolongation involves administration of progesterone or derivatives in ways already discussed. However, care must be taken not to extend the progestational phase for too long as this may have deleterious effects on the uterine endometrium and hence affect conception rates (Roche and Ireland 1984). It is common to administer exogenous progestagens for approximately three-quarters the normal length of the luteal phase: any animal that had just been in heat before the start of treatment would not be influenced. Conversely, animals nearing the end of the luteal phase at the time of administration have an additional three-quarter luteal phase imposed by exogenous progestins, during which follicular development is suppressed. Upon withdrawal of progestins all animals are released from progestin dominance and follicular growth occurs, resulting in synchronized oestrus. Because this method is similar to that for animals without corpora lutea, it is the method of choice if there is the possibility that within the group of animals some have corpora lutea and some do not.

For animals that are known to have corpora lutea, the use of exogenous $PGF_{2\alpha}$ may be preferable. However, there is a drawback. $PGF_{2\alpha}$ is not luteolytic in the early luteal phase, e.g. days 0–4 in sheep or days 0–6 in cattle and as long as days 0–12 in pigs. This is an almost insurmountable problem for pigs, but for other species a double injection regime has been developed. Before using $PGF_{2\alpha}$ it must be established whether the animals are pregnant or not; it would be professionally negligent not to do so as $PGF_{2\alpha}$ is abortifacient during early pregnancy in many species. At the time of the first $PGF_{2\alpha}$ injection all those animals not in the early luteal phase will come into oestrus; those between days 0 and 4 or 6 of the cycle will not be affected. A second injection of $PGF_{2\alpha}$ given 8–10 days later in sheep or goats, or 10–13 days later in cows and horses (Figure 3.4), will result in all animals coming into heat after a few days because (1) those initially in the early luteal phase and unaffected by the first injection will be in a responsive phase at the time of the second injection and (2) those that did respond to the first injection will again be in the responsive phase of the next cycle by the time of the second injection. A more economical but possibly more labour-intensive system than this double injection regime involves a period (approximately 7 days) of intense observation of oestrus and subsequent insemination. A single injection of $PGF_{2\alpha}$ is then given only to those animals not inseminated during the 7-day observation period. In this situation, if the observation of oestrus is very efficient, all the animals given $PGF_{2\alpha}$ should be beyond day 7 of the cycle and hence in the responsive phase of the cycle.

Fairly high doses of oestrogens given on days 0–6 in cattle are known to prevent corpus luteum development; hence a capsule containing oestradiol benzoate is incorporated into the progesterone releasing intravaginal device (PRID) to enhance success rates of this product. However, it is not common practice to inject oestradiol alone in place of $PGF_{2\alpha}$ to cows on days 0–6 as a method of control of oestrus, mainly because of the difficulty of being certain that cows are at that stage of the cycle.

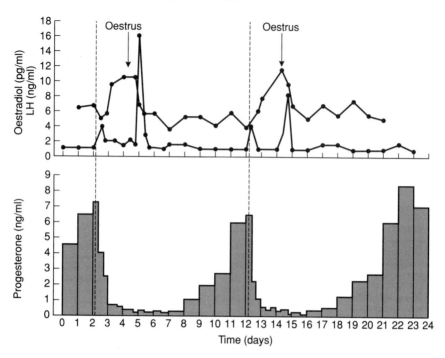

Figure 3.4 Plasma progesterone (histograms), oestradiol (▲) and LH (●) in a heifer given two injections of a PGF$_{2\alpha}$ analogue, cloprostenol (vertical interrupted lines) 10 days apart (from Dobson *et al.* 1975).

Methods of increasing ovulation rate

Unfortunately it is not known how any animal regulates the number of ovulations that occur within each period of oestrus. It is known that waves of several follicles begin growing, with many becoming atretic before antrum formation. However, even after this event a selection procedure takes place during which a number of follicles become dominant and proceed to ovulation, depending upon the species and breed involved. There have been recent suggestions that intraovarian factors are responsible, at least in part, but so far these have not been conclusively identified. In fact, it is probable that a complex interaction of intraovarian factors and possibly gonadotrophins is necessary, for it is known that animals with insufficient circulating FSH concentrations have reduced follicular growth. However, there do not appear to be markedly increased concentrations of FSH in animals with high ovulation rates. The present consensus of opinion is that FSH is a permissive hormone; so long as more than a threshold amount of FSH is available, other factors are involved in determining ovulation rate in normal untreated animals. Having said that, however, it is possible to increase ovulation rates in many animals by exogenous application of FSH. Over recent years progress in techniques of purification of pituitary FSH, and even genetically engineered production of FSH, has meant that purified FSH has been available for inducing superovulation. Nevertheless, there are still many drawbacks: pure FSH has a very short half-life, hence repeated injections at 12-hour intervals for 2–4 days are required; between animals of the same breed there is an extremely variable response in the number of ovulations achieved; FSH purification procedures for some species, e.g. horses, are extremely difficult. Prior to the use of purified FSH the preparation eCG (PMSG) was always used. This has a much longer half-life, and has LH activity but still results in very variable ovulation rates. Both eCG (PMSG) and FSH have been used at high doses to induce superovulation for techniques such as embryo transfer, and they have also been used in much lower doses to overcome antagonistic influences that reduce ovulation rates, e.g. season, lactation, suckling.

An alternative method of increasing ovulation rates, especially in sheep, is now available. This involves immunization against one of a number of steroids, especially androstenedione. Mating 2–3 weeks after a booster immunization results in a greater number of lambs born. For example, normal lambing rates of 1.2 can be increased to 1.7, mainly by increasing the proportion of twin-carriers rather than causing great increases in litter size in a few individuals (Scaramuzzi *et al.* 1987). In spite of a lot of research work it is still not clear how the increase in ovulation rate is achieved.

The pregnant female

Establishment of pregnancy

One major problem facing early conceptuses is that of establishing maintenance of maternal corpora lutea. Early pregnancy (up to day 40) in cattle, goats, sheep, horses and pigs depends on the continued function of corpora lutea. Proteins secreted by the conceptus and/or the endometrium intervene with uterine prostaglandin synthesis and release, thereby inhibiting luteolysis (Thatcher *et al.* 1988).

After release from the zona pellucida the trophoblast surrounding the conceptus comes into close apposition with the uterine endometrium. This presents another problem for the conceptus: being composed of maternal and paternal genetic material it is ostensibly foreign to the dam and an immune rejection might be expected. However, strategies have evolved ensuring that this does not happen and it has recently been discovered that trophoblastic proteins involved in alteration of $PGF_{2\alpha}$ activity have a close similarity to interferon, which itself is known to modify immune reactions (Heap et al. 1988). It remains to be seen whether this will lead to the development of pharmacological preparations that can be given early in pregnancy to increase the efficiency of the establishment of early pregnancy. The greatest proportion of embryo losses occur just after release of the conceptus from the zona pellucida.

Tests for early pregnancy

Continued progesterone production by corpora lutea in early pregnancy has provided the basis for an early test of pregnancy. In most species samples of body fluid (milk, blood or saliva) are taken when the next oestrus might be expected if the animal was not pregnant. Low progesterone values confirm that the animal is not pregnant; high values suggest that the animal might be pregnant. Errors creep in when prolonged corpora lutea occur for reasons other than pregnancy, or when samples have been taken at the wrong time, usually after mistimed inseminations.

Attempts have also been made to test for pregnancy by quantifying proteins secreted by the conceptus. However, so far none has been found in easily accessible body tissues in sufficiently high concentrations to be measurable. The only current hope is the measurement of pregnancy specific protein B (PSPB), which originates from the endometrium and has been found in elevated concentrations in plasma of pregnant cows 24 days after insemination (Sasser et al. 1986). It must be remembered that embryo loss can take place after a positive early pregnancy test.

Placental hormone production

Further development of trophoblast tissue and its reaction with the endometrium leads to the formation of the placenta, which itself becomes an important temporary endocrine gland. In goats and pigs the presence of functional corpora lutea is essential throughout the whole of pregnancy. Although the placenta of the goat is known to produce active progestins such as pregnanediols, synthesis of progesterone by corpora lutea is a prerequisite for maintenance of pregnancy in goats and pigs. In sheep, the placenta begins to provide progesterone from approximately day 50 of pregnancy; in cattle, it is thought that other potent progestins may be produced by the placenta throughout the period 150–250 days of pregnancy. Before that, and for the last 30 days of pregnancy, the cow is dependent on the corpus luteum for progesterone production. The situation is quite different for the horse: in this species progesterone from a primary corpus luteum maintains pregnancy for the first 35 days. Secondary corpora lutea supplement progesterone production from this time until approximately day 150 of pregnancy, after which ovariectomy does not result in abortion. It is possible that other progestins are produced by the placenta and act locally within the uterus to maintain pregnancy beyond day 150. Over the last 30 days of pregnancy peripheral plasma concentrations of progesterone again increase until parturition.

The implications for these species differences in dependency on progesterone from corpora lutea are important when it becomes necessary to choose an abortifacient agent, e.g. for treating cases of misalliance. Treatment with $PGF_{2\alpha}$ will terminate pregnancy when the latter is dependent on corpora lutea, i.e. before day 50 in sheep, throughout the whole of pregnancy in goats and pigs, before day 150 and after day 250 in cattle, and before day 30 in horses.

In addition to progestins the placentae of most of these species also produce oestrogens, usually in the later stages of pregnancy. Oestrone sulphate, an oestrogen with little bioactivity, gradually increases in concentration in peripheral plasma at approximately the same time as the progestin-synthesizing activity of the placenta increases, i.e. from day 50 in sheep and goats, from day 100 in cattle and from day 70 in pigs.

The concentrations of oestrone sulphate in milk or blood after these times in pregnancy are much greater than in non-pregnant animals and this has been utilized in the development of a test to confirm the maintenance of pregnancy (Holdsworth et al. 1982). In all these species, except the sheep and the horse, oestradiol production by the placenta also increases gradually at this time. In the sheep, however, oestradiol only increases, albeit dramatically, during the last 48 hours of pregnancy. In horses, there is evidence to suggest that the oestrogens are produced by the foetal gonads over the period 100–300 days of pregnancy.

Initiation of parturition

The foetus is responsible for initiating the processes that eventually lead to parturition. Maturation of the foetal hypothalamus–pituitary–adrenal axis results in increased plasma cortisol concentrations in the foetus, especially over the last 2–3 days of pregnancy. The increased cortisol influence is responsible for coordinating many of the events required for a successful outcome of parturition. These processes include foetal lung maturation, i.e. production of lung surfactant to enable instant expansion and function upon birth of the foetus, as well as changes in liver glycogen metabolism and gut metabolism. In addition, under the influence of cortisol, placental steroid production is changed, resulting in reduced progestin synthesis (which among other things had been suppressing myometrial muscle contractions) in favour of oestradiol synthesis (Flint and Ricketts 1979) (Figure 3.5). Oestradiol also coordinates many essential body functions at this time, including an increase in coordinated myometrial muscle contractions via increased $PGF_{2\alpha}$ production, softening of the uterine cervix, induction of synthesis of oxytocin receptors to facilitate the Fergusson reflex, release of oxytocin and preparation of the mammary gland for milk production.

Periparturient endocrine therapy

Successful expulsion of a live foetus is the consequence of a series of precisely timed events, some of which can be mimicked by exogenous hormones for either clinical or managerial reasons. Induction of parturition is most successfully achieved when properly planned. Corticosteroids, when administered to the dam, can initiate the natural series of events usually under foetal adrenal control. The further back into pregnancy the corticosteroid is used the less efficacious it becomes and the longer it takes to result in birth. Long-acting synthetic preparations are used if the animal is earlier than 2 weeks from term. This can be followed up to 7–10 days later with short-acting corticosteroids particularly in sheep, or with $PGF_{2\alpha}$ especially in cattle, pigs and goats. If attempting very early induction of

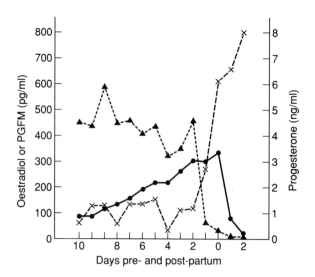

Figure 3.5 Concentrations of oestradiol (●), $PGF_{2\alpha}$ metabolite (PGFM; ×) and progesterone (▲) in the peripheral plasma of a cow in the last days of pregnancy (from Kaker *et al.* 1984).

parturition, it is thought preferable to proceed cautiously with long-acting corticosteroids, to enhance surfactant production by the foetal lung. As normal term approaches the initial stages of this process will have already taken place. Within the last 7–14 days of pregnancy in all species, except the sheep and horse, a favourable response to $PGF_{2\alpha}$ alone will be obtained.

There is increasing evidence to suggest that many clinical problems at parturition are the result of erroneous hormone production. For example, failure of the cervix to soften or dilate may be due to inadequate oestradiol and/or prostaglandin activity, incoordinated muscle contractions may result from impaired oxytocin or prostaglandin production or action, births before term may be the result of inadequate progesterone production by placenta or corpora lutea, or, alternatively, may be the consequence of foetal compromise resulting in increased foetal adrenal activity and hence precocious initiation of the whole event.

Unfortunately, there is relatively little that can be done therapeutically in many of these situations. Treatment with oestrogens or $PGF_{2\alpha}$ to help cervical dilatation takes too long (about 36 hours) to be of any use to a distressed foetus (Dobson 1988). Similarly, by the time a clinician is aware that a foetus has been compromised by reduced progesterone production, too many other events have been set in motion so that treatment with progesterone to prevent birth before term may do more harm than good. The same may be said of attempts to delay parturition with ß-adrenergic agents that temporarily abolish uterine contractions. However, there is evidence that one such drug, clenbuterol, has been used successfully in cattle, sheep and pigs, causing delays of approximately 12 hours. The indications for delaying parturition include final softening of the cervix, avoidance of night-time delivery, or as an aid to obstetrical manoeuvres, i.e. malpresentation or malposture. In other situations the opposite effect may be desired, i.e. to hasten the progress of labour. Once satisfied that the cervix is dilated, that obstructive dystocia is absent and that there is no abnormal uterine distension, oxytocin preparations can be given. Due to the powerful effects of this hormone, especially on an oestrogen-primed uterus, continual observation must be maintained, especially with horses. While deep intramuscular administration is often recommended, it may be more prudent to use approximately one-quarter the dose intravenously. Use of lower doses will result in a less violent if slightly longer labour. In some situations in ruminants and bitches subclinical hypocalcaemia may be responsible for the uterine inertia, in which case calcium borogluconate may be more appropriate treatment.

Postpartum period

Throughout pregnancy final maturation of ovarian follicles is prevented probably by progesterone domination of gonadotrophin synthesis and release. The foetus, and consequently the uterus, grow at a considerable rate especially in the last few weeks of pregnancy. Suddenly, after parturition, everything is different and quite remarkable changes have to take place to return all systems to a correctly functioning non-pregnant state. In domesticated species it is usually expedient to re-establish the next pregnancy as soon as possible. The seasonal breeders, sheep and goats, are the exception to this if only one offspring crop per year is required; however, in some intensive systems even for these species early rebreeding is necessary.

In the approximately 3-week period after birth, vast changes in tissue remodelling have to take place. The maternal anatomical adaptations made during placental development have to be destroyed, any remaining foetal placental tissues must be expelled, and during both these necrotic processes defence mechanisms against infection must be maximized. The uterine musculature, which has been gradually stretched throughout pregnancy and has then carried out a massive work programme during birth, needs to readjust to a new role in the non-pregnant animal. Similarly the cervix, kept tightly closed through pregnancy then structurally modified to allow passage of the foetus, has again to revert to an altered role in non-pregnancy. The ovaries are required to spring into action again to provide both fertilizable ova and the hormones involved in the orchestration of reproductive cyclicity. The hypothalamus and pituitary, which are involved in regulation of the ovaries, also need to come out of the quiescent state maintained during pregnancy.

All these processes are modified by influences imposed by domestication and the environment. For example, those dams that suckle their young benefit from the increased influence of hormones (e.g. oxytocin) that evacuate the lumen of the uterus and activate the uterine musculature. However, there are disadvantages to suckling: compounds (possibly oxytocin, cortisol, prolactin and/or others) released during this process suppress regeneration of hypothalamic and pituitary activity leading to reduced ovarian stimulation. Dams that have had their young weaned very early and are then subjected to artificial milk removal face increased uterine compromise but, unfortunately, do not always benefit from early ovarian activity because very often increased elevation of milk yields achieved by genetic selection are not always matched by adequate provision of nutrients. This in turn results in suppression of hypothalamus–pituitary activity. In species such as sheep and goats some of these problems are masked by the intervention of seasonal anoestrus.

Uterine involution

Relatively little is known about the rate-controlling mechanisms of this process: obviously the quicker it occurs the better. It is known that animals that have problems at parturition tend to have delayed involution, which in turn often occurs simultaneously with uterine infection. The latter results in delayed conception of the next pregnancy (Borsberry and Dobson 1989).

Placental separation

Even before the onset of parturition, gradual processes have begun within the placenta that accelerate alongside maturation of the foetus, leading to rapid expulsion of placental tissues within hours of birth. In fact evidence is accumulating to show that abnormalities in placental expulsion are preceded by abnormal endocrine events, e.g. altered ratios of oestradiol and progesterone concentrations. The delivery of an increased number of offspring, especially with the usual accompanying decrease in gestation length, also predisposes to placental retention and is probably associated with deranged endocrine activities. It is thought that hormones control the early degenerative changes around the boundaries of maternal and foetal membranes. The failure to expel the placenta immediately after birth could either be due to a malfunction of these degenerative changes, or due to lack of adequate muscular activity to force the now unwanted material out of the uterus. Until more is known about the precise changes that take place before birth, it would be very dangerous to consider prophylactic treatment at this time—the risk to the offspring would be too great. Hence postpartum therapy is the only choice.

Uterine activity around birth is influenced by oxytocin release from the posterior pituitary and is associated with $PGF_{2\alpha}$ release from the uterus. The concentrations of both hormones increase around parturition and exogenous administration will enhance muscular contraction. In common with the action of all other hormones, receptors for oxytocin and $PGF_{2\alpha}$ are required within target tissues and, although it has been assumed for some time that such receptors diminish in number very rapidly after birth, more evidence is now accumulating that both hormones can be quite effective for some time post partum. However, the nearer after birth these hormones have been administered the larger the effects that have been seen in inducing muscular activity and expulsion of placental membranes. Even 6 hours after birth the effectiveness may become diminished, i.e. before a problem has become clearly established because it is usually considered that membranes have only been abnormally retained 12–24 hours after birth. However, if a predisposition to placental retention is suspected, prophylactic treatment with oxytocin or $PGF_{2\alpha}$ may be considered.

Uterine infection

Once involutionary changes have taken place in the cervix (by approximately 48–72 hours) it becomes physically more difficult to expel larger pieces of tissue from the uterus and it may be more prudent to allow necrotic processes to take over. This then brings into question the use of antibiotic therapy. Without hesitation, if the dam is showing any signs of systemic illness then administration of parenteral antibiotic is necessary. Otherwise, intrauterine administration of antibiotics may be contra-indicated for the rapid progress of necrosis. Very often, without pharmacological treatment, by 7–10 days after birth, sufficient degeneration has taken place to permit seepage of uterine contents through the partially involuted cervix, especially if the activity of uterine musculature is enhanced. In some species, especially the dairy cow, reports are now accruing to suggest that one treatment with $PGF_{2\alpha}$ within 30 days after calving can be beneficial in terms of calving-to-conception intervals (Young and Anderson 1986). Although this has not yet been well proven, it may be that enhancing uterine muscle activity contributes to more rapid normalization of the uterine environment.

The bacterial flora of the uterus changes constantly during the postpartum period and is, on the whole, harmless. However, there is a suggestion that a lot of damage can be caused by the facultative anaerobe *Actinomyces pyogenes*, especially if associated with the obligative anaerobe *Fusobacterium necrophorum*. Improved efficiency of treatment may be achieved if either of these organisms could be identified at the time of clinical examination and then an appropriate antianaerobic therapy instituted (Pepper and Dobson 1987).

If, at any time, external entry to the uterus is necessary, e.g. during dystocia or caesarean operations, then it would be wise to apply intrauterine antibiotic therapy, mainly to overcome any inadvertent contamination. Similarly, every attempt should be made to reduce opportunities for infection: only enter the uterus if absolutely necessary; provide clean hygienic areas for parturition, outside on grass if at all possible; and if membranes are retained no attempt should be made at manual removal by force, but rather exteriorize a cleaner portion from the vagina and excise the membranes to limit the chances of ascending infection.

At later times after parturition (>4 weeks) it is also possible for the uterus to succumb to uterine infections. Again, intrauterine antibiotic therapy may not be most appropriate. Usually considerable uterine involution has taken place, with a rejuvenated musculature and active ovaries. In this situation the animal's own defence mechanisms should be promoted rather than relying on antibiotics. When under progesterone dominance the uterine cellular defence system is suppressed; alternatively oestrogen enhances macrophage and lymphocyte activity. Consequently, if corpora lutea are present in the ovaries, treatment with $PGF_{2\alpha}$ will remove progestational influences, resulting in increased oestradiol production from the ovaries, enhanced uterine muscular activity and improved immune responses. However, if corpora lutea are not present in these animals then exogenous parenteral treatment with oestradiol may be beneficial.

Finally, it must be stressed again if an animal is systemically ill, even with evidence of uterine infections, it would be professionally negligent not to treat with systemic antibiotics.

Resumption of ovarian cyclicity

This is very dependent upon a fully functional hypothalamus–pituitary interaction. Having been suppressed for the whole of pregnancy, on the first day after parturition there is a diminished release of gonadotrophins from the pituitary in response to exogenous GnRH. This is partially due to reduced stores of gonadotrophins in the pituitary, as well as a lowered sensitivity to GnRH. By approximately 14 days after parturition the response to GnRH is much improved. Similarly, the ability of the hypo-thalamus–pituitary to release a preovulatory surge of LH in response to oestradiol only gradually resumes normality after parturition, possibly lagging behind the GnRH response by 7–14 days. There is even a suggestion that all responses do not actually return to optimum until after at least one normal cycle of luteal activity (Alam and Dobson 1987).

The ovaries also take time to adjust. Often the first wave of ovarian follicles to grow does not produce enough oestradiol to bring about full expression of oestrous behavior, and the resultant corpora lutea formed after the first ovulation often produce lower progesterone output for a shorter life-span (Figure 3.6). However, this diminished progesterone phase is often sufficient to result in better functioning of the hypothalamus–pituitary axis, as well as perhaps improved intraovarian communication to provide ideal conditions during the next wave of follicular growth that results in the second ovulation and normal luteal life-span. (Such a gradual resumption of activity occurs after other periods of anoestrus, e.g. at puberty, after seasonal or nutritionally induced anoestrus.) Resumption of ovarian cyclicity also undoubtedly leads to improved uterine endometrial and myometrial function. With each succeeding cycle all these factors are reflected in improved expression of oestrous behaviour, increased

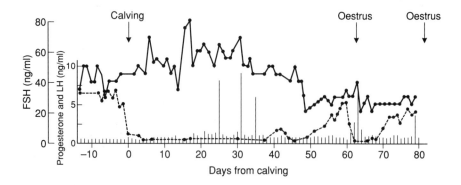

Figure 3.6 Plasma concentrations of FSH (▲), progesterone (●) and LH (vertical bars) during the postpartum period of a dairy cow (from Dobson 1978).

ovulation rates in multiple ovulators, and better single-service conception rates.

As stated before, other factors can influence the re-establishment of normal cyclicity, e.g. suckling, season, nutrient (especially energy) availability, rate of body growth and/or milk production. The success of pharmacological techniques to overcome any of these factors largely depends on the intensity of the suppression. Partial withdrawal or alternative food supplementation of suckling offspring will have little effect 4–6 weeks after birth, but in later stages of lactation it is easier to stimulate cyclicity. Similarly, the effects of season, energy availability, body growth and milk production are graded. Especially in some breeds of species in which genetic selection has led to excessive demands for milk production, a situation can occur when normal cyclicity has resumed and the animal has been inseminated but the (energy) demands of lactation become so great that hypothalamus–pituitary–ovarian axis activity stops again until the crisis is over. In economic terms this can be disastrous, especially if the owner thinks the absence of oestrous behaviour is indicative of pregnancy.

Subfertility and treatment

Anoestrus

Anoestrus can be treated either by GnRH (in a high-dose injection, or by low-dose continuous application) or, more effectively, by progesterone treatment of luteal duration (Ball and Lamming 1983), as already outlined. However, the predisposing situation that resulted in the aberration in the first place should also have been corrected, otherwise if the animal does not conceive at the first induced period of oestrus, anoestrus will probably take over again.

Cystic ovaries

Another abnormality that takes place in the postpartum period is that of ovarian cysts. There is now strong evidence to suggest that a follicular cyst develops due to the failure of a correct preovulatory LH surge—in fact most probably due to the absence of a hypothalamic positive feedback response to oestradiol (Dobson and Alam 1987). The cyst either continues to produce oestradiol for prolonged periods resulting sometimes in nymphomaniacal behaviour, or the cyst may gradually luteinize ultimately producing a luteinized follicular (or luteal) cyst. Follicular cysts may be treated with GnRH or LH (commercially available as hCG) in which case a normal luteal phase follows in 90% of cases. In some hCG preparations progesterone is also included; this ensures suppression of oestrous behaviour. Luteal cysts respond to $PGF_{2\alpha}$ just as normal corpora lutea. However, clinically it is not always easy to distinguish between the two types of cyst and to give the incorrect treatment would be fruitless. Consequently combined treatment with GnRH or hCG followed 14 days later by $PGF_{2\alpha}$ leads to a greater subsequent fertility rate and lower recurrence rate (Nanda et al. 1988). It is possible to successfully treat follicular cysts with progesterone administration, but again if misdiagnosis occurs (as it can in up to 40% of cases) this type of treatment of luteal cysts will be of no avail.

The number of cases of cystic ovaries that occur in the first 4 weeks after parturition is quite high, undoubtedly due to the stabilization period required for correct functioning of the hypothalamus–pituitary–ovarian axis. As many of these cysts resolve spontaneously treatment is often best delayed until a confirmatory diagnosis >30 days post partum (Morrow et al. 1969).

Delayed ovulation

In some species, especially horses, a delay in ovulation can occur and this may result in lowered fertility. Appropriately timed application of GnRH or hCG will cause ovulation 24 hours later. In species with very short follicular phases (2–3 days), e.g. sheep, goats and cows, the correct timing of this injection becomes critical. If injected too soon, insufficient maturational changes within the nuclei of the ova will have taken place before signals are provided by gonadotrophins for resumption of meiosis (Wassarman et al. 1981). This will lead to ill-prepared ova and, although fertilization may appear to have occurred successfully, further conceptus development may be impaired leading to embryo losses. However in many situations veterinarians are called to examine animals in oestrus that have repeatedly failed to conceive on previous occasions for unknown reasons. One course of action is to consider delayed ovulation and administer GnRH or hCG. If the animal has reached the stage of producing oestrous behaviour it is quite likely that this will do no harm, but there is very little scientific evidence currently available for sheep, goats and cows to prove that the administration of gonadotrophins in this situation is truly efficacious.

Repeat breeders

In many species repeat breeders are a problem and 'holding injections' as above are often prescribed. However there is evidence to show that the uterine environment may be abnormal in these animals, especially between days 8 and 12 of the cycle (Ayalon 1978), a time when the embryo is hatching from the zona pellucida and expanding rapidly. Until more is known about these processes, successful therapy of such abnormalities is impossible.

Persistent corpora lutea

Cases of persistent corpora lutea do exist, especially in the presence of endometritis, presumably because the source of luteolytic $PGF_{2\alpha}$ is malfunctioning. Treatment with exogenous $PGF_{2\alpha}$ is very effective in the majority of these cases. In the horse endometritis shortens the luteal phase.

Detection of oestrus

In all the above clinical situations the aim is to revert the animal to normal cyclicity. Unfortunately even in animals that have not had prior corrective treatment there can still be problems when the ovaries are cycling normally. The biggest trouble occurs when AI programmes are used, especially when no males of the species are present to help detection of oestrus. Indeed, in the cattle industry heat detection is the major single cause of failure to maximize efficient fertility and many aids have been developed to overcome the problem, including heat mount detectors (KAMARs, tail-paint), milk temperature monitors, and, as in other species, vasectomized or penile-deviated males. In the absence of clear symptoms of oestrous behaviour, breeding in all species is severely hampered. Sometimes it is not always clear to the clinician whether ovarian cyclicity is proceeding normally or true anoestrus is occurring. In this situation it is advantageous to take either plasma, blood or milk samples at least once a week for 3–4 weeks; if there is a high progesterone concentration in at least two of these samples, then the animal must be cycling (Dobson and Fitzpatrick 1976). Further progesterone monitoring could be carried out to pinpoint the likely time of oestrus. In addition, progesterone analysis on the day of insemination may help to confirm or refute accurate heat detection. Alternatively, being assured that there is no possibility of pregnancy, treatments discussed earlier could be instituted and if necessary fixed-time insemination arranged at the end of treatment, thus removing the necessity for detection of oestrus.

A final word of warning

A greater understanding of reproductive physiology and endocrinology will no doubt lead to improved clinical awareness. However, successful treatments of subfertility depend on a partnership between the animal(s), the owner and the vet. The last two especially must work together and the use of drugs will not always provide the best answers. In many situations alterations in management or less interference with the animals' natural instincts may be more appropriate.

4

CATTLE BREEDING AND INFERTILITY

P J HARTIGAN MA, BSc(Vet), MVM, PhD, MRCVS

Reproductive record systems
Examination of the female reproductive tract
Examination of the bull
The physiology and pathology of puberty
The oestrous cycle
Pharmacological regulation of the oestrous cycle
Mating
Pregnancy
Parturition
The postpartum period
Investigation of the individual infertile cow

Veterinary expertise in the reproductive biology of cattle can be utilized to best advantage in the context of a reproductive herd health programme. An essential component of any such programme is the critical analysis of the reproductive records compiled by the stockperson. The record system must be accurate and up to date and it must be capable of alerting the stockperson and the veterinarian to the management decisions that are imminent.

Reproductive record systems

There is a considerable literature on record systems that range from simple notebooks to wall charts to computers. Here, attention will be restricted to an outline of the essential features of a simple efficient record system, together with a brief account of the criteria that are used to evaluate reproductive efficiency.

The record system should provide a ready source of information on the following items:

1. cows ready for service;
2. cows that should be observed closely for signs of oestrus (i.e., anoestrous cows calved more than 25 days; cows 17 to 25 days after service);
3. cows ready for pregnancy diagnosis;
4. cows pregnant;
5. cows due to calve.

To meet these requirements the following information should be recorded:

1. identification of the animal;
2. calving date;
3. periparturient disease/treatments;
4. dates of oestrus before the beginning of the breeding season;
5. service dates and sire(s);
6. results of pregnancy diagnosis;
7. other veterinary problems.

Irrespective of whether the system used to store the permanent record is simple or complex, the stockperson will find it convenient to use two simple working documents: a pocket notebook and a heat expectancy chart. The pocket notebook is used to record data on heat detection as the observations are made in the field, thus reducing the risk of inaccuracy due to faulty recollection. In the heat expectancy chart (Figure 4.1) dates are arranged in parallel rows of 21 days; this enables the stockperson to

HEAT EXPECTANCY CHART

Date	Cow numbers	Date	Cow numbers	Date	Cow numbers
Jan. 1	24̶	Jan. 22		Feb. 12	
2		23	18̶	13	16 (18)
3	18̶ 18̶ 25̶	24	18̶ (24)	14	
4		25	(23) 18̶	15	(15)
5	18̶ 18̶	26		16	19
6	(10)	27	18̶	17	

Figure 4.1 Heat expectancy chart. The dates are arranged in columns of 21 days. The purpose of the heat expectancy chart is to prompt the stockperson to watch certain cows more carefully at the time of expected oestrus. All oestrus periods are recorded whether or not the cow is served. The previous oestrus period is crossed out when the cow returns to heat. If the cow is served at a given oestrus, her number is circled.

see at a glance which cows ought to be observed carefully on a particular day because they were in oestrus 18–24 days ago.

Analysis of breeding records

Target fertility indices

Mean calving interval (days)	365
Mean calving-to-conception interval (days)	85
Mean calving-to-first-oestrus interval (days)	<45
Mean calving-to-first-service interval (days)	<60
Submission rate	85%
Intervals between services (days)	18–24
Mean number of services/conception	1.6
Non-return rates: 30–60-day	75–85%
60–90-day	68–70%
Involuntary culling due to infertility	<10%

The calving interval (the period from calving to calving; target: less than 365 days) is the criterion of reproductive efficiency for each individual cow; less than 5% of the cows in a herd should be outside the range of 11–13 months.

Calculation of the calving-to-conception interval ('days open', 'days non-gravid') has certain advantages over the calving interval in that it can be calculated several months earlier and it includes cows sold before calving. Less than 5% of the cows should have calving-to-conception intervals longer than 95 days.

The submission rate, the percentage of the calved cows in a herd that are inseminated during the first 4 weeks of the breeding season, has a very significant effect on the calving pattern. In Table 4.1 the first row relates to a herd in which cows were not presented for service before 60 days after calving; the conception rate was good but the benefit was lost because of the poor submission rate. The second row refers to a herd in which breeding began on a predetermined date after which every cow in oestrus was served, irrespective of the interval from calving. The conception rate was reduced because some cows were served too soon after calving but the beneficial effect of the high submission rate was evident. The third row

Table 4.1 Interaction of submission rate (SR) and conception rate (CR) on the calving pattern (after O'Farrell, 1975)

Herd policy	SR (%)	CR (%)	Percentage calving in the first 4 weeks of calving season
Service delayed until after day 60 post partum	50	68	34
Service at first oestrus in the breeding season	85	54	45
Very compact early breeding pattern	85	68	55

refers to a herd that already had a very compact early calving pattern, which favoured both a high submission rate and a high conception rate.

The calving interval and the calving-to-conception interval can be computed accurately only for previous breeding seasons. Since the repeatability of breeding efficiency is extremely low, an assessment of the current situation requires other indices, such as the intervals between services and the number of services per conception. Calculation of the intervals from calving to first oestrus and to first service and the submission rate will give a good indication of the commitment of the stockperson to heat detection and recording.

The artificial insemination industry monitors current levels of fertility by calculating 30–60-day and 60–90-day non-return rates. These indices are based on the assumption that a cow is pregnant to first insemination if she has not been submitted for a second insemination within the specified interval. The non-return rates can overestimate the calving rate by 10–15%. Much of this difference can be accounted for by loss of cows from the herd (sale, death), foetal loss and return to service later than 90 days after insemination. The real value of the non-return rates is to the insemination service—as an index of the fertility of the bulls or the efficiency of the inseminators.

Conception rate to first service (as confirmed by rectal palpation between days 42 and 60) is often given as 60–68% but the actual calving rate to that service may be 50–64%. Fertilization failure and embryonic mortality each account for 12–15% of reproductive failures in dairy cattle. Much of the embryo loss occurs gradually between days 8 and 16, with the result that the cows return to oestrus at the normal 18–24-day interval. Such cows may eventually conceive and carry the conceptus to full-term. However, if an average conception rate of 60% to each service is accepted, approximately 6% of apparently normal cows will not be pregnant after three services (Table 4.2). These cows will be classified as 'repeat breeders' and in herds that maintain compact calving seasons they may be culled as

Table 4.2 Pregnancy rates after repeated services in a herd of 100 clinically 'normal' cows (conception rate to each service: 60%)

	Cows
Presented for first service	100
Pregnant to first service	60
Presented for second service	40
Pregnant to second service	24
Presented for third service	16
Pregnant to third service	10
Pregnant after three services	94
'Repeat breeders'	6

infertile, especially if they calved towards the end of the previous calving season.

When so many apparently normal cows are culled simply because they have not been bred often enough, there is a serious risk that involuntary culling due to infertility will exceed 10%, which should be the upper limit in a well-managed dairy herd. The best way to avoid this predicament is to have a reproductive management plan that has four main objectives:

1. to ensure that young stock reach puberty at the appropriate time to provide an adequate number of high-quality replacement heifers that deliver their first calves near the beginning of the calving season;
2. to ensure that the detection of oestrus is efficient and accurate, and there is a high submission rate during the first month of the breeding season;
3. to monitor the course of uterine involution and the resumption of cyclic ovarian activity during the postpartum period, so that the cow is capable of initiating pregnancy early in the breeding season;
4. to diagnose and treat any specific disease that may impair fertility.

Examination of the female reproductive tract

Before performing a physical examination of the female reproductive tract, the veterinarian should study the herd records and consult the stockperson on the history of the animal, with particular emphasis on the calving date, periparturient disorders, oestrous cycles, service dates and any previous treatment.

Physical examination should include visual inspection of the perineum, vulva, base of the tail, back and flanks. Then the vagina and cervix should be inspected through a speculum. For palpation per rectum the operator should wear a latex obstetrical sleeve or a disposable plastic sleeve that has been lubricated with a water-soluble non-irritant jelly. The fingers and hand are inserted into the rectum in the form of a cone. If the rectum contains a quantity of faeces, this should be removed before the hand is advanced gently and carefully beyond the level of the organ to be palpated.

The cervix is a very firm cylindrical structure about 5–10 cm long and 2–5 cm in diameter. In young non-pregnant cows it is located well within the pelvic cavity but in older pluriparous cows it lies at the pelvic brim or within the abdominal cavity.

The uterine body is 3–4 cm long but on rectal palpation it appears to be longer because the caudal parts of the horns are held in close opposition by the intercornual ligaments. The horns are 35–40 cm long. At the point where they separate they are 3–4 cm in diameter but they taper as they coil outward and downward then backward and upward before each horn meets its uterine tube (oviduct, fallopian tube) at the uterotubal junction (Figure 4.2).

It may be necessary to retract the genital tract to palpate the horns throughout their lengths. The essential requirement is to achieve complete retraction without lodging the uterus beneath the broad ligament, where it is difficult or impossible to palpate properly. The exploratory movements are made with the edge of the opened hand rather than with the fingertips, which might damage the rectal mucosa. The hand may be inserted in front of the uterus, which then is cupped in an angle formed by the arm and hand and is gently retracted into the pelvis. Alternatively, the cranial end of the cervix may be grasped firmly and pulled gently into the pelvic cavity. Tilting the long axis of the cervix so that the internal os is higher than the external os will facilitate the process and allow the operator to apply traction on the lateral border of the uterine broad ligament or on the ventral intercornual ligament.

In non-pregnant animals both horns are palpated, from the base to the tip, in order to assess the size and symmetry of the two horns, the thickness and tone of the uterine wall and the nature of the luminal contents. Conditions in which significant changes in these attributes can be detected include segmental aplasia of the Müllerian duct ('white heifer disease'), delayed involution, metritis, pyometra, hydrometra and mucometra. For the diagnosis of pregnancy the operator will seek the 'membrane slip' of the chorioallantoic membrane, the amniotic vesicle, the placentomes or the foetus itself. Retraction of the uterus becomes very difficult or impossible in cows pregnant more than 90 days. However, by that time it should be possible to palpate placentomes, membranes and/or foetal parts without retracting the uterus.

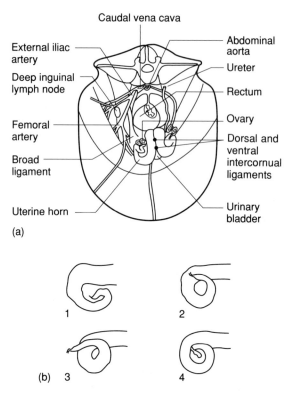

Caudal vena cava

External iliac artery

Deep inguinal lymph node

Femoral artery

Broad ligament

Uterine horn

Abdominal aorta

Ureter

Rectum

Ovary

Dorsal and ventral intercornual ligaments

Urinary bladder

(a)

(b)   1   2   3   4

Figure 4.2 The genital tract of the cow. (a) Anterior view of the female genital tract at the pelvic inlet. Note the dorsal and ventral intercornual ligaments, the coiled and tapering uterine horns, the uterine tubes and the ovaries. (b) Diagrammatic representations of the lateral view of the bovine uterus on the basis of ultrasonographic visualization; horns maximally curled under luteal dominance (4), less curled during follicular dominance (1) (adapted from Pierson, R.A. and Ginther, O.J. (1987) *Journal of the American Veterinary Medical Association* **190**: 996).

When the examination of the uterus has been completed, the genital tract should be released and allowed to resume its original position. Then it can be pushed laterally to one side or the other so as to tense the broad ligament and make it easier to locate the ovary on the contralateral side.

In the adult cow the right ovary tends to be the more active and larger gonad. Normal follicles are smooth, convex, thin-walled, fluctuant structures. The smallest palpable follicles are about 6–8 mm in diameter and the largest follicles are about 20 mm in diameter. Shortly before ovulation, the preovulatory follicle becomes less tense. Atretic follicles also become soft.

After ovulation the corpus luteum may grow to occupy more than half of the substance of the ovary. Most corpora lutea have a papilla or crown-like projection above the surface of the ovary. However, a corpus luteum may lack a papilla and be embedded within the substance of the ovary; careful palpation may be required to detect it but in many cases it is possible to find a 'waistline' between the base of the corpus luteum and the underlying stromal tissue.

When the ovary has been examined, the ovarian bursa may be explored. The ovary is held firmly as two or three fingers are slid down along the lateral surface of the ovary into the bursa, which can lifted and stretched across the fingers while the thumb is used to check for adhesions, cysts and distension of the uterine tube. This exploration should be done sparingly and with great care and gentleness.

The uterine tubes (oviducts) are about 20–35 cm long and they follow a convoluted course in the mesosalpinx. A skilful operator can palpate the oviduct in the mesosalpinx but, in my opinion, the risks of iatrogenic damage greatly outweigh the potential benefits.

Examination of the bull

A veterinary examination to assess the breeding capacity of a bull is done in three phases: an inspection of the general health of the animal, a study of his physical conformation and a specific investigation of his reproductive system. A bull with poor conformation of the hind limbs is predisposed to the development of musculoskeletal problems that will inhibit his ability to function as a sire. Foot problems, lesions of the stifle and tarsal joints or back problems will impair sexual activity. Inherited conditions that reduce the breeding potential of a bull are hip dysplasia, spastic paresis and progressive hereditary ataxia.

The specific examination of the reproductive system involves an assessment of the sex drive of the bull as well as a physical examination of his genital organs. Sex drive may be diminished because of musculoskeletal problems but in some bulls a weak sex drive appears to be an inherited characteristic, particularly in beef bulls. The bull's performance should be observed at test matings.

The scrotum

When the cremaster muscles and the dartos are relaxed the scrotum should be pendulous and, when viewed from behind, it should have convex lateral contours with a definite neck at the base. Abnormal conformation of the scrotum is often associated with poor fertility. For instance, the straight-sided scrotum owes its shape to a pad of fat at the base that is thought to disturb the thermoregulatory mechanisms in the testes, which usually are smaller than average. Again, the thermoregulatory mechanisms may be disturbed when the scrotum is short and tapered ventrally; in this case the testes are held too close to the body wall and they are likely to be small or hypoplastic.

The scrotal skin should be thin and pliable. The testes should be firm but not hard, they should be approximately equal in size and they should be freely movable within the scrotum. During the examination each testis, in turn, should be pushed dorsally to facilitate the palpation of the other testis and epididymis.

The epididymis consists of head, body and tail (Figure 4.3). These parts can be detected as structures of firmer consistency than the adjacent testicular tissue. The head is a flattened U-shaped structure that lies over the proximal pole and upper third of the front of the testis. The body is a slender structure that runs down the posterior border of the testis; it can be palpated when the contralateral testis has been pushed dorsally. The tail is attached to the lower pole of the testis and projects below it; in the adult bull it is about the same size as the distal phalanx of the operator's thumb.

The size of the testicles and scrotum varies with the breed, size and age of the bull. Maximum testicular size is reached at about 4 years old. It has been established that total sperm cell production, testicular size and scrotal circumference are highly correlated in young bulls. Therefore, the measurement of scrotal circumference can be used, with confidence, as an indicator of the spermatogenic potential of a bull until he is about 5 years

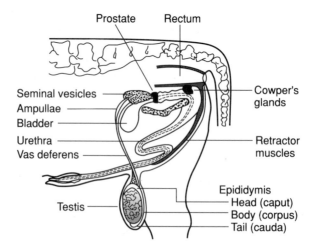

Figure 4.3 The genital tract of the bull.

Abnormalities detected during palpation of the scrotum and its contents

- scrotal dermatitis
- rotation of the scrotum
- scrotal hernia
- varicosities of the pampiniform plexus
- cryptorchidism ('rig')
- testicular hypoplasia (unilateral or bilateral)
- testicular degeneration
- adhesions between the scrotum and testis
- orchitis
- hydrocoele
- testicular tumours
- segmental aplasia of the epididymis
- spermatocoele
- spermatic granuloma
- epididymitis

---

old; after that age the amount of seminiferous tissue may decline without a comparable loss in testicular size. It can be used in yearling bulls as a criterion for the selection of stud bulls: a bull that has small testes at 14–16 months old will still have small testes at 2 or 3 years old. Yearling bulls of different breeds have scrotal circumferences of 30–36 cm, whereas a 3-year-old bull with well-developed testes could be expected to have a scrotal circumference greater than 40 cm.

The procedure for measuring scrotal circumference is as follows. The testes are pushed into the lower part of the scrotum by firm downward pressure exerted by grasping the base of the scrotum with the thumb and fingers at the sides of the scrotal neck. This eliminates wrinkling of the scrotal skin in the region to be measured. The position of the hand is very important. If the thumb and fingers are located in an anterior–posterior relationship they may slip between the testes, force them apart and give a false reading. The measurements should be made with a flexible tape formed into a sliding loop, which is pulled snugly around the widest diameter of the scrotal contents. Differences in scrotal circumference between breeds have been recorded (Coulter *et al.* 1987).

Infectious causes of orchitis-periorchitis and epididymitis

- *Actinomyces pyogenes*
- streptococci
- staphylococci
- *Chlamydia* and *Mycoplasma*
- *Brucella abortus*
- *Mycobacterium bovis*

A soft consistency of the testes is often related to poor quality of the semen and to poor conception rates. A tonometer has been developed to provide an objective measure of testicular consistency. It has been claimed that tonometer measurements are repeatable, heritable and related to semen quality and fertility (Coulter and Foote 1979).

The prepuce and penis

The bull should be observed during service to assess his ability to erect the penis. The prepuce and penis should be examined for physical factors that impair or prevent natural mating or ejaculation into the artificial vagina.

Physical abnormalities of prepuce and penis

- eversion of the prepuce (particularly in polled bulls)
- prolapse of the prepuce
- phimosis
- persistence of the penile frenulum
- balanoposthitis (IBR/IPV virus, non-specific opportunist bacteria)

- adhesions
- fractured penis
- hair rings
- fibropapillomata
- short penis
- corkscrew penis
- ventral deviation of the penis

Rectal examination

At rectal examination, the seminal vesicles, the ampullae of the vasa deferentia and the body of the prostate gland can be palpated (Figure 4.3).

The seminal vesicles are found on the floor of the pelvis, near the brim; they are compact glandular structures with lobulated surfaces. Frequently, the two vesicles are asymmetrical in size and shape; in the adult bull each measures approximately 10–12 cm by 5 cm by 3 cm. Increases in size, changes in shape and lobulation, and changes in consistency can be detected when the seminal vesicles are infected (seminal vesiculitis). The organisms most commonly isolated from diseased seminal vesicles are *Actinomyces pyogenes, Escherichia coli, Pseudomonas aeruginosa,* and α-haemolytic streptococci. *Brucella abortus, Mycoplasma, Ureaplasma, Chlamydia* and several viruses may also be involved in the pathogenesis of seminal vesiculitis.

In the acute phase of the disease, rectal palpation may elicit signs of severe pain, perhaps related to a localized pelvic peritonitis. The affected gland(s) may be enlarged (generalized or local), have lost the lobulations and be firm in consistency. Abscesses may form as a consequence of blockage of the ducts by exudate. The tentative diagnosis of seminal vesiculitis based on findings by rectal palpation can be confirmed by the detection of neutrophils in a fresh sample of semen. The semen contains purulent material consistently in acute cases, intermittently in chronic cases. The inflammatory reaction may extend to the ampullae (which lie between the seminal vesicles) but ampullitis is not easily detected by rectal palpation. Similarly, inflammation of the body of the prostate is not likely to be detected clinically.

The physiology and pathology of puberty

Puberty is defined as the time at which the young animal acquires the ability to reproduce offspring. The heifer is considered to have reached puberty when she experiences the first spontaneous ovulation that is accompanied by overt signs of oestrus. The criteria for puberty in the young bull are the ability to extrude a fully erect penis from the prepuce and the production of an ejaculate that contains more than 50 million spermatozoa with at least 10% forward motility. These events allow calculation of 'age at puberty', which for cattle is most frequently between 9 and 15 months old, but they are not proof of full sexual maturity.

Hormonal and morphological changes at puberty

In the prepubertal animal the hypothalamic–pituitary–gonadal axis is prevented from functioning in the adult fashion by two different mechanisms that suppress the release of gonadotrophins, principally luteinizing hormone (LH):

1. an intrinsic inhibitory neural mechanism that is steroid independent;
2. exquisite sensitivity of the hypothalamus to the negative feedback effects of small amounts of circulating oestrogen or testosterone from the gonads.

The approach to puberty is marked by an attenuation of the intrinsic neural inhibition and by a gradual decline in the sensitivity of the hypothalamus to negative feedback. In the heifer the frequency of LH pulses increases gradually (from one every 8 hours at about 3 months before puberty to one every hour just before first ovulation), follicles develop to more advanced stages and, eventually, sufficient oestrogen is produced to activate the positive feedback mechanism that releases a surge of LH capable of inducing ovulation.

In the young bull pulses of LH are detectable at 8–10 weeks of age, the Leydig cells begin to secrete androgens at about 3 months old, and serum concentrations of both LH and testosterone increase in a linear fashion from 7 months to at least 13 months of age.

In the calf the penis is firmly adherent to the prepuce and cannot be extruded. When testosterone is produced by the testes, it stimulates the growth of the penis and the progressive separation of the glans penis and prepuce. This process is completed by 8 or 9 months of age, so that the pubertal bull can protrude the penis. The testes grow rapidly from 6 months old to puberty, at which stage the scrotal circumference should be approximately 28 cm regardless of breed, size or age of the individual bull. Thereafter, the testes should continue to grow and they should have reached approximately 90% of their mature size by the end of the second year of life. During that time the quality of the ejaculate (sperm number, motility, morphology) continues to improve. In some animals the continuous curve of testicular growth is interrupted around the time of puberty; if this set-back is sufficiently large to result in underdeveloped gonads at 2 years old, there is little likelihood that the testes will develop to full maturity.

Factors that influence the age at puberty

There are inherent breed variations in the age at puberty. In all breeds the process of maturation is subject to modulation by factors such as season of birth, level of nutrition, growth rate, body size, photoperiod, high ambient temperatures, intercurrent diseases and social environment.

It has been reported that heifers born in spring attain puberty at younger ages than those born in autumn. However, the effects of season of birth and of seasonal changes are complex and, in general, their overall influence is to increase the probability that heifers will give birth to offspring in spring or summer, regardless of their own date of birth.

The effects of season on age at puberty may be mediated by average daily gains in weight. Animals reared on high planes of nutrition are younger and heavier at puberty than those on restricted planes of nutrition; however, the evidence does not support the idea that heifers treated alike reach puberty at a common ('critical') body weight.

Obviously, the prepubertal and pubertal animal requires a diet that contains sufficient protein, vitamins, minerals and energy to enable it to make the daily gains in weight that are compatible with early activation of the adult pattern of gonadotrophin releasing hormone (GnRH). Manipulation of food intake can be of particular advantage in the management of young bulls for optimal fertility, since it can be used to ensure that the interval between the onset of puberty and the introduction of the bull to stud duties is sufficiently long to derive the maximum benefit from the continuing improvement in semen quality that occurs in the months immediately after puberty. However, there is evidence that prolonged feeding of very high energy diets has a deleterious effect on the quality of semen and on the sexual activities of the bull.

Delayed puberty

Most cases of delayed puberty are due to poor management. Serious errors in management are likely to result in several affected animals in the group; nevertheless, the role of management should be given careful scrutiny even when the condition is apparent in only one or two animals, particularly if there are significant differences in the age and size of animals housed together during the prepubertal period. All affected animals should be given a thorough clinical examination, with particular emphasis on the detection of congenital defects of the reproductive tract or chronic conditions that affect utilization of nutrients and depress growth rate. If the basic problem is nutritional, dietary adjustments should be implemented before there is any attempt to induce puberty by hormone therapy, especially in heifers that may not yet have built up sufficient reserves to meet the demands of pregnancy and lactation.

Ideally, hormone therapy should attempt to mimic the hormonal pattern at spontaneous puberty. In most pubertal heifers, first ovulation is silent and gives rise to a short-lived corpus luteum. The short luteal phase primes the system so that the next surge of LH is associated with oestrus, ovulation and the formation of a normal corpus luteum. This sequence can be mimicked by the insertion of a progesterone-releasing intravaginal device (PRID) for 9 days followed by an ovulatory dose of LH or GnRH.

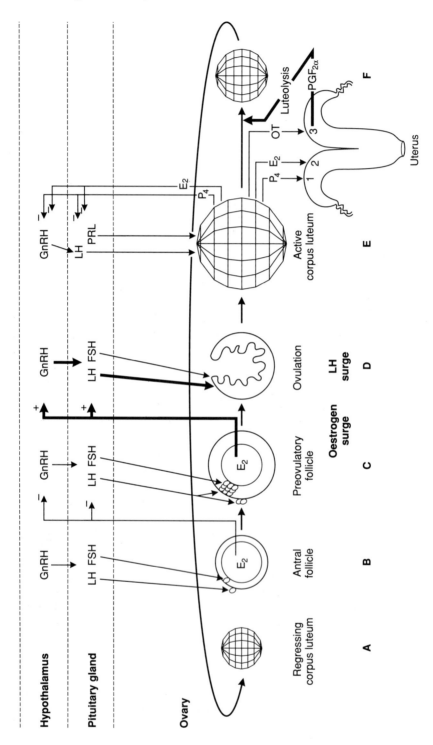

The oestrous cycle

Physiological background

The mean length of the oestrous cycle is 20 days in the heifer and 21 days in the cow (with a range of 18–24 days being considered normal). Most of the variation in the length of the cycle is due to variations in the duration of the luteal phase, which can vary by several days even in successive cycles in the same animal. The newly formed corpus luteum begins to secrete progesterone on day 3 of the cycle and by day 7 it has raised the plasma concentration to a level (6–10 ng/ml) that exerts a strong negative feedback on the release of gonadotrophins. Thus, although there is sufficient trophic stimulation of the ovaries to induce three separate waves of follicular growth (each with a dominant follicle) during the luteal phase, a preovulatory surge of gonadotrophins is inhibited. Eventually, the progesterone-primed uterus produces enough prostaglandin $F_{2\alpha}$ ($PGF_{2\alpha}$) to induce regression of the corpus luteum. Luteal regression may begin as early as day 15 or as late as day 19 of normal (18–24 day) cycles. As the corpus luteum regresses the circulating levels of progesterone decline and inhibition of the hypothalamus and pituitary gland is attenuated (Figure 4.4). The resultant increase in gonadotrophin activity stimulates the dominant follicle present at that time to grow to the preovulatory stage and to secrete increasing quantities of oestrogen that, in 2 or 3 days, will activate the positive feedback mechanism that elicits the preovulatory

Figure 4.4 Interrelationships between the hypothalamus, pituitary gland, ovary and uterus during the oestrous cycle. When the corpus luteum (CL) regresses at the end of a cycle (A), the hypothalamus and pituitary gland are released from the strong negative feedback exerted by progesterone (P_4) throughout the luteal phase of the cycle. FSH and LH stimulate the growth and secretory activity of a dominant ovarian follicle (B) that secretes increasing quantities of oestradiol (E_2). The initial low concentrations of E_2 have a negative feedback effect until the preovulatory follicle produces a surge of oestrogen (C) that exerts a positive feedback and results in a surge of LH that causes ovulation (D). A new CL develops under the trophic influence of both LH and prolactin (PRL). It secretes P_4 and E_2 that re-assert a strong negative feedback effect on the hypothalamic–pituitary axis. In addition, the P_4 causes an accumulation of fatty acid precursors in the endometrium (1). After day 10, E_2 induces the synthesis of prostaglandin from the stored precursors (2). Finally, oxytocin (OT) causes the release of the $PGF_{2\alpha}$ (3), which is transferred from the uterus to the ipsilateral ovary by a countercurrent mechanism and induces luteolysis (F) (after Hartigan, P. J. (1992). In Andrews, A. H., Blowey, R. W., Boyd, H. and Eddy, R. G. (eds) *Bovine Medicine*. Blackwell Scientific Publications, Oxford, p. 418).

surge of LH and follicle stimulating hormone (FSH). This surge lasts about 8 hours and leads to ovulation at approximately 25–30 hours after the onset of oestrus (or 10–12 hours after the end of oestrus).

Behavioural oestrus results from the actions of both progesterone and oestrogen in physiological concentrations and in the proper temporal sequence: progesterone domination followed by a rapid decline in progesterone concentrations as oestrogen levels rise.

Oestrus

The duration of oestrus ranges from 2 to 30 hours, the 'average' lying between 15 and 18 hours. The duration of oestrus may vary slightly according to breed, season, the number of animals in oestrus at the time, or the presence of a bull.

The intensity of the signs of oestrus varies greatly amongst individual animals. The most reliable sign is that the cow will stand firmly to be mounted. She will attempt to mount other cows, often after sniffing and licking the vulva and testing the reaction by rubbing or resting her chin on the rump. If the cow being solicited is in oestrus also, the sexually active cow may show 'flehmen'. Cows in oestrus tend to be restless and they show a tendency to form groups that are more active and mobile than the remainder of the herd. The vulva may be swollen and congested and there is a flow of elastic mucus ('bulling string'), which hangs from the vulva or is smeared on the tail and buttocks. Other less reliable signs include increased frequency of urination, tail raising and switching, excessive bellowing and sensitivity to palpation of the rump (which elicits depression of the back and raising of the tail). The tail-head and rear of the animal in oestrus may be soiled and excoriated due to mounting by other cows.

Detection of oestrus

Good breeding management demands efficient and accurate detection of oestrus. Each oestrus that is missed increases the risk that a potentially fertile cow may not be served often enough to become pregnant before the end of the breeding season. 'False-positive' detection of oestrus can also cause serious problems. For instance, a cow that is already pregnant may abort if she is inseminated. Insemination of a non-pregnant cow during the luteal phase of the oestrous cycle wastes semen, time and money; furthermore, if the semen is deposited in the uterus there is a risk of uterine infection, endometritis and impaired fertility at subsequent services.

It is generally agreed that frequent and careful visual observations are necessary, including a final check in the late evening. The accuracy of the observations will depend on the knowledge, skill and motivation of the observer and on the choice of the correct times, frequency, duration and location of the observations.

The most important source of knowledge for the observer is a simple, accurate recording system, such as a 21-day calendar (see Figure 4.1). Every observation of oestrus should be recorded, whether or not the cow is served. This information will enable the stockperson to predict when individual cows are likely to be in oestrus again so that they can be subject to careful observation at that time. It will also draw attention to cows with abnormalities in frequency or duration of oestrus. Of course, the accuracy of the records will depend on the ability of the stockperson to identify correctly each of the animals in the herd.

There may be periods during oestrus when standing behaviour is temporarily absent, particularly during the morning and evening milking times; hence the importance of observing the cows when they are not being distracted by feeding or milking activities. The literature on the timing, frequency and duration of visual observations indicates that the herd should be inspected at regular intervals from early morning to late evening. Most authors advise three periods of observation every day but the precise times vary somewhat depending on local conditions. O'Farrell (1982) reported a detection rate in excess of 90% when the stockperson moved through the herd for 20 minutes five times a day (at intervals of 4 hours from 08.00 to 22.00).

Aids to detection of oestrus

Heat detection aids should be used to supplement visual observation, not to replace it.

Mounting activity can be detected by pressure-sensitive devices or by paint on the tail-head, which is rubbed off when the cow is mounted. They should not be used as the sole means of detecting oestrus; both types of detector may give false-positive results on cows that are not in oestrus. Checking for other confirmatory signs of oestrus (vaginal mucus, swollen vulva, restlessness, dirt marks on the flank or back) is important.

Vaginal resistance probes have been used to detect the fall in electrical resistance in the vagina during oestrus. The problem with this method is that cows must be probed once or twice daily, which is time-consuming and can be irritating to the cow. Also, the oestrus-induced changes in resistance are similar to the between-cow variation and this makes it necessary to have an individual profile for each cow.

Teaser animals (vasectomized bulls, androgenized heifers, androgenized steers) fitted with 'chin-ball' markers have been used to identify cows in oestrus. There are drawbacks: the males may transmit venereal diseases and they may become dangerously aggressive; if there are a number of cows in oestrus at the same time they may concentrate on some cows and ignore the others.

In herds where milk progesterone assays are used for early detection of pregnancy a diagnosis of non-pregnancy should facilitate heat detection by focusing the attention of the stockperson on the cows that are likely to return to oestrus. However, if the test for pregnancy is made on day 24 after service most of the non-pregnant cows should have been in oestrus already. If it is to be of significant value as an aid to heat detection, the progesterone assay should be made no later than days 20 or 21; day 19 is probably the optimal time for 'advanced warning' of impending oestrus.

Anoestrus

The heifer or cow that fails to show oestrus during periods when she might be expected to do so is described as being anoestrous. This can happen in the heifer when there is a delay in the onset of puberty (pubertal anoestrus). In both heifers and cows it often happens after parturition (postpartum anoestrus). In both of these situations the basic problem may be total inactivity of the ovaries (true anoestrus) or it may be the failure to exhibit the behavioural signs of oestrus although the ovaries are undergoing the normal cyclic changes of follicular growth, ovulation and formation of the corpus luteum (suboestrus; also called silent heat or silent ovulation). Anoestrus may also be associated with a persistent progesterone-secreting structure, such as a luteinized follicular cyst or a persistent corpus luteum, that inhibits cyclic ovarian activity by negative feedback on the secretion of gonadotrophins.

Silent ovulations must be distinguished from undetected oestrus, where the stockperson fails to observe the behavioural signs. Oestrus may pass unnoticed if the signs are either weak or of relatively short duration; up to one in five cows may exhibit oestrus for less than 6 hours and this may include the hours of darkness. Moreover, cows that exhibit oestrus of normal intensity and duration may be missed if the observations are not frequent enough, if they are cursory or perfunctory, or if they are done in the wrong environment (e.g. in yards when cows are assembled for milking and feeding). Cows may be misdiagnosed as anoestrous when recording errors arise either because the stockperson does not make immediate entries in a notebook or because the animals do not have identification marks that are read easily.

Silent ovulations are common in the early postpartum period. In a high-yielding dairy herd up to 80% of cows may have a silent first ovulation; the figure drops to 55% at the second ovulation and to 35% at the third ovulation. About 5% of dairy cows do not resume ovarian activity within 50 days of calving while a small proportion (about 5%) of the animals that resume cyclic ovarian activity within a few weeks of parturition become anoestrous during the second and third months post partum. This may happen in the absence of obvious pathology in high-yielding cows and in primiparous heifers that are still growing; it seems reasonable to assume that nutritional or metabolic factors are responsible for the anoestrus. A similar pattern may be seen in cows that develop severe metritis due to *A. pyogenes* in the second and third months after calving. In this instance, the inflamed uterus does not release sufficient $PGF_{2\alpha}$ to induce luteolysis and the persisting corpus luteum predisposes to the development of pyometra accompanied by anoestrus.

The beef cow has a more extended period of postpartum anoestrus. Published figures for the interval from parturition to first oestrus range from approximately 46 to 104 days. Suckling delays the onset of ovarian activity and early weaning of calves reduces the interval to first oestrus.

Conditions that may prolong the period of postpartum anoestrus

- inadequate nutrient intake
- mineral deficiencies (aphosphorosis, hypo-cupraemia, subclinical cobalt deficiency)
- metabolic disturbances (ketosis, the 'fat cow syndrome')
- marked weight loss
- stress
- winter season
- high milk yield
- suckling
- retained placenta
- metritis
- delayed uterine involution
- lameness

Induction of ovulation in the anoestrous animal

The first task is to eliminate the precipitating factors, be they nutritional, metabolic or infectious. Treatment of the specific disorders combined with an increase in energy intake should allow normal ovarian function to resume. However, it may be desirable to accelerate the process by hormone therapy.

Hormone therapy must

1. stimulate a cohort of ovarian follicles, one of which will enter the preovulatory phase;
2. ensure that there is a surge of LH to ovulate the preovulatory follicle.

Follicle growth can be stimulated by gonadotrophic hormones (LH, FSH, pregnant mare's serum gonadotrophin (PMSG), human chorionic gonadotrophin (hCG)) or by GnRH. A disadvantage with exogenous pituitary gonadotrophins is that they need to be given in repeated doses. A single dose of PMSG will stimulate ovarian activity: 1500–2000 iu should induce follicular growth and the oestrogen from the follicles should induce oestrus and exert a positive feedback to release a preovulatory surge of LH. However, if the cow is not served or if she fails to conceive she is likely to return to anoestrus; in the latter case, it may be assumed (incorrectly) that she is pregnant. If PMSG is given to a cow that already has follicular activity it may induce superovulation with the attendant risk of multiple pregnancies.

The ovarian response to the GnRH-induced release of LH is dependent on the maturity of the follicles present in the ovaries at the time of treatment. A follicle larger than 15 mm is likely to ovulate but follicles smaller than 15 mm may not respond. GnRH may be even less successful in attempts to initiate cycles in suckled beef cows, where the suckling stimulus significantly delays the onset of follicular growth. Webb *et al.* (1977) reported that 500 µg GnRH given as a single injection to suckled cows at 13–32 days post partum resulted in follicular growth and ovulation but the life-span of the corpus luteum was short (6–8 days). However, a second dose of 500 µg GnRH 10 days later, when the transient rise of progesterone had subsided to basal concentrations, induced cyclic ovarian activity.

A transient increase in plasma progesterone is necessary for the initiation of normal cyclic ovarian activity and it seems that the most logical treatment for postpartum anoestrus might be to use a combination of a progestogen and a luteolytic agent.

The most convenient method of administering a progestogen is in the form of a PRID. This consists of a stainless steel coil covered by a layer of silastic impregnated with 1.55 mg progesterone. Attached to the inner surface of the coil is a small gelatin capsule containing 10 mg oestradiol benzoate. The coil is inserted into the vagina by means of a special speculum and after 7, 9 or 12 days in place the device is removed by pulling on a string that is left hanging at the vulva when the coil is inserted. Both of the hormones are absorbed readily through the vaginal wall. The oestradiol acts as a luteolytic agent if a natural corpus luteum exists. The progesterone generates plasma concentrations that simulate a natural luteal phase. The cow should show oestrus 2 or 3 days after the PRID is withdrawn.

An alternative source of progestogen is a subcutaneous implant containing 3 mg norgestamet, which is placed behind the ear for 9 days. On the first day, the animal is given an intramuscular injection containing

3 mg norgestamet plus 5 mg oestradiol valerate, which acts as a luteolytic agent.

With either method it is prudent to give an injection of $PGF_{2\alpha}$ or an analogue at the end of the progestogen treatment (or a day or two before the end). In beef cows the response has been enhanced by an injection of 750 iu PMSG at the end of a 9-day progesterone treatment, with up to 15% of twin births.

Defects in ovulation

If the surge in LH is inadequate or at the wrong time, ovulation will be delayed or absent. Until very recently, the detection of delayed ovulation and anovulation had been by repeated rectal palpation of the same follicle over a period of days after the expected time of ovulation. These procedures might have a deleterious effect on the follicle or they might cause premature rupture. Therefore, data on the incidence of either condition must be interpreted with caution; however, the advent of transrectal diagnostic ultrasonography has allowed a more reliable assessment of follicular dynamics and it is to be expected that more accurate data will emerge soon.

Delayed ovulation

There are several reports to indicate that the incidence of delayed ovulation is no more than 2–3%. However, Van Rensburg and de Vos (1962) found that ovulation did not occur at the expected time in 140 (26%) of 536 oestrous cycles. In many cases (85%) the delay was less than 48 hours but in some cases it was as long as 7–9 days and in 47 cycles (9%) ovulation did not occur. The authors recommended that the cows should be served again if ovulation had not occurred by 24 hours after the first service. This resulted in pregnancy in 32 (63%) of 51 cows while there was no pregnancy in the group of 18 cows that were given the single service. An alternative approach is to use hormone therapy to hasten ovulation: for instance, an intramuscular injection of 150 µg GnRH or an intravenous injection of 3000–4500 iu hCG.

Anovulation

Occasionally, a fully developed follicle secretes sufficient oestrogen to induce behavioural oestrus but does not ovulate. The wall of the follicle may undergo luteinization but the structure does not grow to cystic proportions and it undergoes atresia. The cow returns to oestrus at the expected time and, more often than not, ovulates normally. However, the anovulatory cycle has wasted 3 weeks of the breeding season. The most important condition in which there is oestrus without ovulation is cystic ovarian disease.

Ovarian cysts

Three types of cystic structures may be found in the bovine ovary: the cystic corpus luteum, the follicular cyst and the luteal cyst. One type, the cystic corpus luteum, arises when the developing corpus luteum incorporates a central fluid-filled cavity. It has an ovulatory papilla and the luteal cells that surround the cavity are capable of synthesizing and secreting adequate amounts of progesterone. It is susceptible to the luteolytic action of endogenous $PGF_{2\alpha}$ and it does not alter the length of the oestrous cycle. The other two types, the thin-walled follicular cyst and the thick-walled luteal cyst, arise following failure to ovulate but they differ in histological structure and steroidogenic activity. The follicular cyst is lined by granulosa cells that secrete oestrogens whereas the cells of the luteal cyst secrete progesterone. Inevitably, ovarian cysts alter the balance of steroid hormones in the peripheral circulation but in the majority of affected cows the absolute values for the individual hormones remain within the ranges found during the oestrous cycle. The mean plasma concentrations vary considerably both between affected cows and in affected cows over time.

Some follicular cysts may undergo luteinization over a period of time, so that structures that began as follicular cysts may become luteal cysts. Since both structures are pathological and both are treated the same way, it is not necessary to be able to distinguish every follicular cyst from every luteal cyst by rectal palpation. I propose to include both types under the general title of ovarian cysts, which I then define as smooth, fluctuating, follicle-like structures of at least 2.5 cm in diameter that persist for at least 10 days in the absence of a corpus luteum.

Ovarian cysts occur principally in dairy cows but they occur occasionally in heifers and in beef cows. It has been reported that 6–18% of dairy cows may develop ovarian cysts in any breeding season but it is recognized that these figures grossly underestimate the true incidence. It is known that many ovarian cysts develop within 6 weeks after calving; furthermore, over 60% of the cows that develop ovarian cysts recover spontaneously before the first ovulation post partum and are not included in the statistics. Nevertheless, the undetected cysts are of economic significance because they extend the interval from calving to first oestrus and delay conception in 10–30% of dairy cows.

Aetiology

A small proportion of cases may be due to mechanical interference with ovulation in cows with ovarobursal adhesions. In the majority of cases the immediate cause of ovarian cysts is an endocrine dysfunction that results either in a premature LH surge at a time when the growing follicle is unable to ovulate or in a release of insufficient LH at the normal time of ovulation.

A hypothesis to explain the formation of ovarian cysts before the first postpartum ovulation is based on the evidence that the pituitary gland is not responsive to oestrogen until 4–6 weeks after calving. Because follicular development begins within the first 2 weeks post partum, the oestrogen secreted by the growing follicles is unable to induce the LH surge required to ovulate these early follicles, and they then become cystic. This hypothesis does not explain the sudden development of an ovarian cyst in a cow that had resumed regular ovarian cycles. It is probable that there is not a single cause of all ovarian cysts.

Many factors have been proposed as contributory mechanisms in the causation of ovarian cysts: heredity, high milk yield, fatty liver syndrome, high nutrient intake, winter conditions, phyto-oestrogens (red clover, alfalfa, mouldy hay, mouldy brewer's grain), β–carotene deficiency and uterine infection. A relatively high incidence of ovarian cysts occurs in cows with clinical problems such as metritis, milk fever, ketosis or mastitis in the early postpartum period; it has been suggested that stress associated with these conditions causes an increase in the secretion of cortisol that blocks the release of LH. Intrauterine infections soon after calving may predispose to the development of ovarian cysts before first ovulation whenever the preovulatory release of LH is suppressed by adrenal secretion of cortisol, induced either by the direct action of endotoxin from Gram-negative bacteria in the uterus or by products of endotoxin activity (e.g. prostaglandin).

Clinical signs

Most cysts that form before first ovulation are asymptomatic and regress spontaneously; about 60% of affected cows re-establish normal cyclic ovarian activity during the breeding season. If ovarian cycles are not re-established it does not mean that the original cyst has persisted; it is more likely that it has regressed but at a time when there was an associated wave of follicular growth that provided another anovulatory follicle as its replacement.

According to the early literature the most common sign of ovarian cysts was nymphomania, which was attributed to abnormally high levels of oestrogen secreted by the cyst(s). More recent literature indicates that over

80% of affected cows are anoestrous and that when nymphomania occurs it may be a response to an extended period of oestrogen domination of the endocrine balance rather than, necessarily, to excessively high oestrogen production.

Nymphomaniacal cows show intense oestrous behaviour persistently or at frequent but irregular intervals. There is frequent and copious discharge of clear mucus from the vulva, which may be oedematous. There is relaxation of the sacrosciatic ligaments and a raised tail-head. The excessive sexual activity (mounting and standing to be mounted) renders cows with relaxed pelvic ligaments prone to pelvic and hip fractures. The excessive activity causes loss of body condition and decreased milk yield; it also disturbs other cows in the herd and interferes with accurate heat detection.

Cows with luteal cysts of long standing may become virilized: they develop a masculine conformation and they will attempt to mount other cows but will not stand to be mounted.

Treatment

There is evidence of a hereditary predisposition to develop ovarian cysts, which poses the ethical question of whether or not to treat such an animal. If it is decided to treat the condition, there are two approaches:

1. manual removal of the cyst(s);
2. administration of hormones aimed at causing luteinization of the cyst(s).

Manual rupture of the cystic structures by rectal palpation has been reported to give a recovery rate of up to 45%. The procedure may cause haemorrhage and ovarobursal adhesions.

The aim of hormone therapy is to establish a period during which negative feedback by progesterone allows the hypothalamic–pituitary–ovarian axis to re-establish normal cyclic activity.

1. hCG can be used to provide an exogenous source of LH-like activity which will cause luteinization of the cystic structure(s);
2. GnRH can be used to stimulate the release of endogenous LH;
3. exogenous progesterone can be used to create an artificial luteal phase.

The literature reveals that approximately 80% of affected cows responded to a single intravenous injection of hCG. The interval from treatment to oestrus averaged about 23 days and the pregnancy rates to service at first oestrus varied from 38 to 58%. There are some disadvantages associated with the use of hCG. It is a relatively large foreign protein (molecular weight 38 000) that is antigenic in the cow; if treatment has to be repeated the antibodies may induce an anaphylactic response or they may attenuate the physiological effects of the second treatment. Also, if there is an error in diagnosis so that hCG is given to a cow with a fully active corpus luteum, it will prolong the life-span of the corpus luteum and delay the next service. The recommended dosage of hCG for treatment of ovarian cysts varies from 3000 to 4500 iu in Europe and from 5000 to 10 000 iu in the USA.

The literature indicates that approximately 80% of dairy cows with ovarian cysts began cyclic ovarian activity within 30 days of treatment with 100 µg GnRH by intramuscular injection. A luteolytic dose of $PGF_{2\alpha}$ on the ninth day after GnRH treatment reduced the mean interval between treatment and oestrus to 12 days, without affecting the level of fertility. Pregnancy rates to first service ranged from 37 to 55% and the overall recovery rates ranged from 62 to 97%.

Exogenous progesterone has been administered as a single dose of 750–1000 mg repositor progesterone, repeated doses of 100 mg by intramuscular injection on three occasions at intervals of 48 hours, or as an intravaginal device for 12 days. Some authors have reported marked delays in the resumption of oestrous cycles after treatment. Recovery rates of 61–72% have been recorded, with an overall pregnancy rate of about 50%.

Prophylactic use of hormones

It has been reported that a single injection of 200 µg GnRH at day 12–14 post partum will reduce both the incidence of ovarian cysts and the number of cows culled because of infertility. It appears that the benefit derived from this treatment is dependent on the induction of ovulation. GnRH does not induce ovulation before day 12, and then only when there is a follicle of adequate size; therefore, some cows may not respond to the treatment. Benmrad and Stevenson (1986) reported that fertility was improved in all cows but especially in those with puerperal problems (dystocia, retained placental membranes, uterine infections, purulent discharges, milk fever, ketosis). They suggested that the early re-establishment of oestrous cycles of normal length allowed the cows to have an average of three heats before first service and that this was a major factor in reducing the number of services per conception and the mean interval from calving to conception.

Pharmacological regulation of the oestrous cycle

Synchronization of oestrus

'The single most significant factor frustrating improvements in reproductive efficiency is the failure to improve the rate of detection of oestrus' (McMillan 1988). This has stimulated the development of therapeutic regimes that provide more precise control over the timing of ovulation; the so-called oestrous synchronization regimes are based on two different strategies:

1. the use of a luteolytic agent to terminate a natural luteal phase;
2. the use of exogenous progestational compounds to create an artificial luteal phase that can be terminated by withdrawal of treatment.

Induction of luteolysis

Between day 5 and day 17 of the cycle, a single injection of exogenous $PGF_{2\alpha}$ or one of its analogues results in premature luteolysis and a prompt fall in plasma progesterone concentrations to basal levels within 30 hours. The interval from injection to the onset of oestrus can vary depending on the stage of the cycle and, to some degree, on the lactational status and age of the animal.

There are, on average, 8 days from day 18 of one cycle to day 4 of the next cycle when there is no specific target for $PGF_{2\alpha}$. Several treatment regimes have been devised to avoid the necessity of doing repeated rectal examinations to determine which animals have a vulnerable corpus luteum. The most successful regimes are based on the expectation that cyclic cattle that are given two injections of $PGF_{2\alpha}$ 11 days apart will have a responsive corpus luteum present on at least one of the occasions. Those animals that are responsive at the first treatment may be served but, if not, they should be responsive again 11 days later (day 6–9 of the induced cycle). Those animals that are not responsive at the first treatment (day 18 to day 4) should be responsive at the second treatment (day 8 to day 15 of a spontaneous cycle). However, delayed responses to the first injections could result in the second injections being ineffective.

In cyclic heifers two injections 11 days apart give acceptable pregnancy rates either to service at observed oestrus or to fixed-time artificial insemination (AI) at 72 and 96 hours after the second treatment. However, in lactating dairy cows the results from fixed-time AI tend to be very variable and it is recommended that service should be at observed oestrus.

Simulation of the luteal phase

Exogenous progesterone or a progestagen can be used to suppress the release of gonadotrophins and to delay follicular growth. However, the treatment does not have any significant effect on the life-span of a natural corpus luteum. Therefore, there is a risk that the natural corpus luteum might outlive an artificial luteal phase of less than 16 days. Unfortunately, the use of exogenous progesterone for as long as 16 days is associated with a depression in fertility at first oestrus after termination of the treatment. Duration of treatment needs to be restricted to 9–12 days and this necessitates the use of luteolytic agent in conjunction with the progestational compound. The PRID incorporates a capsule containing oestradiol benzoate. A luteolytic injection of $PGF_{2\alpha}$ or an analogue may be given either on the day the PRID is withdrawn or a day or two earlier.

If an ear implant of norgestamet is used, an injection of 5 mg oestradiol valerate should be given on the first day of treatment. Dairy cattle are inseminated at 48 and 72 hours after removal of the implant. Beef cattle are injected with 400–600 iu PMSG when the implant is removed and inseminated between 48 and 56 hours later. Pregnancy rates of 60% have been reported for both dairy and beef cattle.

Fertility following synchronization of oestrus

Many factors influence the response of a group of animals to attempts to synchronize oestrus. There is evidence that the results are affected by breed, nutritional status, postpartum interval, milk yield, inadequate handling facilities, poor heat detection and mistiming of insemination.

In theory, hormonal therapy to synchronize oestrus and ovulation should make it possible to dispense with heat detection in favour of 'fixed-time insemination'; for instance, when prostaglandins are used to synchronize a group of cows or heifers it should be possible to get satisfactory conception rates to a single service at 80 hours after treatment or to two inseminations at 72 and 96 hours after treatment. In practice, the common experience is that in lactating dairy cows the intervals from treatment to oestrus and ovulation are so variable that a significant number of treated cows may not respond until several days after the fixed-time insemination(s). Some of the variation in results is related to the stage of the cycle at which the cow is injected. McMillan (1978) summarized his experiences as follows:

1. Few cows treated at day 0 (oestrus) to day 5 of the cycle will be synchronized.
2. Although 60% of cows treated on day 6 will be in oestrus within 96

hours, the remaining 40% will either experience a silent oestrus or not show oestrus for a further 12–18 days.

3. Approximately 85% of cows treated on days 6–17 will be observed in oestrus within the following 6 days but others will not show oestrus for a further 5 days. The interval from injection to oestrus is longer for some cows treated during the mid-luteal phase (days 10–13).

These data clearly show that the treatment regimes fall very short of the principal requirement for successful fixed-time AI, which is that the vast majority of the treated animals should be synchronized within a period of 24–30 hours. The most precise synchronization is achieved when treatment is timed to take advantage of one of the waves of follicular growth that occur during the luteal phase of the oestrous cycle, i.e. cows are injected on day 7 or on days 15–16. In practice, it is seldom possible to do this; therefore, fixed-time AI needs to be supplemented by post-service observation for oestrus and by reinsemination of all cows that show a delayed response.

Mating

The fertile life of the spermatozoon is said to be 30–48 hours, while the fertile life of the ovum is 20–24 hours. Natural mating is during oestrus, i.e. semen is ejaculated into the anterior vagina at least 10–12 hours before ovulation. This provides adequate time for transport and capacitation of spermatozoa within the fertile life-span of the ovum. Problems with timing of service may arise when AI is used.

Timing of service

Research has shown that the best fertility is obtained when cows are inseminated during the second half of standing oestrus, with good results up to 6 hours after the end of oestrus. Therefore, insemination services recommend that cows seen in oestrus in the morning (before 10.00) should be bred that day, whereas cows that come into oestrus in the afternoon should be bred before noon the following day. However, in practice problems can arise because of the great variation in the overall duration of oestrus (reported range: 2–30 hours) and in the length of time that may elapse from the onset of oestrus to detection, particularly in herds where the frequency of observations or the efficiency of the observer are below standard.

Artificial insemination

Semen collection

Semen can be collected with an artificial vagina or by electroejaculation. The artificial vagina (Figure 4.5) consists of a strong outer rubber cylinder and a thin inner latex liner that is turned back over each end of the rubber cylinder and tied to form a watertight jacket. A collection funnel that drains into a graduated collection tube is fitted to one end of the artificial vagina. When prepared for use the jacket is filled with warm water and the inner lining is lubricated with sterile soft paraffin. At the time of collection the temperature of the water in the jacket should be between 42 and 45°C.

For collection, the bull is allowed to mount a 'teaser' cow, preferably a cow in oestrus, but a non-oestrous cow, a steer or a mechanical 'dummy cow' may be used. The operator holds the vagina close to the teaser, in parallel with the expected path of the penis, and when mounting occurs grasps the sheath and directs the penis into the artificial vagina. If the temperature, pressure and lubrication are appropriate, the bull will thrust and ejaculate into the artificial vagina.

The collecting tube should be warmed and insulated to protect the spermatozoa from cold shock. The aim should be to maintain semen at 30–35°C at all times from collection until it is diluted in extender. Semen must not be exposed to temperatures in excess of 50°C, which are lethal to spermatozoa. It may be necessary to fit an inner liner of a particular texture or to have it at a particular temperature to get an individual bull to give of his best. Every precaution should be taken to prevent adulteration of semen with biological or physical contaminants during collection and processing.

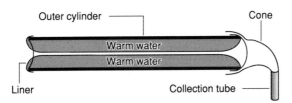

Figure 4.5 Artificial vagina for the bull. Diagrammatic longitudinal section through an artificial vagina with collecting tube attached.

Semen can be collected routinely from a bull on a daily basis week after week without an adverse effect on fertility. In practice, commercial breeding centres collect from an individual bull either twice a day on two days a week or once a day on three alternate days each week. In such a routine, the average number of spermatozoa in each ejaculate will be lower (by about 25%) than it would be in the first few ejaculates after a period of sexual rest.

Sexual stimulation

When semen is collected from a bull several times a week, the period of sexual stimulation should be extended beyond that needed for mounting and ejaculation. The bull that is subject to restraint and prolonged sexual stimulation will provide a greater volume of semen and a larger number of spermatozoa than a bull that is allowed to serve at will. The procedures for sexual preparation include walking the bull around the teaser, restraining him a few feet away from the teaser, allowing a few preliminary false mounts (he is allowed to mount but not to ejaculate), introducing a second bull or changing the location of the teaser. An effective combination of false mounting and restraint can increase the number of spermatozoa in the ejaculate by up to 100%; even one false mount may increase the sperm density by 50%.

If these procedures are to be effective, care must be taken to eliminate various distractions that interfere with sex drive. Excitement, mishandling, sudden vigorous movements by the operator or helpers, loud noises or a restive teaser can distract the bull from his main task. Furthermore, bulls can become uninterested when the same procedure is followed exactly at each collection. Novelty is needed if sex drive is to be maintained over a long period on a routine schedule of semen collection. Novelty can be obtained by changing the teaser or the location of collection.

Special care should be taken to avoid distractions while the bull is becoming accustomed to the new surroundings. One unhappy experience may cause a bull to refuse to work ever again in that location.

Electroejaculation

Electroejaculation is useful for bulls with physical disabilities that seriously inhibit or prevent mounting activity. The electric current is applied to a rectal probe. The electrodes are located over the ampullae and seminal vesicles so as to stimulate both the nerves that control the release of semen into the urethra and those that control the ejaculation of semen from the urethra. The ejaculate is collected into a graduated tube through a funnel held below the prepuce.

Evaluation of semen

After collection, the semen is maintained at 30–35°C while it is examined grossly and microscopically.

An immediate check can be made on the volume, colour and quality of the semen. The volume can vary from 3 to 15 ml, with averages of approximately 6 ml for dairy bulls and 4 ml for beef bulls. The normal colour is creamy white and the consistency should be fairly uniform. The semen is checked for the presence of hair, blood, faeces, urine or pus.

The microscopic examinations include those for sperm motility, the proportion of live spermatozoa, the proportion of spermatozoa with morphological abnormalities, and the concentration of spermatozoa in the semen. An ejaculate with less than 70% forward motility is considered unsuitable for use in AI.

The percentage of live spermatozoa in the ejaculate is estimated on a thin smear made after mixing a drop of semen with two drops of warm nigrosin–eosin stain on a warm slide. The dead spermatozoa take up the eosin whereas the live spermatozoa exclude it; the nigrosin provides the dark background against which the dead and live cells can be seen easily. The ratio of dead to live spermatozoa is expressed as percentage counts. An ejaculate that contains up to 25% dead cells would not be considered unsuitable for use in AI.

To assess the morphology of the spermatozoa, a thin smear is made after a drop of semen is mixed with two drops of India ink at body temperature. Under the oil immersion objective, 200 or 300 spermatozoa are examined and classified according to their shape and appearance. A number of abnormalities of heads, midpieces and tails have been described in the literature. Several of the defects have not been correlated with infertility but there seems to be general agreement that fertile bulls show about 90% normal spermatozoa. Semen that contains more than 20% abnormal spermatozoa would not be used for AI.

Methods for determining concentration of spermatozoa include:

1. using a haemocytometer to perform a direct visual count of the number of spermatozoa in a standard volume when samples of semen are diluted at a constant rate;
2. using a calibrated spectrophotometer to compare the optical density of a sample of semen diluted at a standard rate with that of a sample of semen whose concentration of spermatozoa has been determined by direct count;
3. using a photometer to compare the optical density of semen diluted at a standard rate with the optical density of a density standard that has been calibrated against a direct count.

Semen with a concentration of spermatozoa less than 8×10^8/ml is not suitable for use in AI.

Dilution of semen

Semen for use in AI is diluted in an extender that sustains and protects the spermatozoa during storage and distribution. The extent to which the original ejaculate can be diluted is dependent upon the concentration of spermatozoa. While satisfactory conception rates can be achieved at dose rates of 6–12 million motile spermatozoa per insemination, AI services commonly use 20 million 'total' spermatozoa, or more, at each insemination. If the 'average' ejaculate yields 6 ml of semen containing 1000 million spermatozoa/ml and the standard inseminate required 20 million spermatozoa in a plastic straw of 0.25 ml capacity, the required dilution rate would be 12 times. Bull semen can be extended between 10 and 75 times.

A satisfactory extender has several functions in addition to dilution. It must provide the spermatozoa with energy and nutrients, including essential minerals. It must protect the spermatozoa from cold shock and act as a cryoprotectant during freezing. It must buffer the toxic end-products of metabolic processes in the spermatozoa. It must be isotonic with the spermatozoa and must inhibit bacterial growth.

The common extenders contain egg yolk or milk to protect against cold shock and glycerol and/or dimethyl sulphoxide as cryoprotectants. Citrate, phosphate and Tris buffers are used to counteract the lactic acid produced by sperm metabolism. Simple sugars (fructose, glucose) can supply energy without upsetting the osmotic balance between the extender and the spermatozoa. Antibiotics (penicillin, streptomycin, lincomycin) are added to prevent the transmission of bacteria.

Packaging and freezing of semen

The standard packaging system is a plastic straw of 0.25 ml capacity (0.5 ml in the USA), which contains 20 million spermatozoa in extender and is stored at $-196°C$ in liquid nitrogen. The spermatozoa are protected from the lethal effects of freezing by the glycerol (final concentration: 7%) in the extender. The filling of the straws is a highly automated process. Once they are filled they are cooled to 5°C and allowed to equilibrate for 6 hours. Then, they are brought down at a controlled rate to $-110°C$, before storage at $-196°C$.

Thawing of semen and insemination

The usual procedure for thawing semen on the farm is to immerse the straw in water at 35°C for 7 seconds. After thawing, the plug is cut off and the straw is inserted into a special metal gun, which will be used to propel the contents of the straw into the cow's reproductive tract. The inseminator grasps the cervix per rectum, pushes it forward to straighten and extend the vagina and then by downward pressure on the perineum with the operating arm opens the vulva and inserts the gun as far as the internal os of the cervix before injecting the semen into the uterine body.

Transport of spermatozoa

Fertilization takes place in the oviduct, close to the junction of the isthmus and the ampulla. Transport of both the spermatozoa and the ovum is achieved by muscular and ciliary activity and the flow of fluids in the female genital tract. At the beginning of oestrus the direction of flow is from the cervix towards the oviduct, at the end of oestrus the direction is reversed. These processes are regulated by oestrogen and progesterone.

Spermatozoa have been recovered from the ampulla of the oviduct within 3–5 minutes after service but most of these cells are dead or damaged and they do not include the sperm that will fertilize the ovum. Viable sperm are transported more slowly. It takes 8–12 hours to establish an adequate population of viable spermatozoa in the caudal isthmus, where they are sequestered, in a quiescent state, for a further 18–20 hours before they become activated and begin to migrate to the site of fertilization. Activation of quiescent spermatozoa in the functional sperm reservoir in the caudal isthmus is in response to the arrival of follicular fluid and the ovum in the oviduct.

Capacitation of spermatozoa

During transport through the female genital tract the spermatozoa undergo physiological changes that make them competent to penetrate the zona pellucida and fuse with the ovum. This process, known as capacitation, does not involve any visible change in the morphology of the spermatozoa. However, it does involve the loss of proteins from the plasma membrane that facilitates the influx of calcium required for the activated form of motility that takes the spermatozoa to the site of fertilization and for the acrosome reaction, an essential prerequisite for fertilization.

The acrosome reaction

The acrosome reaction (Figure 4.6) begins as point fusions between the cell membrane of the spermatozoon and the outer acrosomal membrane over the front half of the sperm head. These fusions create gaps through which the acrosomal enzymes escape. The escaping enzymes, particularly

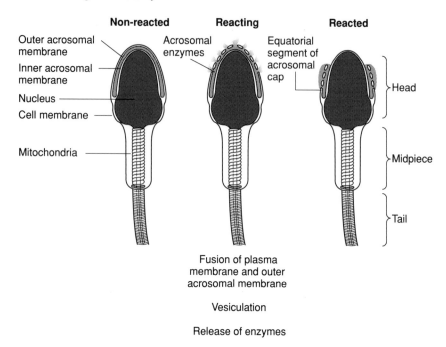

Figure 4.6 The acrosome reaction of the spermatozoon. The acrosome-reacted spermatozoon has lost all of the components of the acrosome except the equatorial segment and the inner acrosomal membrane. The reaction renders the spermatozoon capable of attaching to and passing through the zona pellucida and of fusing with the plasma membrane of the ovum.

hyaluronidase, are responsible for both the progressive disintegration of the acrosomal covering over the head of the spermatozoa and the passage of the sperm through the corona radiata that surrounds the zona pellucida of the ovum. Spermatozoa that have not undergone the acrosome reaction cannot bind to the external surface of the zona pellucida.

Fertilization

After spermatozoa have undergone capacitation and the acrosome reaction they can bind to the zona pellucida and then pass through it into the perivitelline space. The sperm tail propels the spermatozoon across the perivitelline space and fusion with the plasma membrane of the ovum begins in the equatorial or post-acrosomal regions of the sperm head where the plasma membrane has remained intact after the acrosome reaction. The sperm head and part of the tail are incorporated into the egg, the male and female pronuclei are formed and they come together to form the zygote.

The fusion of the egg and the sperm triggers a series of reactions that prevent polyspermy by making both the zona pellucida and the plasma membrane of the ovum impenetrable to other spermatozoa.

Pregnancy

Early development of the conceptus

The zygote (or conceptus) spends 3–4 days in the oviduct before it enters the uterus. During that time it undergoes a series of mitotic divisions (cleavage), each doubling the number of daughter cells (blastomeres). It enters the uterus at the 8-cell or 16-cell stage as a solid mass of blastomeres (the morula) still within the zona pellucida. Subsequently, the blastomeres begin to secrete fluid that accumulates in a central fluid-filled cavity, the blastocoele. In cattle, the blastocoele appears on day 7. At that stage the conceptus is described as a blastocyst. It consists of an outer layer of cells, the trophoblast, that surrounds the blastocoele and an aggregation of cells, the inner cell mass, at one pole. In due course, the trophoblast will form the chorion and the inner cell mass will become the embryo. The blastocyst 'hatches' from the zona pellucida some time between day 7 and day 10; between day 12 and day 14 it begins to elongate greatly.

By day 17 or 18 the elongated blastocyst (or blastodermic vesicle) occupies about two-thirds of the gravid horn, by day 18–20 it fills the horn and by day 24 it has expanded into the contralateral horn. At that stage the embryo is contained within the fluid-filled amniotic sac inside the elongated vesicle formed by the expanding chorion (Figure 4.7). The chorion is derived from the avascular trophoblast but it acquires a rich blood supply when the allantois, a vascular outgrowth from the developing hindgut, expands to line the chorionic vesicle by days 24–28. The newly formed, richly vascular chorioallantois is the foetal component that attaches to the maternal tissues at implantation.

Implantation

The process of attachment begins at day 19 or 20 when there are definite areas of adhesion between the chorionic epithelium of the conceptus and the endometrial epithelium; implantation is completed between days 35 and 42. Placental attachment involves specialized areas of both the endometrium and the chorioallantois. On the maternal side, the endometrium

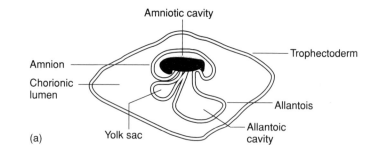

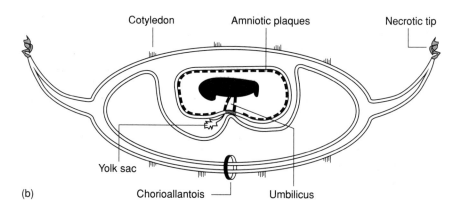

Figure 4.7 Early bovine embryo and associated membranes. Diagrams of relationships (a) before and (b) after the expansion of the chorionic sac. Note the appearance of the amniotic plaques, the regression of the yolk sac, the formation of the chorioallantois, the development of placental cotyledons and the necrotic tips of the chorioallantois.

has about 120 caruncles arranged in rows. The luminal surface of the caruncle is convex but during gestation it develops a large number of crypts that give the caruncle a sponge-like appearance. At approximately day 30 special areas on the chorioallantois develop opposite the caruncles (see Figure 4.7). These areas, known as cotyledons, are formed by proliferation of cones of trophoblast cells (chorionic villi). At implantation these two specialized structures come together to form the functional unit of attachment, the placentome, in which the chorionic villi fit into the caruncular crypts like fingers into a glove. As gestation proceeds the primary villi of the cotyledons give rise to secondary villi and tertiary villi that project into corresponding crypts in the caruncle.

Maternal recognition of pregnancy

The survival of a conceptus in the uterus depends on the continued function of the corpus luteum over at least 200 days of pregnancy. The critical period for the extension of the functional life-span of the corpus luteum in the cow is between day 15 and day 17; if there is a viable conceptus present at that time the dam will 'recognize' that she is pregnant and luteolysis will not occur. Since maternal recognition of pregnancy occurs several days before there is any attachment of the conceptus to the endometrium, it is evident that the preimplantation conceptus is using biochemical signals to inform the dam of its presence and well-being. The bovine conceptus can synthesize a number of products (steroids, prostaglandins and proteins) that could act as signals to the maternal utero-ovarian axis. A hypothesis consistent with the current information is that the bovine conceptus initiates both antiluteolytic and luteotrophic activities. It is thought that a group of proteins, called bovine trophoblast protein-1 but now identified as isotypes of α-interferon, are secreted by the conceptus between days 16 and 26 and prevent regression of the corpus luteum because they inhibit the synthesis of $PGF_{2\alpha}$ by the endometrium. Putative luteotrophic factors include products produced by the conceptus itself (e.g. a lipid-like substance released by the conceptus between days 13 and 18) or by the endometrium in response to a signal from the conceptus (e.g. PGE_2).

The endocrinology of pregnancy

The corpus luteum is absolutely essential for the maintenance of pregnancy up to about day 200; thereafter, the adrenal glands seem to be able to produce enough progesterone to maintain pregnancy in ovariectomized cows. In the intact pregnant cow the corpus luteum remains functional up to full term. The principal luteotrophin appears to be LH, assisted by prolactin.

Plasma progesterone concentrations of about 10 ng/ml (range: 6–15 ng/ml) are maintained until a decline begins about 3 weeks before parturition and culminates in a sharp drop to less than 2 ng/ml about 24 hours before delivery. Oestrone sulphate from the placenta is the principal oestrogen in the maternal circulation during pregnancy. The concentrations in the peripheral circulation show some fluctuation but the general trend is a prolonged rise from about 80 ng/ml at day 72 to approximately 3000 ng/ml at day 225; it then rises rapidly to approximately 4000 ng/ml at day 270. There is a three-fold to four-fold increase in total corticosteroid concentrations in peripheral blood over the last 2 days before delivery (almost coincident with the final decline in progesterone concentration) and it has been suggested that the corticosteroids may play an active role in the initiation of parturition. Release of $PGF_{2\alpha}$ from the uterus, as deduced from measurements of the metabolite PGFM in the peripheral blood, begins to increase about a week before delivery and shows a sharp rise in the 24 hours before delivery (concomitant with the sharp decline in plasma progesterone concentration).

Functions of progesterone during pregnancy

1. In the first 6 or 7 weeks after conception it stimulates the endo-metrial glands to secrete the uterine fluids that sustain the preimplantation embryo;

2. throughout pregnancy it exerts a strong negative feedback on the hypothalamus and pituitary gland to suppress the release of gonado-trophins and prevent the preovulatory surge of LH and ovulation;

3. it exerts a 'block' on uterine muscle in that it depresses the amplitude of contractions, suppresses the reactivity to oxytocin and prostaglandin and prevents the development of synchronous coordinated contractions that might expel the foetus prematurely.

Pregnancy diagnosis

Cows that are not observed in oestrus between 18 and 24 days after service are assumed to be pregnant. However, since heat detection is seldom 100%, this assumption will be incorrect in relation to several cows and, therefore, their calving-to-conception intervals are likely to be extended by at least 3 weeks. In some herds up to 10% of pregnant cows may show signs of behavioural oestrus. Service by AI during such an oestrus is likely to lead to death of the conceptus. Therefore, there are strong economic reasons for a more accurate method of diagnosing pregnancy and, perhaps, even stronger reasons for identifying those cows that are not in-calf: the earlier a non-pregnant animal can be identified, the sooner a repeat service can be given.

Progesterone assays

Non-pregnant cyclic animals return to oestrus every 18–24 days and at that time the concentrations of progesterone in plasma or milk are at basal values. Since pregnant cows maintain high concentrations of progesterone throughout this period, enzyme-linked immunosorbent assay (ELISA) for

Method of pregnancy diagnosis in the cow

Length of gestation	Method
Days 18–24	Failure to return to oestrus; persistence of the corpus luteum
Day 24	Progesterone assays (milk, plasma)
Days 30–65	Palpation of amniotic vesicle
Days 35–90	Fluctuation of uterine contents; disparity in size of uterine horns; palpation of the chorioallantois
Day 90+	Palpation of placentomes; fremitus in ipsilateral middle uterine artery
Day 150+	Fremitus in contralateral middle uterine artery

the detection of progesterone in blood or milk can be used to diagnose pregnancy. The optimal time to use these assays as a means of pregnancy diagnosis is day 24 after the oestrus at which the cow was served. Day 24 is chosen rather than day 21 in order to eliminate the risk of a false-positive result whenever a cow has a longer than average cycle (say, 24 days); however, it does carry a risk that a non-pregnant cow with a shorter than average interval (say, 18 days) between two ovulations, the second of which is silent, may have a functional corpus luteum and elevated progesterone concentration at day 24.

Sources of false-positive results to progesterone assay

1. early embryonic mortality, when the embryo dies after the test;

2. a persistent corpus luteum or a luteal cyst, both of which cause elevated concentrations of progesterone in non-pregnant cows;

3. an active corpus luteum formed following a silent ovulation.

When properly performed, the progesterone assay is virtually 100% accurate in the detection of non-pregnant animals but only about 85% of the positive tests for pregnancy are accurate. Cows that give a positive test for pregnancy at day 24 should be examined by rectal palpation at a later date. An alternative, non-invasive method of confirmation is to assay the oestrone sulphate concentration in milk at day 105 or later.

Ultrasonic methods

Pregnancy can be diagnosed by means of a real-time B-mode ultrasonic instrument fitted with a rectal transducer. High-frequency scanners (5.0 or 7.5 MHz) give sufficient resolution to enable an experienced operator to detect an embryonic vesicle in the bovine uterus as early as days 13–15. The embryo can be visualized within the vesicle between day 27 and day 30 and the rhythmic pulsations of the embryonic heart beat can be seen on the first day that the embryo is observed. According to Kastelic *et al.* (1988) it is possible to achieve 100% accuracy in the diagnoses of both non-pregnancy and pregnancy with a 5.0 MHz transducer from day 22 onwards. Low-frequency transducers (3.0 or 3.5 MHz) do not approximate that level of accuracy until after day 45.

Palpation of the amniotic vesicle

The diameter of the amniotic vesicle increases progressively from about 1 cm at day 35 to 5 cm at day 50 and 10 cm at day 65. It is present in the uterine horn adjacent to the ovary that contains the corpus luteum, but it cannot be palpated before day 30 (it is too small) or after about day 65 (it is too large and soft). Between these dates gentle palpation of the entire uterine horn between the thumb and two fingers will detect the vesicle as a distinct turgid structure in the allantoic fluid. This is not recommended as a routine procedure because of the risk of rupturing the vesicle itself or of rupturing the embryonic heart; in either case the pregnancy is lost.

Palpation of the chorioallantois ('membrane slip')

From about day 30 to day 35 the pregnant horn increases in size. The uterine wall feels thinner and it fluctuates when palpated; this is because of the presence of the allantoic fluid in the enlarging chorioallantois. Experienced clinicians can diagnose pregnancy at about day 35 by palpating the chorioallantois. The method of detection is based on the fact that attachment of the membrane to the endometrium occurs only at the cotyledons and the intercotyledonary part of the membrane is free. Therefore, when a portion of pregnant uterine horn is grasped between the thumb and a finger and squeezed so that the contents of the horn slip away, the chorioallantois is felt to 'slip' in a characteristic manner just before the wall of the uterus is lost from grasp. In early pregnancy, the chorioallantois is very thin and the most readily detectable part of the membrane is the connective tissue band that contains the blood vessels; therefore, in the early stages the whole width of the uterus should be grasped so as to include the connective tissue band.

As pregnancy advances the chorioallantois extends to fill both horns; the pregnant horn becomes turgid and after day 70 it is often easier to detect the membrane slip in the non-pregnant horn. A false diagnosis of pregnancy can be made by an inexperienced clinician who grasps the broad ligament with the uterine horn and feels it slip away.

Palpation of the foetus

The turgidity of the amniotic sac declines when the fluids begin to flow between the amniotic sac and the allantoic sac via the urachus. The less tense sac allows the clinician to palpate or ballot the foetus from about day 65 to about day 112. However, as the foetus grows and the volumes of foetal fluids increase, the uterus is drawn down by the weight of the contents towards the abdominal floor and by approximately day 120 it has become entirely abdominal in location. Between day 150 and day 210 the foetus will be palpable in less than half of the pregnancies: in some cows the uterus will have 'disappeared' into the abdomen and the foetus will be out of reach of the arm of the clinician, while in other cows the foetal head and/or the flexed limbs can be palpated just anterior to the pelvic brim. Touching the foetus often produces reflex movement. From day 210 to term, the foetus will be detected in the vast majority of cases.

Palpation of the placentomes

The placentomes can be detected by a skilled and experienced clinician at 70–80 days of gestation but most operators find it difficult to identify them as distinct structures before about day 90. The size of the individual placentomes varies with the stage of gestation and with location within the uterus. As pregnancy advances they become progressively larger, pedunculated and mushroom-like. In general, the placentomes in the middle of the pregnant horn (in the region of the foetus) are larger than those in either extremity of that horn or those in the non-pregnant horn. When the uterus drops into the abdomen during the fifth to the seventh month it may not be possible to palpate the placentomes.

Palpation of the ('middle') uterine arteries

Each uterine horn receives the bulk of its arterial supply from the uterine artery, a branch of the internal iliac artery that runs a tortuous course to the concave surface of the uterine horn near its middle. During pregnancy both uterine arteries increase in size and exhibit a diagnostically significant change in the character of the arterial pulse. It is not always easy to identify the uterine arteries in the non-pregnant cow or during the early weeks of pregnancy. Estimates made at rectal examination put the diameter of the uterine artery in the non-pregnant cow at 0.2 cm. After 6 weeks of gestation, the size increases progressively to reach 1.2 cm near full-term. The increase in size becomes evident earlier in the artery that supplies the pregnant horn; the difference in size between sides can be detected per rectum at about day 100. In a bicornual twin pregnancy the two uterine arteries will be enlarged to a similar degree.

The change in character of the arterial pulse also occurs earlier in the artery that supplies the pregnant horn (at day 90 to day 100) than in the artery of the non-pregnant horn (at approximately day 150). On rectal palpation the flow of blood through the enlarged artery is felt as a thrill (fremitus) rather than the usual arterial pulse. Roberts (1986) described the fremitus of late pregnancy as feeling 'much like a stream of water surging intermittently through a thin rubber hose'.

There is considerable variation between animals in the time at which fremitus is detected for the first time and, also, in the time at which it becomes continuous. To a degree, the reported variations may be related to the technique of the different clinicians. Up to day 135, light pressure on the arteries may elicit fremitus whereas heavy pressure may give the tactile sensation of a pulse. In general, fremitus becomes continuous from approximately day 175 onwards; prior to that, it is a common experience to detect fremitus when the artery is grasped only to find that it soon gives way to pulsation.

These changes in the uterine arteries can be particularly valuable in diagnosing pregnancy during the period when the uterus has dropped into the abdominal cavity and the foetus cannot be palpated, i.e. the fifth and sixth months of gestation.

As pregnancy advances, the uterus sinks towards the abdominal floor and the uterine artery is pulled caudally until it lies 2–10 cm anterior to the shaft of the ilium. It is the only large pulsating artery, ventrolateral to the rectum, that can be picked up by the fingers per rectum and moved. If the fingertips are drawn back along the lateral pelvic wall, the first large artery encountered is the external iliac artery, which lies on the abdominal side of the shaft of the ilium and is fixed in position. The movable uterine artery is caudal to the external iliac artery.

Errors in pregnancy diagnosis by rectal palpation

In general, errors are of three types:

1. those due to faulty procedure;

2. those due to incorrect interpretation of findings;
3. those in which the correct interpretation is invalidated by subsequent developments.

The principal error in procedure is failure to retract the uterus into the pelvic inlet. This is particularly important in large pluriparous cows in which the uterus may be located out of reach in the abdomen.

False-positive errors in rectal pregnancy diagnosis

Organ/Condition	Mistaken for
Urinary bladder	A pregnant horn
Ovaries	Placentomes
Uterine neoplasms	Early pregnancy
Incompletely involuted uterus	Pregnancy
Hydrometra	Pregnancy
Mucometra	Pregnancy
Pyometra	Pregnancy

Occasionally, the clinician has to differentiate a poorly involuted uterus from a pregnant uterus. Here the distinguishing features are the contrast between the relatively thin-walled fluctuant pregnant horn and the thick-walled fluid-filled uninvoluted horn that feels 'doughy' and sometimes has longitudinal grooves on the dorsal surface.

Sometimes the clinician makes the correct interpretation of findings at rectal examination only to have the diagnosis invalidated by subsequent events. This may happen when the embryo or foetus dies after a positive diagnosis has been made (in time, this will be seen as a false-positive diagnosis). Occasionally, an error may arise when a cow is pregnant to a service at a later date than is shown on the records. If the pregnancy to the unrecorded service is too recent to produce positive signs of pregnancy, the clinician will make a diagnosis of non-pregnancy; however, as the pregnancy becomes evident, the initial assessment will be seen as a false-negative diagnosis.

Pregnancy wastage induced by palpation

If palpation is done gently and carefully, it should not cause a significant loss of pregnancy; nevertheless, where pregnancy diagnosis by rectal palpation is adopted as a routine in a herd the owner should be told that some pregnancies are lost after the date of the examination and that losses up to 5% are likely to be due to natural wastage rather than to errors in diagnosis or to damage by palpation. Abbitt *et al.* (1978) stated that palpation for fluctuance alone was the safest method, while palpation of the amniotic vesicle was associated with fewer losses than was membrane slip. They also reported a greater loss after all three methods when palpation was carried out between days 35 and 51 (overall loss: 8.5%) rather than between days 52 and 70 (overall loss: 3.7%).

Termination of pregnancy

Indications for termination of pregnancy

- pregnancy in very small or young heifers;
- pregnancy in heifers entering a feedlot;
- misalliance;
- pathological pregnancies (hydrallantois, hydramnios, macerated foetus, mummified foetus, pathologically prolonged gestation).

The procedure to be used depends largely on the stage of gestation. If the aim is to prevent a heifer or a cow from establishing a pregnancy to an unwelcome service there are two approaches that can be adopted during the preimplantation phase:

1. the conceptus can be destroyed by the intrauterine infusion of an irritant solution;
2. the corpus luteum of the cycle can be destroyed by the injection of an exogenous luteolysin.

An intrauterine infusion will not be effective until after the conceptus enters the uterus on day 4 and it is likely to prolong the oestrous cycle if it is made after day 11. Between those two dates a 50-ml volume of 2% Lugol's iodine, 70% ethyl alcohol or 500 mg tetracycline in saline should kill the preimplantation conceptus.

When misalliance has been observed, pregnancy can be prevented by an intramuscular injection of 4–8 mg oestradiol valerate within the first 2 days. This treatment interferes with the transport of the ovum and alters the biochemical milieu in the uterus.

After day 5, the intramuscular injection of 25 mg $PGF_{2\alpha}$ or 500 µg cloprostenol will cause the corpus luteum of the cycle to regress. Both of these drugs are effective against the corpus luteum of pregnancy up to day 150, but from day 150 to day 250 the prostaglandin should be used in combination with a glucocorticoid (e.g. 25 mg dexamethasone).

From day 40 to day 60 abortion can be induced following rupture of the amniotic vesicle by manual pressure exerted per rectum. Manual enucleation of the corpus luteum during the first 200 days of gestation would induce abortion but the risks of death from haemorrhage or of infertility due to ovarobursal adhesions make this an unacceptable form of treatment. Manual decapitation between day 65 and day 90 has been described as an effective method but I have no practical experience of the procedure.

Spontaneous pregnancy wastage

Between conception and parturition, the normal conceptus passes through three stages: the zygote (from day 1 to day 14 of gestation), the embryo (from day 14 to day 45, approximately) and the foetus (from the end of embryonic differentiation to full-term). Pregnancy may be lost during any of the three stages. When the conceptus dies before maternal recognition of pregnancy at day 16–17, the cow is likely to return to oestrus after a normal cycle, without any clinical evidence that a pregnancy had existed. Embryonic mortality at a later stage will be associated with a delayed return to oestrus, quite often without any other clinical evidence of reproductive disorders. If the conceptus dies during the foetal stage it may be mummified, macerated, aborted or stillborn.

Foetal death

Mummification occurs when the foetus dies in a uterus that is free of bacteria. If the cervix remains closed and the corpus luteum remains functional, the foetal skin can resist autolysis and, over a period of several weeks, the foetal fluids are resorbed and the membranes become closely wrapped around the desiccated foetus. Typically, the mummified foetus is retained within the uterus well beyond full-term. Evacuation may be induced by a luteolytic dose of a prostaglandin preparation or it may require a caesarean section. When a foetus dies in an infected uterus it may undergo decomposition ('maceration') accompanied by endometritis, metritis or pyometra. If the cervix opens, gas-producing bacteria may gain access and induce foetal emphysema.

Abortion

An abortion is the expulsion before full-term of a foetus that is incapable of independent life (days 45–240). It has been estimated that the average rate of success in diagnosing the causes of abortion is between 25 and 40%. Reasons for failure to identify the cause of abortion (Kirkbride 1982) include:

1. frequently abortion is the result of an event that occurred weeks or months earlier and the cause of the event, if ever it was present in the conceptus, is often undetectable by the time of abortion;
2. the foetus is often retained *in utero* for hours to days after death, resulting in autolysis that hides lesions;
3. frequently the foetal membranes, which are commonly affected first and most consistently, are not available for examination;
4. toxic and genetic factors that cause foetal death or abortion are not discernible in the specimens available for examination;
5. many causes of bovine abortion are unknown, or there are no effective routine diagnostic procedures for identifying them;
6. interpretation of serological tests (on maternal serum, foetal serum or foetal thoracic fluid) can be difficult (see p. 131).

The list of potential causes of abortion is extensive but a thorough history of the herd can be an invaluable aid in limiting the possibilities. It should enable the veterinarian to decide whether or not the cause is likely to be infectious, traumatic, genetic, toxic or nutritional. That decision will influence the choice of specimens to be submitted to the diagnostic laboratory. If it is possible, the entire foetus and placenta should be submitted without delay. If this cannot be done the veterinarian should conduct a necropsy during which specimens will be collected for immediate dispatch to the laboratory. If at all possible, these should include fresh specimens (preferably packed in ice) of a cotyledon and any foetal organ or tissue that appears abnormal together with a sample of abomasal contents, pieces of lung, liver, heart, intestine, spleen, thymus, eyelid and adrenal gland, and samples of foetal blood or foetal thoracic fluid. Despite the difficulties it may entail under field conditions, the brain should be exposed and examined; gross evidence of cerebellar hypoplasia would arouse suspicion of infection with bovine viral diarrhoea (BVD) virus. The specimens from the placenta and the gut should be packaged individually in separate containers. A second specimen from each of the sampled sites should be fixed in 10% formalin.

If the facilities are available, samples for bacteriological study should be obtained from abomasal contents, liver, lung and cotyledon. On occasion, it may be worth while to identify the bacteria in the dam's genital tract (vagina, cervix or uterus), particularly if the samples can be taken immediately after the abortion. The bacteriological samples may be submitted to the laboratory as swabs, in transport medium, or on plates (blood agar or MacConkey's medium) that have been incubated at 35°C for 48 hours.

One serum sample (10 ml) from the dam should be submitted for serological investigations and it should be followed by another sample 3–4 weeks later. The purpose of the second sample is to check for rising titres of the putative causal organism. This is necessary because antibodies often persist long after an infectious agent is gone and their presence at the time of an abortion may be of no significance. However, the expectation of an elevated titre in the second sample may not be fulfilled because in most cases the cow has been infected at least 2 weeks before the abortion, the serum antibodies will be near or at their maximum when the first sample is taken and they may be on the decline when the second sample is taken. Therefore, it is prudent to take serum samples from several cows in the herd at the same times. This may provide significant information on whether or not a particular infection is active in the herd.

The history may indicate the desirability of submitting samples of maternal blood for haematological, biochemical or toxicological studies. The full history should be sent with the samples; it may contain highly relevant information that might determine which laboratory procedures should be used.

Some common infectious agents that cause abortion in cattle

Bacteria
Brucella abortus
Campylobacter fetus
Leptospira interrogans var. hardjo
Listeria monocytogenes
Haemophilus somnus
Actinomyces pyogenes
Salmonella dublin
Bacillus licheniformis

Viruses
Bovine viral diarrhoea virus
Infectious bovine rhinotracheitis virus
Akabane virus
Bluetongue virus
Bovine parainfluenza-3-virus

Fungi
Aspergillus fumigatus
Mortierella wolfii

Mycoplasma
Mycoplasma bovigenitalium
Acholeplasma laidlawii
Ureaplasma diversum

Protozoa
Trichomonas foetus
Sarcocystis cruzi
Neospora caninum

Unknown
Epizootic bovine abortion

Gross examination of the foetus and/or the placental membranes

Most of the gross changes seen in aborted foetuses are non-specific and of little diagnostic significance. Frequently, there is the added complication that autolysis is advanced by the time the foetus is expelled. Nevertheless, careful examination of the foetus may be rewarding. For instance, ring-worm-like lesions of the foetal skin are suggestive of aspergillosis, arthrogryposis with or without hydranencephaly (in an abortus or at full-term) indicates the need to consider Akabane virus, while cerebellar hypoplasia might point to the BVD-MD virus.

Frequently, the placental membranes are retained after abortion and only a small segment may be available for detailed inspection. Published accounts of the changes to be expected in specific diseases have been based on careful examination of fresh membranes obtained by pathologists under carefully controlled conditions. Much of this detailed information is of little diagnostic value to the clinician faced with incomplete and autolysed membranes from a field case. However, some pointers may be detected. In brucellosis the intercotyledonary chorioallantois is thickened, oedema-tous, opaque and tough ('resembles yellowish grey morocco leather') and it is covered with a patchy exudate. Affected cotyledons are necrotic, soft, yellow-grey in colour and they may be covered with a sticky exudate ('resembles soft caramel candy'). In mycotic abortion due to *Aspergillus fumigatus* the lesions in the foetal placenta are similar but they are often much more severe. The chorioallantois is leathery with extensive areas of necrosis; the placentomes are greatly enlarged and necrotic with swollen margins and the foetal and maternal tissues are firmly adherent.

The discovery of areas of necrosis at the tips of the chorioallantois or multiple small plaques on the inner surface of the amnion should not be misconstrued as pathological changes—these are normal features of the bovine placental membranes. The necrotic tips are due to lack of vascular supply to the extremities of the chorioallantois. The amniotic plaques are foci of squamous epithelium that are always conspicuous during the third to the seventh months of gestation.

Major infectious causes of 'abortion storms'

The major causes of herd 'abortion storms' are:

- *Brucella abortus*
- *Campylobacter fetus* var. *venerealis*
- *Trichomonas foetus*
- *Listeria monocytogenes*
- *Leptospira interrogans* var. *hardjo*
- *Haemophilus somnus*

Brucellosis

In cattle, infection with *Brucella abortus* is acquired most frequently by ingestion of contaminated material from an aborted foetus, placental membranes or genital discharges. Other portals of entry are the vagina, the conjunctiva and the skin. Once it gains entry, the organism passes rapidly to the regional lymph nodes and then spreads within the body, mainly by the haematogenous route. It tends to localize in tissues that contain erythritol. As a facultative intracellular bacterium it can survive for long periods within macrophages and epithelial cells, principally in the spleen, mammary lymph nodes and udder; from these foci bacteraemia may recur intermittently. The non-pregnant uterus does not contain sufficient erythritol to sustain *B. abortus* but when bacteraemia occurs in a pregnant female the organism shows a particular affinity for the foetal placenta, a rich source of erythritol. Once the infection becomes established in the pregnant uterus it remains active until the foetus and placental membranes are delivered.

Brucella abortus induces necrotic placentitis and ulcerative endometritis that usually cause abortion, most frequently during the sixth and seventh months of gestation. Thus, the interval from infection to abortion can vary enormously. The foetus may be oedematous with serosanguinous fluid in the body cavities. Frequently, there is gross evidence of bronchopneumonia. The abomasal contents are described as turbid, pale yellow in colour and flaky. Some cows carry to full-term and deliver calves that may or may not be viable. Commonly, the placental membranes are retained and, together with the associated discharges, they are highly infective; they constitute a serious health hazard both to animals and to humans (potential victims of undulant fever). The organism may survive for several months in a cold, moist environment but it is readily destroyed by sunlight, drying and disinfectants. After passage of the membranes, the concentration of erythritol in the uterus declines rapidly and *B. abortus* is eliminated within a few weeks. Infected cows excrete the organism in colostrum and they may excrete it in milk, continuously or intermittently, throughout lactation, in the absence of clinical mastitis.

Abortion and/or retained placental membranes are often followed by a period of infertility but this is transient and when an infected cow conceives again she is unlikely to have another abortion due to *B. abortus*.

In the bull *B. abortus* causes orchitis, epididymitis and seminal vesiculitis. Under natural conditions infected bulls play a minor role in the transmission of brucellosis but it is important to realize that venereal infection can occur and that the disease can be transmitted by AI with contaminated semen.

Diagnosis of abortion due to *Brucella abortus*

Microbiology

Isolation from: placenta, foetal abomasum, foetal lungs, vaginal discharges, colostrum or milk.

Serology

Rose Bengal plate test (Brewer Card test), serum agglutination test (SAT), the complement fixation test (CFT), Coombs anti-bovine globulin test (CABGT), ELISA.

Leptospirosis

Cattle are known to be susceptible to infection by six major *Leptospira* serovars: *hardjo, pomona, grippotyphosa, icterohaemorrhagiae, canicola* and *szwajizak*. Of these, the two that have the greatest impact on reproduction are *hardjo* (which is maintained in cattle) and *pomona* (which is maintained in pigs and some free-living species): both can cause abortion and *hardjo* can cause infertility, possibly due its persistence in the uterine tubes.

Leptospires are transmitted amongst cattle by infected urine, placenta, uterine discharges or semen and by infections *in utero*. They survive outside the host in mild moist conditions at a pH close to neutral. Although *hardjo* does not appear to be a great survivor in the environment and most infections arise from direct contact with infected urine, placenta or uterine discharges, *pomona* is able to survive for extended periods in surface water in ponds, stagnant pools, muddy or marshy paddocks; contamination with effluent from a piggery is a particular hazard. All leptospiral serovars are readily destroyed by heat, sunlight, drying, acid and disinfectants. Leptospires enter the body by active penetration through mucous membranes or through abraded or water-softened skin. They multiply rapidly in the liver for 4–10 days before they establish a leptospiraemia, which is associated with acute symptoms. Often the first obvious signs of *hardjo* infection is the 'milk drop syndrome', characterized by a sudden drop in milk yield, a flaccid udder in all four quarters and a thick colostrum-like secretion that may contain clots of blood. With either serovar the leptospiraemia is terminated when specific antibodies appear in the blood. The organisms then localize in the convoluted tubules of the kidneys and in the female genital tract. They may be excreted in the urine for many months, perhaps for a lifetime. Localization in the genital tract of the pregnant cow is followed 1–3 months later by abortion, stillbirth, birth of premature live calves or full-term weak calves. Abortion can occur at any time from the fourth month of gestation to full-term. Advanced autolysis is seen in foetuses aborted before 6 months.

In clinical *hardjo* infection the total herd exposure and the strong humoral immunity render it a largely self-limiting condition; nevertheless a small proportion (3–10%) of pregnancies will continue to result in the birth of premature live, weak full-term or stillborn *hardjo*-infected calves.

Lesions in the placental membranes or in the foetus are not pathognomonic. Similarly, maternal blood samples will not always provide diagnostic serological evidence either immediately after abortion or at 2–3 weeks later. For instance, in *hardjo* infection the titres may be low or undetectable at the time of abortion and they seldom rise after the abortion. Best results are obtained from a combination of foetal serology, immunofluorescence and culture.

The serovars that infect cattle can be transmitted to humans. Infection can be acquired from handling an aborted foetus, removing infected retained placental membranes or being splashed with urine in the milking parlour.

Trichomoniasis

Bovine trichomoniasis causes infertility, abortion and pyometra. It is a true venereal infection: the causative protozoan, *Trichomonas foetus*, is transmitted almost exclusively by coitus. Infection is confined to the reproductive tract: the penis and prepuce in the bull, the vagina, cervix, uterus and uterine tubes in the cow. It is asymptomatic in the bull who acts only as a carrier of *T. foetus*. Carrier cows exist also but they are rare; most cows eliminate the parasite within 100 days of infection. During that interval there may be some mucopurulent discharges due to mild vaginitis and/or endometritis. These lesions do not prevent conception but they tend to be associated with embryonic mortality some time after maternal recognition of pregnancy, thus giving rise to an abnormally long interoestrous interval which, in turn, is followed by a period during which the inflammatory reaction prevents either conception or implantation. However, death of the conceptus can occur at any time up to 5 months of gestation and a small proportion of infected cows (less than 5%) abort or develop pyometra associated with a macerated foetus and a retained corpus luteum. It is rare for the placental membranes to be retained.

Clinical samples for diagnosis consist of preputial washings, cervicovaginal secretions, foetal fluids, and abomasal fluids from aborted foetuses. Diagnosis is based upon direct observation and/or culture of the parasite. Field samples should be sent to the laboratory in a suitable transport medium (e.g. lactated Ringer's solution). The number of organisms in cervical mucus fluctuates during the oestrous cycle; the peak is found a few days before oestrus.

Listeriosis

Listeria monocytogenes is acquired by ingestion and causes sporodic abortion in cattle but occasionally it may be responsible for herd outbreaks, particularly amongst animals fed on silage. Abortions usually occur in the second half of pregnancy. In cattle aborting during the seventh to the ninth months the foetus may be well preserved and it may be possible to see tiny, yellow necrotic foci in the liver. When foetal death occurs before the seventh month the foetus undergoes extensive autolysis over a period of 5–7 days before it is expelled. Retention of the placental membranes is common.

Although the foetal organs may teem with *L. monocytogenes* it is often difficult to culture the organism. The foetus (or the tissue specimens) should be chilled during transport to the laboratory. The recovery rate is improved when specimens are refrigerated at 4°C and recultured at weekly intervals.

Campylobacteriosis ('vibriosis')

Campylobacter fetus subsp. *venerealis*, an obligate parasite of the genitalia, causes infertility and abortion following transmission during coitus or by AI with infected semen. *Campylobacter fetus* subsp. *fetus*, an inhabitant of the intestines of sheep and cattle, causes sporadic cases of abortion in cattle following ingestion of contaminated material.

In the bull *venerealis* is confined to the prepuce and penis where it is asymptomatic; infected bulls over 4 years old tend to become lifelong carriers. Transmission to other bulls may occur indirectly through contact with contaminated bedding or with contaminated equipment used for semen collection. The organism multiplies rapidly in the vagina of a susceptible female animal served by an infected bull; it enters the uterus during the mid-luteal phase (days 10 to 14) and in approximately 25% of the infected animals it may extend to the uterine tubes. It induces mild to moderate endometritis and salpingitis that persists for several weeks to a few months. The inflammatory responses are associated with infertility; in the first instance this effect is probably due to early embryonic mortality, subsequently it may be due to either failure of fertilization or death of the embryo. Returns to oestrus are irregular: some are at normal intervals (18–24 days), others are at extended intervals (24–40 days). There is no palpable abnormality of the genital tract but the mucus shed at oestrus may be cloudy.

Occasionally, but rarely, the pregnancy may be maintained for 4–7 months before it ends in abortion. Most of the infected animals regain fertility within 5 or 6 months but some of those that develop bilateral salpingitis may be sterile.

Agglutination tests (cervical mucus, serum) may indicate a diagnosis but definitive laboratory diagnosis depends on detection of the causative agent, by immunofluorescence or cultural procedures, in preputial washings, vaginal mucus, placental membranes or foetal abomasal fluids. Specimens should be sent to the laboratory in a selective transport and enrichment medium (e.g. Oxide CM 391)

Parturition

The changes in the hormonal profile associated with parturition are depicted in Figure 4.8. The cow shows a number of signs of impending parturition. The sacrosciatic ligaments become slack and sink a few days before delivery; once they are fully relaxed, parturition can be expected to begin within 12 hours. The vulva becomes swollen and strings of mucus are shed from it. The udder fills, becomes swollen and the secretion takes on the characteristics of colostrum. If the cow is free to do so, she may wander away from the herd to give birth in seclusion.

First stage of labour

In stage 1 the myometrium begins to contract rhythmically, initially at the rate of about one contraction every 15 minutes. As the stage advances the contractions increase in frequency, amplitude and duration. In some pluriparous cows the onset of these coordinated contractions may not elicit any external signs of unease but many cows (and practically all heifers) begin to show signs of discomfort and mild colic. The animal is restless, she may bellow, kick at the abdomen, strain occasionally, raise her tail and arch her back, repeatedly lie and stand.

The cervix begins to relax; initially the dilatation of the cervical canal is most evident in the region of the external os but as the uterine contractions bear down on the distended chorioallantois the internal os relaxes also. The chorioallantois engages in the cervix and in some cows it may be visible at the vulva when the cow lies down. By this stage the calf has adopted the normal birth position with the forelegs extended and the head lying on them. When the cervix is completely dilated, the birth canal is a continuous

Cattle breeding and infertility

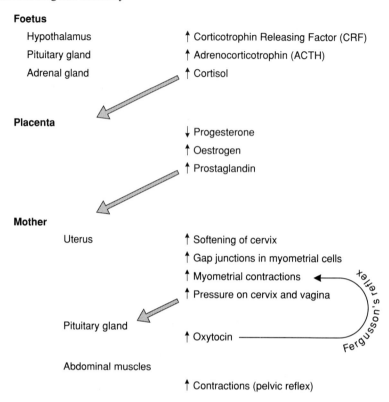

Figure 4.8 Hormonal control of parturition. The hormonal changes are initiated when the foetal hypothalamic–pituitary–adrenal axis releases increased amounts of cortisol. The cortisol induces the placenta to release increased quantities of oestrogens. The oestrogen:progesterone ratio is switched strongly in favour of oestrogen and the inhibitory effect of progesterone on the uterine muscle ('progesterone block') is abolished. The oestrogens promote uterine contractility by stimulating the synthesis of contractile protein and of receptors for both oxytocin and $PGF_{2\alpha}$ and by facilitating the formation of gap junctions between adjacent myometrial cells. Gap junctions enable the uterine muscle to develop spontaneous rhythmical contractions. The more powerful contractions during parturition are generated in response to $PGF_{2\alpha}$, augmented during the second stage of labour by oxytocin.

tube from which the physical constriction at the cervix has been ablated. This marks the end of stage 1.

This stage may last up to 24 hours but it is usually somewhere between 2 and 6 hours. The chorioallantoic sac (the first water bag) ruptures towards the end of stage 1 or early in stage 2 and from then onwards it is the tense amniotic sac and the foetus that exert pressure on the walls of the birth canal.

140

Second stage of labour

Externally, the start of stage 2 is marked by the onset of abdominal contractions. During this stage the cow is usually in sternal recumbency and during the most vigorous phases of muscular activity she will tend to assume lateral recumbency. Internally, the start of stage 2 occurs when the tense amniotic sac is pushed through the fully dilated cervix towards the vagina. The distension of the cervix and vagina as the foetus is forced into the pelvic cavity elicits a neuroendocrine reflex (Fergusson's reflex) in which oxytocin from the posterior pituitary gland stimulates further uterine contractions that force the amniotic sac into the pelvic inlet thereby causing an increase in sensory stimuli that will elicit further secretion of oxytocin.

The myometrial contractions increase in frequency up to 24–48 contractions per hour. As the enhanced myometrial activity forces the foetus into the pelvis, the pelvic reflex is activated and the cow develops strong contractions of the abdominal muscles (straining). The straining forces the amniotic sac against the cervix and anterior vagina, initiating further Fergusson's reflexes and thus further contractions of the myometrium and, in turn, further pelvic reflexes that elicit further straining. Straining tends to occur in bouts of activity, each separated by a few minutes' rest. There may be eight to ten abdominal contractions superimposed on the onset of each myometrial contraction. As the moment of delivery approaches, the frequency of myometrial contractions can go up to 48 per hour.

The amniotic sac (the 'second water bag') usually ruptures when the feet of the calf appear at the vulva; this does not happen in every case and the calf may be delivered within the amnion.

During delivery the greatest effort is when the foetal head is expelled through the vulva. This is often followed by a short rest before the foetal chest is pushed through the vulva, to be followed by another vigorous effort to propel the foetal hips to the exterior. As the calf passes through the vulva it tends to follow a downward arch, which helps relax the foetal abdominal muscles so that the hips and hindlegs extend backwards to complete the arc. This posture facilitates the passage of the foetus through the bony pelvis because it reduces the dorsoventral diameter of the foetal pelvis and it keeps the foetal pelvis high in the maternal pelvis where the transverse diameter is greatest (Figure 4.9). When traction is applied during assisted delivery the direction of pull should follow this natural arc; failure to do so can increase the severity of an existing dystocia or create a dystocia where none existed.

The umbilical cord usually breaks spontaneously during delivery but sometimes the calf is born with an intact umbilical cord and some minutes may elapse before the cord is ruptured by movement of the calf or the mother. This should be allowed to happen naturally because premature

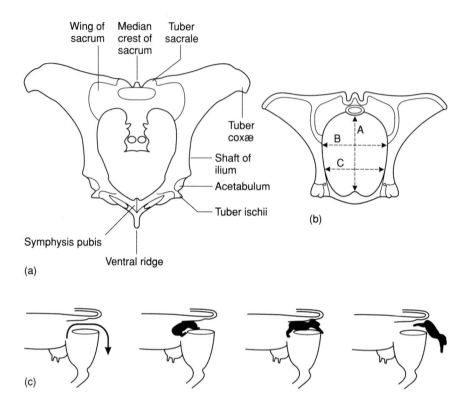

Figure 4.9 The passage of the foetus through the maternal pelvis. (a) Pelvic bones of the cow, viewed from in front and somewhat from below (after Grossman, J. B. (1953). In *The anatomy of the domestic animals*, 4th edn. W. B. Saunders, Philadelphia, p. 152). (b) Diagrams of pelvic inlet showing A, sacropubic diameter; B, dorsal transilial diameter; C, ventral transilial diameter. (c) Diagram to illustrate the arc traversed by the calf during birth in anterior presentation and the appropriate direction of traction at different stages of delivery: slightly ventral until the foetal shoulder has passed the pelvic inlet and the head is outside the vulva, then horizontal until the head, neck and forelegs are outside the vulva. At that stage the calf may be rotated about 90° so that its hips pass through the widest diameter of the maternal pelvis (A in (b)). After that traction should be ventral in direction (after Schuijt, G. and Ball, L. (1980). In Morrow, D. A. (ed) *Current therapy in theriogenology*. W. B. Saunders, Philadelphia).

manual rupture (or ligation) of the cord may deprive the calf of a large volume of blood that normally passes to it from the placenta.

The second stage of labour should be completed in about 0.5–4 hours in pluriparous cows; in primiparous animals it may take up to 12 hours. When the foetus has been delivered, the abdominal contractions cease but the myometrial contractions persist. Their main function at this stage is to assist in the separation and expulsion of the placental membranes.

Third stage of labour

During stage 2 of parturition, the strong uterine contractions squeeze much of the blood out of the placentome and into the foetus. The removal of the rich supply of blood causes shrinkage of the foetal villi and relaxation of the maternal crypts. In other words, there is a 'loosening' of the attachment between the foetal and maternal components of the placentome. Separation begins at the apex of the chorioallantois in response to opening up of the crypts by waves of myometrial contraction that are stimulated by oxytocin. The separated end of the chorioallantois becomes inverted and rolls down within the more caudal attached segments. As it does so, it pulls the foetal villi out of the crypts and eventually a large mass of inverted placenta reaches the maternal pelvis and elicits a pelvic reflex; the induced contractions of the abdominal muscles combine with the myometrial contractions to expel the placenta. Suckling, which induces a reflex release of oxytocin, assists in creating conditions that favour the early expulsion of the placental membranes. This third stage of labour should be completed within 0.5–6 hours; however, retention up to 12 hours is not considered abnormal.

Induction of parturition

Occasionally, it may be necessary to induce parturition when dealing with a pathological pregnancy or with an injured or debilitated cow in late pregnancy. However, the most frequent indications for induction of parturition are concerned with the management of normal pregnancy in commercial dairy herds and beef herds. In those circumstances, the treatment is expected to lead to the birth of a healthy, viable calf and it must not impair the health of the dam, her milk yield or subsequent fertility. This is well illustrated by the situation in suckler herds where the cows are bred to bulls of the larger continental breeds (Charolais, Simmental, Limousin, Blonde d'Aquitaine). Here the economic returns are derived from the sale of the calves and the greatest source of lost revenue is likely to be dystocia due to fetomaternal disproportion. The immediate objective of treatment is to have the calf delivered before exponential growth at the end of gestation creates a major calving problem. However, profitability will depend on the cow providing enough milk to produce a well-grown calf at weaning and on her ability to be in-calf in time to produce another calf early next season.

Pharmacological induction of parturition may be a valuable aid to management in dairy herds where the aim is to maximize the use of pasture for milk production: it could be used to advance the calving dates of cows that conceived late in the breeding season and it may be used to condense the entire calving season.

Parturition can be induced in cattle with corticosteroids, prostaglandins or a combination of these drugs. Treatment may be in the form of a single injection or a two-injection regimen.

The corticosteroid drugs can be divided into two groups: the short-acting steroids in the free alcohol or soluble ester form that generally induce parturition within 3 days and the long-acting preparations in the form of insoluble esters that generally induce parturition within 2–3 weeks. The corticosteroids are effective only when there is a live foetus.

Single injection of short-acting corticosteroids

Parturition can be induced from about day 255 of pregnancy onwards by a single intramuscular injection of a short-acting formulation such as dexamethasone (20–30 mg), flumethasone (10 mg) or betamethasone (20 mg). The interval from injection to parturition is stated to be 24–72 hours, with an average of 48 hours. The treatment does not appear to have any major effect on the viability of the newborn calf and those born after day 268 are unaffected. The colostrum may contain less immunoglobulin than does the colostrum at natural birth but this is not reflected in the plasma levels of the calves. There may be some slight delay in reaching the maximum milk yield but the total milk yield for the lactation is practically normal.

The only consistent difference between induced births and natural births is the very high rate of retained afterbirth following induction (greater than 80%). This may lead to an increase in the interval from calving to conception and in the number of services per conception but the overall effect on reproduction is not significant. The frequency of retained afterbirth declines the closer the treatment is to the date of expected delivery. The treated cows do not have the peak concentrations of oestrogens that normally occur before natural calving. This may be a contributory factor in retention of the placenta; however, the administration of exogenous oestrogens, either at the same time or at 12 hours before and 12 hours after the injection of corticosteroid, does not reduce the rate of retention to any significant extent. Morrison *et al.* (1983) reported that 500 mg dimenhydrinate given 24 hours after injection of a short-acting dexamethasone formulation reduced the incidence of retained placenta (from 73% to 33%); it also compacted the calving pattern.

Single injection of long-acting corticosteroids

Long-acting corticosteroids are given by intramuscular injection about 1 month before the expected calving date. The dosage rates are: dexamethasone trimethylacetate 20 mg; triamcinolone acetonide 30 mg; betamethasone suspension 20 mg; flumethasone suspension 10 mg. The response is more variable than it is with the short-acting preparations. The further the cow is from full-term, the longer she will take to respond. It may take from 15 to 23 days before parturition is induced.

The incidence of retained afterbirth is considerably lower (less than 20%) than after the short-acting formulations. Often there is a high incidence of stillbirths and neonatal losses. Calves delivered before day 250 tend to be weak and to consume inadequate quantities of colostrum, which in any case is likely to have a reduced concentration of immunoglobulins and, therefore, the (weak) calf may not receive adequate passive immunity to provide protection from the pathogens encountered in the early weeks of life. The earlier treatment is started, the lower the concentration of immunoglobulins in the colostrum. Furthermore, early treatment with long-acting corticosteroids provides sufficient time for the steroids to induce 'closure' of the foetal gut to the absorption of the protective antibodies. It is probable that the stillbirths are due to premature separation of the placenta.

Another difficulty that arises, particularly when long-acting formulations are used, is the premature distension of the udder with secretion within a week of treatment although parturition may not occur for at least another week. It may be necessary to milk these cows before calving to relieve the pressure on the secreting tissue and to reduce the risk of trauma and, possibly, mastitis. This will reduce the antibody content of the milk available to the calves at birth.

Single injection of prostaglandin

In the last 2 weeks of gestation most cows will calve within 48 hours after receiving either $PGF_{2\alpha}$ (25–30 mg) or cloprostenol (500 µg). Prostaglandins have one advantage over the short-acting corticosteroids in that they can induce parturition even if the calf is dead; therefore they can be used to evacuate mummified or macerated foetuses.

Two-injection regimens

The long-acting corticosteroids give variable and unpredictable results: the interval from treatment to calving may vary from 4 to 26 days. The timing of the responses can be condensed by using a two-injection regime in which the first injection is a long-acting corticosteroid and the second injection, given 7–12 days later, is either a short-acting corticosteroid or a prostaglandin. Most cows will calve within 2–3 days after the second injection. The precision is greatly improved but, unfortunately, calf mortality rates are not improved. Nevertheless, if a calf has to be delivered more than 3 weeks before the due date the pharmacological use of a long-acting corticosteroid that stimulates the formation of pulmonary surfactant is preferable to caesarean section.

Tocolysis

Drugs that stimulate the β_2-adrenoceptors of the myometrial cells cause relaxation of the uterine muscle. They have been used for that purpose in non-pregnant cows undergoing embryo transfer and in pregnant cows at full-term to delay parturition (tocolysis) or to facilitate obstetrical operations such as foetotomy, caesarean section, or replacement of uterine prolapse. The duration of the tocolysis depends on the position of the foetus at the time of treatment. When a single therapeutic dose of clenbuterol (300 µg) is given early in stage 1 of labour it can delay parturition for 5–8 hours but if it is given after the cervix has been fully dilated, the delay may be as short as an hour or two.

Dystocia

Published surveys indicate that the overall prevalence of dystocia is within the range of 2–12 cases per 100 births. The prevalence is higher in heifers than in cows, in twins than in singletons, and with male calves than with female calves.

Causes of dystocia can be classified as maternal or foetal in origin. Maternal factors can be subdivided into (1) anatomical or pathological defects in the birth canal and (2) insufficient expulsive forces. The foetal factors can be subdivided into (1) oversize, (2) faulty disposition and (3) foetal death.

The more common anatomical or pathological defects of the birth canal are immature pelvis, pelvic fractures, persistence of various parts of the median wall of the Müllerian duct, fibrosis and stricture of the vagina, undilated cervix, fibrosis of the cervix, and torsion of the uterus.

Inadequacies of expulsive forces may relate to the activities of either the uterine muscles or the abdominal muscles. Deficiency of uterine contractions (inertia) may be described as being primary or secondary. Primary inertia can arise due to an inherited predisposition (e.g. in the Ayrshire breed), to overstretching of the myometrium by an excessively large foetus or by hydrallantois, to toxic degeneration of the myometrium, to hypocalcaemia, or to an inappropriate oestrogen:progesterone ratio. Secondary inertia usually occurs as a result of fatigue during a prolonged stage 2 of labour (i.e. it can be a significant factor in prolongation of the delivery but is not the primary cause of the problem). Deficiency of abdominal contractions may be due to advanced age, debility, ventral hernia or ruptured prepubic tendon.

Foetal oversize, the most common cause of dystocia in cattle, includes relative oversize (the foetus is of normal size but the maternal pelvis is too small), absolute oversize (the foetus is normal but very large and the maternal pelvis is normal), and pathological oversize (e.g. foetal giantism, hydrocephalus, fetal anasarca, foetal emphysema, schistosoma reflexus, double monsters).

Faulty disposition of the foetus may involve errors in presentation, position or posture. Presentation refers to direction of the spinal axis of the foetus relative to that of the dam and to the portion of the foetus presenting at the pelvic inlet; presentations may be longitudinal and either anterior or posterior, or transverse and either dorsal or ventral. Position refers to whether the calf is upright (dorsal), on its side (lateral) or upside-down (ventral) in longitudinal presentation and, in transverse presentation, to the position of the head in relation to the components of the maternal pelvis (e.g. right or left cephalo-ilial). Posture signifies the relation of the head and neck or limbs to the body of the foetus (flexed, extended, retained, above, or to left or right of the foetal trunk).

Normal presentation in cattle is anterior longitudinal with extended forelimbs on which the head and extended neck rest. At the beginning of the sixth month of gestation the majority of foetuses are in posterior presentation but by the middle of the seventh month the majority are in anterior presentation. Obviously, the size of the foetus and uterine space must influence the ease with which a foetus can reverse its polarity within the uterus; the number of posterior presentations is above average in twins or in excessively large singletons. Dystocia and stillbirth are much more likely to occur in posterior presentation than in anterior presentation. Errors of position or posture arise during stage 1 or early stage 2 of labour.

Guidelines for when to assist parturition

Abnormal parturition must be distinguished from normal calving and be managed as appropriate. There should be supervision of the parturient animal during stage 1 of labour but this should be as discreet as possible. Frequent, indiscreet direct observations or repeated palpation of the cervix during that stage will tend to delay parturition and increase the number of assisted births. If parturition is proceeding normally, the cow can be left to calve unassisted for about 2 hours after the first appearance of the 'water bag' or foetal limbs at the vulva. Approximately 90% of dairy cows will have calved by then. If there are no signs of difficulty, heifers may be left to calve naturally for up to 3 hours. Cows and heifers of the larger beef breeds may proceed more slowly and, if there are no indications of difficulty, they may be left for up to 5 hours, by which time most of them will have calved naturally (Hartigan 1979).

Ultimately, the decision of when to assist parturition must be based on an assessment of the physical condition of the dam and on the course of parturition up to the time the veterinarian is called.

The birth canal should be explored to ascertain the position and viability of the foetus, the size and degree of dilatation of the pelvic opening, the degree of dilatation of the cervix, and the presence of strictures. Also, a thorough search should be made for damage to the birth canal, especially where lay assistance has been attempted or where labour has been unassisted but very prolonged. The disposition of the calf should be examined carefully. The choice of obstetrical procedure to be used will be influenced by the vital status of the foetus. A live foetus should be delivered either by mutation and forced extraction or by caesarean section. A dead foetus will be delivered by mutation and forced extraction or by foetotomy. Therefore, testing the foetal reflexes can provide important guidelines as to the most suitable obstetrical procedure. The feet may be pinched to produce a withdrawal reflex, the mouth and tongue may be palpated or pinched to elicit suckling or tongue withdrawal reflexes, the eyes may be palpated for a blink reflex. When the viability of the calf declines these reflexes disappear in the order listed above. A positive response to these reflexes indicates that the calf is still alive; however, a negative response does not always mean that the foetus is dead.

History taking in cases of dystocia (Arthur *et al.* 1989)

- Is she at full-term?
- What is her previous breeding history?
- When did straining begin and what was its nature?
- Has a water bag appeared and, if so, when?
- Has there been an escape of foetal fluids?
- Has any part of the foetus appeared at the vulva?
- Has assistance been attempted and, if so, by whom and what was its nature?

Care of the newborn

The newborn calf must establish normal respiratory function, maintain body temperature and resist infections (principally of the alimentary tract, lungs and umbilicus).

Survival depends on the prompt onset of normal spontaneous respirations. The immediate task is to ensure that the nostrils are not occluded by the amnion or by mucus and that the airways are clear. During assisted delivery with the cow standing and the foetus in anterior presentation it is convenient and beneficial to relax the traction when the head and thorax have passed the vulva; this will allow the fluid to flow by gravity from the nostrils and trachea before delivery is completed. After delivery, mucus in nose and mouth can be propelled to the exterior by applying sliding pressure by the thumbs along the bridge of the nose while the flattened fingers of each hand move in the same direction in the intermandibular space. A traditional method of removing the fluids has been to suspend the calf across a gate. It should be noted that if this is not done carefully it can cause serious injury; for instance, there have been reports of rupture of the bladder, particularly in the heavier calves of the continental breeds. The calf may be suspended from its hind legs by means of a pulley or hoist. Other mechanical aids that may be used are an aspirator to remove the fluids by suction, or an endotracheal tube and a cylinder of oxygen for artificial ventilation. Drugs to stimulate respiratory function are available in droplet or injectable forms. Their efficacy in resuscitation of calves has not been proven. Once the calf is breathing regularly, it should be dried and kept warm. The umbilical stump should be sprayed with Lugol's iodine and colostrum should be fed. Weak calves may require glucose by intravenous injection.

The postpartum period

Myometrial contractions persist for several days after parturition and they play a significant role in the reduction of the size of the uterus and in the expulsion of lochia during the initial phase of uterine involution. Prostaglandin $F_{2\alpha}$ is released at high levels from the uterus over the last day or two before parturition and up to about day 5 post partum, then it begins to decline gradually until it reaches baseline between day 10 and day 20. Ovulation is unlikely to occur before the prostaglandin levels return to basal concentration; furthermore, the speed of uterine involution is influenced positively by both the magnitude and the duration of release of $PGF_{2\alpha}$. (This relationship is reversed in cows with uterine pathology; see below.) Thus, it is possible that the high concentrations of $PGF_{2\alpha}$ in the postpartum cow act both as a stimulus for uterine involution and as a signal to delay ovarian cyclicity until involution is well advanced.

Focal points in a reproduction management plan in the post-partum period

- Uterine involution
- Resumption of oestrous cycles
- Detection of oestrus
- Submission rate
- Conception rate

Uterine involution

Immediately after parturition, the uterus is a large floppy sac, nearly 1 m long, which contains up to 1.5 l of fluid and weighs approximately 9 kg. There is considerable shrinkage over the next 10 days: it contracts to half its gravid diameter (40 cm to 20 cm) by day 5 and to less than half its gravid length (100 cm to 40 cm) by day 15; by then the uterine fluid is reduced to about 10% of its original volume. The cervix closes rapidly after parturition; within 12 hours of a normal parturition it is almost impossible to insert a hand through it and by day 4 only two fingers can enter the external os.

At rectal examination during the first 3 or 4 days post partum, the uterine wall is thick and corrugated and it is extremely difficult to identify the soft cervix. At about day 4 or 5 the cervix is becoming firm and it is possible to distinguish it from the uterus; it lies in the midline in the region of the pelvic brim. By days 8–10 the cervix has become quite firm and in heifers and young cows it now lies within the pelvis. At this time the entire uterus can be palpated: it feels soft and smooth, caruncles can be palpated, the contents of the previously gravid horn are fluctuant and the non-gravid horn is much smaller than the gravid horn. From day 10 to day 18 the uterus remains smooth and soft, the caruncles and the fluid contents are greatly reduced in size, and the cervix is hard and readily identified. From day 18 to day 25, the myometrium regains its tone and the uterine horns become similar in texture although the previously gravid horn remains somewhat larger than the non-gravid horn. It will remain larger even into the next pregnancy.

Estimates based upon observations made at rectal examinations put the interval from parturition to completion of uterine involution within the range 25–40 days.

Histological changes

The sequence of events in the regression of the caruncles is: degenerative vascular changes, peripheral ischaemia, necrosis and sloughing. As the caruncular mass is sloughed away it leaves protruding remnants of the blood vessels, from which blood oozes into the luminal fluids for at least 10 days. The caruncular stalk disappears by day 15 leaving the caruncle level with the endometrium and new epithelium grows out from the surrounding intercaruncular areas to cover the surface of the caruncle by day 25. The myometrium undergoes a reduction in mass over the first 20–30 days post partum by reduction in both cell size and cell number.

Lochia

In the first 2 days after parturition the flabby uterus may contain up to 1.5 l of fluid (lochia), derived from residual foetal fluids, blood from the ruptured umbilical vessels and shreds of foetal membranes. As involution and regression of the caruncles progress, quantities of sloughed caruncular tissue are added as is the blood that seeps from the exposed ends of the caruncular vessels. The volume of lochia that is discharged via the vulva and the nature of the discharge can vary greatly from animal to animal. Usually, the discharge begins on day 3 or 4, and ends between days 14 and 18. During the first day or two the colour of the discharged lochia is yellowish brown or reddish brown, then as increasing amounts of blood and necrotic tissue are shed from the regressing caruncles, the colour of the fluid becomes darker and there are chunks of white necrotic tissue afloat in it. The amount of blood in lochia reaches its maximum between days 9 and 12. As the volume of the discharge declines at the end of the second week, the lochia becomes lighter in colour and, eventually, it becomes a clear fluid. Provided the discharge does not become purulent or fetid there is no cause for alarm or for therapy during the first 18 days post partum.

Factors that affect uterine involution

Involution occurs more rapidly in heifers than in pluriparous cows. It has been reported to be more rapid in animals that calve in spring and summer than in those that calve in autumn and winter; however, it is delayed in animals subjected to heat stress. It may be more rapid in suckled beef cows than in milked dairy cows, due to the increased myometrial activity elicited by the frequent release of oxytocin in response to suckling. Involution is retarded by hypocalcaemia (primary uterine inertia), dystocia or twins (secondary uterine inertia), ketosis, retained placental membranes, uterine infection, metritis, subclinical diseases and poor physical condition.

Non-specific bacterial infection of the uterus

The principal physical barriers to ascending infection of the uterus are relaxed during parturition. After delivery of the calf there is a negative pressure within the uterine lumen and bacteria are aspirated into the uterus in every cow at some stage within the first 2 weeks after calving. The most frequent invaders are *A. pyogenes*, *E. coli*, staphylococci and streptococci (Hartigan 1977): in the vast majority of cows they are transient contaminants that are promptly eliminated by the uterine defence mechanisms, so that only about 30% of cows have bacteria in the uterus during the fifth week post partum. Thereafter, bacteria can be isolated from 30–45% of cows but, in general, this is not due to the persistence of the bacteria in a particular cohort of animals; rather it is due to spontaneous clearance and repeated contamination in most cases. The identity of the infected cows will vary from sample to sample as will the identity of the bacteria that are isolated from individual cows. These transient contaminants are not an important cause of infertility in cows that are free of clinically detectable uterine disease.

There is no evidence that any of the non-specific bacteria, apart from *A. pyogenes*, has a lasting detrimental effect on fertility. Intrauterine infection with *A. pyogenes* invariably induces endometritis. The severity of the endometrial lesions and the effect on fertility are determined by the duration of the infection. Transient infection during the first 3 weeks post partum does not appear to affect subsequent fertility; transient infection at a later period may reduce fertility to one or two services; persistent infection induces purulent metritis or pyometra accompanied by anoestrus, particularly when *A. pyogenes* is accompanied by anaerobes, such as *Fusobacterium necrophorum* and *Bacteroides* spp. that act synergistically with it to depress the phagocytic and bacteriocidal activities within the uterus. These activities are depressed also by progesterone and it is possible that this may provide an explanation for the persistence of the pathogenic bacteria in some cows. A precocious ovulation in an infected cow would provide a source of progesterone that would inhibit the mechanisms that normally eliminate the non-specific contaminants of the uterus; the resultant pyogenic response to the bacteria would depress the release of the endogenous luteolysin $PGF_{2\alpha}$ and a persistent state of mutual interdependence between the bacteria and the corpus luteum would be established and, in time, this would lead to pyometra accompanied by anoestrus.

These data might lead one to suppose that contamination of the uterus by non-specific bacteria that do not induce clinical abnormalities has virtually no effect on reproductive efficiency. That is not necessarily so. There is evidence that some apparently innocuous infections may be of economic importance either because they induce protracted release of prostaglandin that delays the onset of ovarian cyclicity or because they release sufficient endotoxin to induce asymptomatic ovarian cysts. On the other hand, there is also considerable evidence that antibiotic therapy to eliminate bacteria from the uterus during the first 2 weeks post partum may depress fertility.

Clearly, the significance of spontaneous uterine contamination during the postpartum period remains a matter of opinion. There is no evidence that would attribute a lasting effect on fertility to most of the contaminants; nevertheless, those that can cause short-term delays in the onset of ovarian cyclicity may assume significance in herds where the policy is to maintain a very compact calving season. Clinicians should be particularly vigilant to avoid the introduction of bacteria into a progesterone-dominated uterus. They should avoid prolonged intrauterine manipulations that could cause extensive damage to the endometrium, the source of the endogenous luteolysin. Similarly, it is unwise to infuse irritant solutions of antibiotics or antiseptics that depress phagocytosis.

Theoretically, bacterial contamination of the postpartum uterus could interfere with fertility by:

- Directly killing the gametes or the conceptus;
- Altering the uterine 'milk';
- Causing endometritis (generating toxic products, inducing luteolysis);
- Causing chronic histological lesions (metritis, pyometra salpingitis);
- Delaying onset of ovarian cyclicity (with or without the formation of ovarian cysts).

Retained afterbirth

In cattle, the placental membranes are considered to be retained if they have not been shed by 12 hours after parturition. Retention is less common in beef cattle than it is in dairy cattle. It has been estimated that the average prevalence of retention after normal parturition in dairy cows in brucellosis-free areas is approximately 7%. This figure can be exceeded greatly in brucellosis-infected herds or when there are outbreaks of abortion due to campylobacteriosis, leptospirosis or infectious bovine rhinotracheitis (IBR).

Aetiology

Retained afterbirth is commonly associated with premature delivery, whether due to infectious agents, trauma, toxins, allergens or the pharmacological induction of parturition. More than half of the cows that expel the foetus between day 240 and day 270 retain the membranes, whereas less than one in five cows that abort between days 120 and 150 do so. (It is not a problem if the conceptus is lost before day 120.) Retention is likely to occur when there is a pathologically prolonged gestation; for instance, with an anencephalic foetus or when there is severe hypoplasia of the foetal adrenal glands.

The likelihood of placental retention in individual cows is increased by uterine inertia, twin births, hydrallantois, dystocia, prolonged forced extraction of the foetus, foetotomy, caesarean section, uterine torsion, hypocalcaemia, ketosis, fatty liver syndrome, vitamin deficiencies (carotene, vitamins A and E) and mineral deficiencies (iodine, selenium, phosphorus).

In essence, placental retention is due either to failure of *loosening* of the placenta or to failure to *expel* the loosened membrane. Loosening is the process by which the villi of the cotyledon detach from the crypts of the caruncle. The physiological mechanisms responsible for this process are not fully understood but there is evidence that some essential preparatory changes in the histology of both the maternal and foetal components of the placentome occur during the final weeks of gestation in response to the normal sequence of hormonal changes that prepare the dam for parturition. It has been suggested that oestradiol-17β may initiate, and perhaps sustain, the maturation of cotyledonary tissues. Chew et al. (1979) reported that the balance between the plasma concentrations of progesterone and oestradiol-17β at 6 days before parturition was significant. When progesterone was high (greater than 7.9 ng/ml) or when both progesterone (less than 3 ng/ml) and oestradiol-17β (less than 100 pg/ml) were low there was a ten-fold higher rate of retention than when progesterone was intermediate (4–8 ng/ml) and oestradiol-17β exceeded 99 pg/ml.

When the foetus is expelled prematurely, either by spontaneous abortion or following pharmacological induction, the hormonal pattern is disturbed, the placentome is 'immature', there is failure of separation, and the afterbirth is retained. In cases of prolonged gestation, proliferation of connective tissue enlarges the caruncular septa and dehiscence of the foetal villi is impeded. At full-term or earlier, retention may occur if the villi are swollen as a result of hyperaemia (associated with premature rupture of the umbilical blood vessels), oedema (associated with elective caesarean section or with uterine torsion) or inflammatory exudate (placentitis).

Failure to expel the placental membranes may be due to uterine inertia or to physical interference with expulsion. Uterine inertia is associated with hydrallantois, hypocalcaemia and dystocia. It is estimated that retention because of uterine inertia without any disturbance in the loosening process accounts for only 1–2% of cases. Mechanical interference with expulsion is very rare also. It can occur when the membranes are trapped around a large caruncle in a rapidly involuting uterine horn, around a double cervical canal or around a horizontal remnant of the median wall of the Müllerian duct in the anterior vagina.

Clinical signs

The retained membranes may be visible at the vulva or they may be retained completely within the genital tract. Usually, there is no sign of illness. It is estimated that only 1–4% of affected cows have systemic signs and in the majority of these the signs are mild—slight elevation in body temperature, mild anorexia and a drop in milk yield. However, some cows with retained placenta develop acute metritis. If left undisturbed, retained membranes will undergo progressive liquefactive putrefaction over a period of 7–10 days and this will produce a characteristic foul odour.

Treatment

Most of the conditions that interfere with the loosening process are not amenable to treatment by the time the cow with retained afterbirth is presented to the clinician. The traditional treatment has been manual removal, usually on day 3. However, in recent years informed veterinary opinion has discouraged manual removal in all but the most simple cases in which the membranes are loosely attached or are retained by mechanical obstruction. There is general agreement that, even when done quickly and gently, manual removal causes considerable trauma and haemorrhage within the uterus, leaves fragments of the membranes attached to the caruncles, and inhibits phagocytic activities of uterine leucocytes for the next few days. Thus, manual removal creates conditions that are favourable for bacterial growth. It can provoke an acute metritis, septicaemia, toxaemia or perimetritis with abdominal adhesions. If there is evidence of systemic illness already, manual removal should not be attempted. When compared with cows from which the membranes separate naturally, cows from which they are removed manually have delayed involution of the uterus, lower conception rates to first service, lower total conception rates and longer calving-to-conception intervals. The case against manual removal is strong and clients should be persuaded to accept alternative methods of treatment.

If there is uterine inertia, myometrial tone can be improved by parenteral administration of calcium borogluconate and, within 30 hours of parturition, by intramuscular injection of 40 units oxytocin or 1–5 mg ergometrine. Ergometrine has a more prolonged effect. Exogenous oestrogens are not recommended.

If there is any evidence of systemic illness, the cow should be given therapeutic doses of a broad-spectrum antibiotic parenterally.

When a cow shows no sign of illness, treatment may be restricted to the introduction of antibacterial or antiseptic drugs into the uterus to curtail the proliferation of putrefactive bacteria until the degenerating membranes are shed. The drugs will reduce the degree of putrefaction but, in doing so, they will delay lysis of the villi and prolong retention of the membranes. A wide variety of drugs can be used for this purpose. Irritant substances, such as Lugol's iodine, should not be used. Penicillins are unlikely to be effective because the mixed flora present at that stage almost certainly will include organisms that synthesize and release penicillinases. It has been reported that intrauterine therapy with oxytetracycline hydrochloride (2–3 g), either once only or at 48-hour intervals, has given satisfactory results. Treated cows should be examined routinely between days 25 and 30 post partum to detect and treat any residual uterine or ovarian abnormality. It has been claimed that cows treated in this way have fertility rates almost as good as those of herd mates that expel the membranes swiftly.

It should be remembered that antibiotics that are inserted into the uterine lumen will give rise to residues in the milk for 3–4 days after the end of treatment.

Sequelae

Possible sequelae are acute septic metritis, subacute metritis, chronic metritis, pyometra, and endometritis. A relatively rare sequel is tetanus due to the presence of *Clostridium tetani*.

Acute metritis

Acute metritis that develops within the first 10 days after calving produces systemic signs of septicaemia and/or toxaemia and it may be fatal.

Aetiology and pathogenesis

The common pathogens are *A. pyogenes*, coagulase+ staphylococci, haemolytic streptococci, *E. coli*, *Ps. aeruginosa* and, occasionally, *Clostridium* spp. In most cases the pathogens gain entry during parturition or within a few days thereafter. Events that predispose to the introduction of infection include prolonged dystocia, foetotomy, delivery of an emphysematous foetus, and rough or unhygienic manipulations within the uterus either during parturition or in an attempt to remove the afterbirth. Usually the metritis is associated with uterine inertia and is frequently accompanied by retention of at least a portion of the afterbirth. Thus, the uterus becomes a large flaccid vat containing lochia, an ideal medium for bacterial growth and multiplication that is maintained at body temperature under microaerophilic, if not anaerobic, conditions. Toxins released by the pathogens give rise to toxaemia and a necrotizing inflammation of the uterus.

Clinical findings

The cow is acutely ill. In the early stages body temperature may exceed 40°C but in advanced cases the pyrexia subsides and in the terminal stages temperature may be subnormal. The animal is toxic, anorexic, may have diarrhoea, and may be dehydrated. Pulse and respiratory rates are rapid. Usually, there is a fetid, watery, reddish discharge from the vulva. If it is possible to make an accurate diagnosis without an internal examination, the clinician should refrain from either direct or rectal exploration of the genital tract. Manual removal of the afterbirth must not be attempted. If considered necessary, rectal palpation will reveal an atonic, flaccid uterus in which the wall is thin and friable. The cow may exhibit signs of peritonitis if perimetritis and peritoneal adhesions develop, and she may have swollen hock and fetlock joints.

Treatment

The immediate requirements are to counteract the effects of toxaemia and dehydration and to eliminate the causal organisms. The twin aims demand prompt systemic treatment with fluids and antibiotics. Many authors recommend the use of a broad-spectrum antibiotic parenterally but the evidence is that procaine penicillin G is probably a more effective antibiotic against the bacteria involved; therapeutic levels should be maintained for 5 days. If the case is seen within the first 2 days after calving, 5 iu of oxytocin intravenously should cause myometrial contractions and expulsion of infected lochia. Once the life-threatening crisis is over it may be beneficial to siphon off the infected lochia provided it can be done gently and without damage to the genital tract. A soft rubber tube is inserted carefully into the uterus, a large funnel is attached to the free end and a quantity of warm sterile fluid is used to create the siphon. Several litres of flushing fluid can be used to siphon off the fetid lochia. Little value can be derived from local (intrauterine) therapy until the bulk of the lochia has been evacuated.

The use of oestrogens is not recommended. By increasing the blood flow through the uterus, they facilitate the absorption of large quantities of bacterial toxins.

Subacute metritis

During the second and third weeks after calving, cows may present signs of extensive pyogenic infection of the uterus that causes little or no systemic reaction; this condition is called subacute metritis and is associated with retarded involution of the uterus.

Any of the bacteria listed as aetiological agents of acute metritis can be isolated from the pus.

There may be a slight elevation in body temperature, mild anorexia and a decline in milk yield. The tail and perineum of the cow is smeared with purulent discharge and, on rectal examination, the uterus is found to contain a quantity of purulent material that gives it a 'doughy' consistency. Usually, a corpus luteum can be palpated on one of the ovaries.

If there are signs of illness, penicillin or a tetracycline should be given by intramuscular injection. If there is a palpable corpus luteum, prostaglandin should be given. If the decision is to rely on local treatment, as much as possible of the purulent material should be siphoned off gently before the intrauterine infusion of antibiotic. The usual recommendation is to infuse 2–3 g oxytetracycline in 200–300 ml of warm sterile water.

At this stage after parturition, the myometrium does not respond to therapeutic doses of oxytocin. Some authors recommend 1–5 mg ergometrine to increase the tone of the myometrium.

Chronic metritis

Chronic metritis, most commonly caused by persistence of *A. pyogenes* infection, is presented for attention as the breeding season approaches or during the early weeks of the breeding season. The condition should resolve following luteolysis induced by exogenous prostaglandin. For intrauterine therapy, the drug of choice is penicillin (2 million u in 50–100 ml fluid).

Pyometra

In pyometra there is closure of the cervix, an accumulation of purulent material in the uterine lumen, persistence of a functional corpus luteum and anoestrus.

Aetiology

Cultures of the uterine contents reveal that any of a variety of bacteria may be involved. Many of the isolates are incidental contaminants; the significant persistent bacteria are *A. pyogenes*, *F. necrophorum* and *B. melaninogenicus*. These three organisms act synergistically to depress the defence mechanisms of the host and to enhance bacterial growth. Pyometra is also a feature of bovine trichomoniasis caused by *Trichomonas foetus*.

Pathogenesis

Predisposing factors include dystocia, twins, retained placental membranes, abortions, septic metritis. There is evidence that precocious ovulation may be a contributory factor, particularly if the ovulation is from the ovary ipsilateral to the recently gravid uterine horn (Hartigan *et al.* 1974). It is thought that the formation of a corpus luteum at a time when the ipsilateral uterine horn still contains a considerable quantity of infected lochia depresses both the phagocytic and bacteriocidal activities of the leucocytes and the activity of the uterine muscle; as a result, the quantity of lochia will increase within the uterus, the pathogenic bacteria will proliferate, the endometrium will be damaged, the effectiveness of uterine luteolysin will be compromised, the corpus luteum will continue to secrete progesterone, and pyometra will supervene.

Clinical findings

The affected cow does not appear to be ill; the condition is discovered at routine examination of the reproductive tract or when the cow is presented as anoestrous. Rectal palpation reveals a fluid-filled uterus with a thick atonic wall. In the majority of cases, a corpus luteum can be palpated but in some cases the persistent luteal tissue is deeply embedded in the ovary and is not detectable by palpation.

Vaginal examination may reveal a slightly relaxed cervix and the discharge of purulent material, which usually is thick mucoid and may be yellowish, white or brown in colour.

The differential diagnosis includes pregnancy and hydrometra or mucometra.

Clinical features that distinguish pyometra from pregnancy

Feature	Pyometra	Pregnancy
Uterine contents	Heavy (pus)	Vibrant (foetal fluids)
Uterine wall	Thick, atonic	Thin, tonus
Placentomes	Absent	Present
Slip of chorioallantois	Absent	Present
Fremitus in uterine artery	Absent	Present

Mucometra occurs when there is segmental aplasia of the genital tract (e.g. white heifer disease) or in chronic cases of follicular ovarian disease. These conditions can be diagnosed on the basis of the history and the findings by rectal palpation.

Treatment

The primary objective is to cause regression of the corpus luteum since this will result in dilatation of the cervix, increased myometrial activity, evacuation of the uterine contents, and removal of the block on ovarian cyclicity. Manual expression of the corpus luteum is not recommended.

Oestrogens can cause luteolysis. Intramuscular injection of 5–15 mg oestradiol benzoate or 5–15 mg oestradiol cypionate may be followed by evacuation of the uterine contents within 1–3 days but the results tend to be inconsistent. Undesirable side-effects have been reported, particularly adhesions due to spread of infection to the oviducts, ovarian bursae and ovaries. If the treatment has to be repeated there are additional risks of inducing cystic ovarian disease or of causing relaxation of the pelvic ligaments, which may predispose to fractures.

The method of choice is the administration of $PGF_{2\alpha}$ (25 mg) or cloprostenol (500 µg). Evacuation of the uterine contents begins within 24 hours and should be completed within 1 week. Oestrus can be expected within 3 or 4 days after injection. Cows should not be bred at the induced oestrus and it may be prudent to delay service until the second spontaneous oestrus, which should occur at about 7 or 8 weeks after treatment. Most cows with pyometra require that interval to regain fertility.

If there is evidence that the uterine contents have not been evacuated completely, the cow should be treated again at 12–14 days after the first injection. There is little solid evidence to support the recommendation that treatment with prostaglandin should be followed about 10 days later by an intrauterine infusion of an antibiotic. In one trial, the infusion of nitrafurazone did not have a beneficial effect on the uterus and it depressed the conception rates.

Endometritis

In practice the term endometritis is used so loosely that it can convey different meanings to different people. The clinician tends to use it when there is a purulent or mucopurulent discharge from the vulva in the absence of any evidence of ill health or, in many cases, of any palpable evidence of uterine pathology; histologically, the lesion may be an endometritis but it is just as likely to be a mild metritis or, even, cervicitis or vaginitis. To compound the issue further, endometritis is diagnosed frequently on the basis of lymphocytic and plasma cell infiltrations in biopsy specimens taken from clinically normal repeat breeder cows. Since the criteria that would distinguish physiological levels of lymphocytes and plasma cells from pathological levels have not been defined, a pathologist would not endorse the diagnosis of endometritis in many of these cases.

Cows with clinical 'endometritis' may show oestrus but they tend to do so at irregular and extended intervals. Treatment may be by intrauterine infusion of antibiotic or antiseptic solutions or intramuscular injection of antibiotics or luteolysins. Most cases of clinical 'endometritis' involve *A. pyogenes*, which should be sensitive to intrauterine infusion of penicillin or oxytetracycline. The antibiotics give rise to residues in milk and tissues, while the antibiotics or their vehicles may inhibit the phagocytic cells in the endometrium.

Antiseptics, such as povidone-iodine or chlorhexidine, can be used as intrauterine infusions. It has been reported that an infusion of 50–100 ml of a dilute solution (2–4%) of Lugol's iodine is an effective treatment for 'endometritis'. Again, there is evidence that the treatment may interfere with the activities of phagocytic leucocytes. Moreover, the solution is irritant and, at certain times, it may be responsible for alterations in cycle lengths. When it is administered during the plateau of the luteal phase or during oestrus it has no apparent effect on cycle length, when it is given at day 4 or 5 of the cycle it will cause early luteolysis and a short cycle of about 10 or 11 days, but when it is given at day 16 or 17 it will extend the cycle beyond day 25 (an oxytetracycline preparation containing propylene glycol will induce a similar effect). The luteolytic effect seems to be due to the release of $PGF_{2\alpha}$ from the regenerating endometrial cells. The possibility of using repeated intrauterine infusions of Lugol's iodine to induce oestrus at short intervals has been proposed as a therapy for 'endometritis' but I am not aware of any data on its effectiveness. On the other hand, success has been claimed following systemic treatment with $PGF_{2\alpha}$ (or an analogue) repeated once or twice at 11–14-day intervals.

Investigation of the individual infertile cow

The first step is a general clinical examination and assessment of body condition. This is followed by the specific examination of the genital tract, which should be made bearing in mind the following checklist of major conditions that can cause infertility:

1. congenital defects (p.160);
2. vaginitis (p.161);
3. cervicitis (p.161);
4. endometritis (p.159);
5. metritis (p.154);
6. pyometra (p.157);
7. foetal mummification (p.129);
8. maceration of the foetus (p.129);
9. anoestrus (p.102);
10. cystic ovarian disease (p.106);
11. salpingitis and/or bursal adhesions (p.163);
12. the clinically normal repeat breeder cow (p.163).

Physical examination should include visual inspection of the perineum, vulva, base of the tail, back and flanks. Then the vagina and cervix should be inspected through a speculum and the internal genitalia should be palpated per rectum.

Special procedures may include progesterone assays on blood or milk, swabs for bacteriology from vagina, cervix or uterus, stained smears of uterine or cervical mucus, or endometrial biopsies. In certain circumstances blood samples or vaginal mucus may be collected for serological tests.

Congenital defects

The congenital defects encountered most frequently are segmental aplasia of the Müllerian ducts, failure of fusion of the median wall of the Müllerian ducts, ovarian hypoplasia and the freemartin.

Segmental aplasia of the Müllerian ducts results in the absence or rudimentary development of a portion (or portions) of the anterior vagina, cervix, uterus or oviducts. As a rule, the affected animals have normal oestrous cycles accompanied by the usual secretory activity in the tubular tract. In time, the tubular structures proximal to the segmental defect will become distended by the accumulation of secretions. It follows that the more caudal the defect, the more extensive the distension and the more serious the consequences. For instance, when an imperforate hymen is the only lesion the entire tubular tract will become distended and, if the condition is not corrected soon after puberty, the animal will become sterile; on the other hand, in uterus unicornis the absence of an entire uterine horn does not interfere with the flow of secretions from the normal horn or with the transport of either gametes or conceptus and the affected cow is fertile. Segmental aplasia occurs sporadically in all breeds but it is best known as a genetically determined defect in white shorthorns (white heifer disease).

Failure of fusion of the caudal regions of the Müllerian ducts may leave a double vagina, a double cervix, a double os cervix or a double cervix and uterus (uterus didelphys), all of which may be physical impediments to the transport of spermatozoa to the site of fertilization. A smaller remnant of the median walls of the ducts may be found in the anterior vagina as a dorsoventral band (which has been known to 'retain' an afterbirth that formed a loop around it).

In ovarian hypoplasia one or both ovaries are small and inactive; the left ovary tends to be affected more often and more severely than the right ovary. When both ovaries are affected there are no oestrous cycles and the tubular tract is infantile. The condition occurs sporadically (and rarely) in a number of breeds but it is recognized as a genetic defect in Swedish Highland cattle. Again, there appears to be an association with white coat colour.

The freemartin is a genetic female born as a co-twin with a bull calf. Vascular anastomoses of the chorioallantoic sacs occur at about day 30 of gestation and lead to masculinization of the female twin. If the male twin should die subsequently and be resorbed, the female twin may survive to be born as a singleton freemartin. In the masculinized twin various parts of the Wolffian ducts are present and the derivatives of the Müllerian ducts do not develop fully. The external genitalia are recognizably female; as a rule, the clitoris is enlarged and there is an obvious tuft of hair at the inferior commissure of the vulva. The vagina is hypoplastic; usually it is about one-third of the normal length. A traditional field test to diagnose the condition is based on the distance a small (10–12 mm diameter) test tube can be inserted into the vagina; in the normal female it can travel to a depth of 150–200 mm, whereas in the freemartin it cannot penetrate beyond the level of the hymen (at a depth of 75–100 mm).

Vaginitis and cervicitis

Invariably, swabs taken from the vagina or cervix of cows will yield mixed cultures of 'non-specific bacteria' that normally inhabit these sites without any evidence of an inflammatory reaction. Nevertheless, they are the organisms that are most likely to cause vaginitis and/or cervicitis after parturition, particularly when obstetrical trauma, lacerations, retention of the placental membranes, or metritis occur. Occasionally, the infection may cause severe lesions (e.g. the necrobacillary lesions induced when *Fusiformis necrophorum* infects obstetrical lacerations) but in the vast majority of cases the lesions are mild and most of them resolve spontaneously well in advance of the breeding season.

Vaginitis and cervicitis can occur independently but they often occur concurrently as extensions of endometritis or metritis. When the primary focus of infection is in the uterus it is unlikely that the cervicitis and vaginitis will either resolve spontaneously or respond to local treatment until after the uterine infection has been eliminated. Therefore, careful exploration to discover the primary lesion is essential in every case.

In older cows, the vulva may be sufficiently stretched or deformed to cause pneumovagina, thus exposing the vagina and cervix (and, probably, the uterus) to repeated contamination by bacteria in the aspirated air and faeces. When the back of an old cow sags so that the angle of the vaginal floor is tilted below the level of the pelvic brim urine will pool in the anterior vagina, causing vaginitis and cervicitis. The slight but progressive eversion of the caudal cervical rings that occurs with each succeeding pregnancy is a significant predisposing factor in the development of cervicitis. The mucosa of the prolapsed rings is exposed to the microbial population of the anterior vagina and it responds by mounting an inflammatory reaction. The nature of the inflammatory exudate varies according to the causal agent: it may be mucoid, mucopurulent or purulent. There is a tendency for the discharge to accumulate in the anterior vagina, from which it is expelled periodically; thus, the quantity voided at any one time may give a false impression of the severity of the reaction. When discharges from the vulva occur at any time after involution of the uterus has been completed, the clinician should use a speculum to determine the source of the exudate and the extent of the lesion.

Although most cases of vaginitis are due to 'non-specific bacteria' that induce an inflammatory response in tissue that has been devitalized by trauma, lacerations or irritants, there are some significant specific causes of vaginitis or vulvovaginitis. For instance, each of the two herpes viruses that cause infectious pustular vulvovaginitis (IPV) and infectious bovine cervicovaginitis and epididymitis ('epivag') can be transmitted by coitus and have a serious impact on herd fertility. However, it appears that vaginitis is not the principal cause of the infertility. For instance, about one in four females that contract 'epivag' become sterile largely due to chronic bilateral salpingitis that develops when the virus extends rapidly from vagina to oviducts. Similarly, the contagious granular vaginitis induced by *Ureaplasma urealyticum*, the vaginitis induced by *T. foetus* and the cervicitis induced by *C. fetus* var. *venerealis* are not the most probable causes of the infertility that accompanies each of these infections.

In theory, cervicitis might cause infertility by impeding the passage of spermatozoa deposited in the anterior vagina during natural service or by creating an environment that is lethal to the sperm. In practice, there is little evidence that mild vaginitis or mild cervicitis cause infertility in the absence of endometritis/metritis. When AI is used, it is unlikely that even severe cervicitis would reduce the fertilization rate; however, if the inflammation is associated with a patent cervix, the survival of the conceptus might be in jeopardy. Severe chronic cervicitis, particularly if it is superimposed upon obstetrical laceration, may lead (in time) to a malformed, enlarged and indurated cervix, possibly with some degree of stenosis of the cervical canal; again, this could be a physical barrier to fertilization. Many older cows have enlargement, induration and distortion of the cervix as residual lesions that are not amenable to treatment.

If the vaginitis or cervicitis coexists with endometritis, treatment must be directed specifically towards the uterine lesions; otherwise, it will consist of local treatment by douches, emulsions or ointments containing antibiotics or mild antiseptics repeated every 2 or 3 days to effect.

Lesions of the oviducts and ovarian bursae

The oviducts may be blocked because of segmental aplasia, inflammation due to either ascending infection or to passage of irritant therapeutic solutions from the uterus, or adhesions following trauma induced by palpation per rectum. Loss of patency of the tubes, from whatever cause, will lead to accumulation of fluid: watery fluid in hydrosalpinx, pus in pyosalpinx. The most common infectious causes of inflammatory lesions of the oviducts are staphylococci, streptococci, *E. coli*, *A. pyogenes*, *U. urealyticum*, *Mycoplasma bovigenitalium* and *Acholeplasma laidlawii*. The mucosa of the oviduct has a low capacity for restoration after inflammation so that tubal obstruction is a common sequela. The patency of the oviducts may be checked by the phenolsulphonphthaline test (in which the dye passes from the uterus through the oviduct into the peritoneal cavity, from whence it is absorbed and excreted in the urine) and the starch test (in which starch granules are placed on the surface of the ovary, from whence they pass via the oviduct and uterus to the vagina, where they can be detected in the vaginal mucus). Unfortunately, there is no treatment for these conditions.

The repeat breeder cow

A clinically normal cow that exhibits oestrus at normal intervals (18–24 days) but fails to conceive to three or more services is described as a repeat breeder. Based on this definition, one can expect that 6% of normal healthy cows declared fit to breed at the beginning of the breeding season will become repeat breeders (see Table 4.2). Since the cows have oestrous cycles of normal length, the failure to establish a pregnancy must be due either to failure of fertilization or to loss of the embryo before day 16.

Possible problems in repeat breeder cows

Failure of fertilization may be due to:

1. delayed ovulation or anovulation;
2. infertile semen;
3. insemination at the wrong time;
4. physical impediments, congenital or acquired, to the transport of gametes;
5. uterine infection and endometritis;
6. immunological reactions;
7. high ambient temperatures.

Early embryonic mortality may be due to:

1. fertilization of an aged ovum;
2. lethal chromosomal anomalies;
3. high ambient temperatures;
4. deficiencies of specific nutrients;
5. oestrogen:progesterone imbalance;
6. progesterone deficiency;
7. uterine infection and endometritis.

Some of the putative causes of the repeat breeder syndrome cannot be diagnosed in the field, and even if it was possible to do so it would not be possible to correct them. The transport of the fertilized ovum down the oviduct is a finely tuned process in which the proper sequence and balance of progesterone and oestrogen secretion ensures that the conceptus enters a receptive uterus on day 4. If there is an excess of oestrogen (which retards tubal transport) or an excess of progesterone (which accelerates tubal transport), the conceptus will encounter a hostile uterine environment in which it will not survive. Obviously, the clinician is not able to diagnose or correct this imbalance.

It is possible that insufficient progesterone secretion may be a cause of embryonic loss between days 8 and 17. There are conflicting reports as to whether or not the serum progesterone concentrations are higher between days 10 and 18 when the cow is pregnant than they are after an unsuccessful service. Nevertheless, there is a belief that the administration of exogenous progesterone tends to increase the pregnancy rate in repeat breeder cows. This requires pharmacological doses of progesterone, which has the disadvantage that it may inhibit the release of LH, the endogenous luteotrophin. An alternative approach is to use hCG to stimulate the production of endogenous progesterone by the corpus luteum. Again, reports on the efficiency of this treatment are not convincing.

Insemination at the wrong time covers three separate circumstances:

1. insemination during the luteal phase;
2. insemination too early or too late in oestrus;
3. insemination too soon after calving.

A cow might be inseminated during the luteal phase either because the stockperson has mistakenly interpreted her sexual behaviour as oestrus or because the cow has been mistaken for another cow that was in oestrus. It is well known that cows that are served before day 42 post partum are likely to have significantly lower conception rates than those that are served for the first time more than 60 days post partum, an interval that should allow them experience heat on two or three occasions before service.

Both failure of fertilization and early embryonic death have been implicated in the reduced fertility that is seen during periods of high ambient temperatures in tropical and subtropical climates. The effects of thermal stress are more severe on lactating cows than on heifers.

There is an extensive literature on the effects of energy intake and specific nutritional deficiencies on reproductive failure in cattle. Infertility has been attributed to hypoglycaemia and to deficiencies of phosphorus, copper, cobalt, manganese, iodine, vitamin A, β-carotene. These specific deficiencies are responsible for clinical signs of various kinds and there is little to convince the critical reader that any of these elements is responsible for the repeat breeder cow syndrome.

The congenital physical defects that may impede the transport of gametes have been mentioned (see p. 163). The principal acquired lesions that do so are severe ovarobursal adhesions, salpingitis, hydrosalpinx and pyosalpinx. It may be possible to detect the more extreme forms of these conditions by rectal palpation.

The endometrium is capable of producing local antibodies against antigenic components of spermatozoa, seminal plasma, semen diluent, antibiotics and microorganisms. The precise role, if any, of these antibodies in the repeat breeder cow syndrome is not known. Nevertheless, it would seem prudent not to give intrauterine infusions of antibiotics that are standard constituents of the inseminate unless there is a definite indication for their use. Also, when a cow has repeated a number of times to service by AI her chances of conception might be improved if she is mated naturally.

Uterine biopsy specimens from repeat breeder cows often show sufficient numbers of plasma cells and lymphocytes to prompt a diagnosis of chronic endometritis. Usually, the reactions are mild and, in my opinion, are merely evidence of an immunologically competent endometrium that has been challenged by antigenic material in the recent past. The most likely sources of antigens are the bacteria that invade the uterus periodically throughout the period from parturition to conception. Occasionally, some of these 'non-specific bacteria' (especially *A. pyogenes*) induce a clinically detectable uterine response but there is no convincing evidence that any of them is responsible for infertility in clinically normal repeat breeder cows. It follows that there appears to be no justification for the routine use of intrauterine infusions of antibiotics.

Whenever the aetiology of the syndrome cannot be identified I would choose to use an intrauterine infusion of 3–5 ml of Lugol's iodine in 30–50 ml sterile water at approximately 24 hours after insemination. If the cow does not conceive to that service, I would recommend that she should be served again at the next oestrus. The treatment is empirical and there has not been any carefully controlled investigation of its efficacy. However, in my experience, it is as good as any other and it does not have the contraindications associated with the use of antibiotics or exogenous hormones. The timing of the infusion is important. The recommended procedure introduces the fluid into the uterus after the spermatozoa are safely in the oviducts and sufficiently long before the arrival of the conceptus to preclude the risk of a direct embryotoxic effect. It should not be given after day 3 because of the potentially lethal effect on the conceptus and because at day 4 or 5 it can cause premature luteolysis. It should not be given during oestrus for two reasons: (1) it will create a uterine environment that is inimical to the survival and transport of spermatozoa and (2) it may be transported from the uterus to the oviducts and the ovarian bursae where it is likely to induce an inflammatory reaction that may cause ovarobursal adhesions and/or blockage of the oviducts. The volume of the infusion should not exceed 60–70 ml because of the risk of uterine rupture, which would lead to perimetritis with serosal adhesions and obstruction of the oviduct(s).

5 GOAT BREEDING AND INFERTILITY
K Bretzlaff DVM, PhD

Breeding systems

Dairy goats and pure-bred goats of other breeds are frequently kept in confinement where individuals are readily accessible and information on individual animals is available. Under these conditions, selective mating programmes (hand-mating, pen-mating, artificial insemination) are commonly used. Most meat goats and Angora (hair) goats are managed on extensive systems where animals forage large tracts of rangeland (Gall 1981). In these situations, animals are handled relatively infrequently and unsupervised natural service is used during the desired breeding season. In some developing countries, a mix of these systems exists where animals are confined at night and turned out to forage during the day. In these cases there may be no breeding management at all, with all males and females running together year-round.

Dairy goats are commonly manipulated for out-of-season breeding because of the desire for a year-round milk supply. Depending on the producers' preference for milk or kids, dairy goats may be bred for kidding intervals of two years instead of one. Out-of-season breeding is also theoretically desirable with meat and hair goats because more offspring will produce more meat or hair. However, nutrition may be a constraint on reproduction in rangeland animals to the extent that producers are not interested in more than one kid crop per year.

Terms used in goatkeeping include the following:

- Billy   Adult male
- Buck   Adult male (preferred term by many dairy goat producers)
- Doe   Adult female (preferred term by many dairy goat producers)
- Nanny   Adult female
- Doeling   Young female from birth until first freshening
- First freshener   Female that has had one set of offspring
- Freshening   Parturition
- Goatling   Young goat from birth until puberty
- Kid   Young goat from birth until puberty
- Kidding   Parturition
- Wether   Castrated male

Puberty

Goat kids reach puberty any time after 4 months of age depending on body size and season of the year. Kids that are born early in the kidding season and that are well grown will reach puberty at the first breeding season after they are born. Kids born late in the kidding season or those that are small due to poor nutrition may or may not reach puberty at the subsequent breeding season. Generally, young animals should be approximately 65% of their expected adult body weight before they are used for breeding. Undersized doe kids may breed and conceive only to undergo stress abortions in mid to late gestation. Young Angora nannies are often not exposed to males until the second breeding season after they are born. The marginal nutrition they receive together with the demands of mohair growth do not allow them to reach sufficient body size for breeding during their first breeding season. Those young females that do breed and conceive are susceptible to stress abortions.

Selection of breeding animals

Animals should be selected for their ability to produce the desired commodity, to reproduce efficiently, and to survive in the environment in which they are placed. When commodity prices are high, producers are more likely to retain their animals and not cull those that they should. Under these situations, an increased incidence of infertility problems may be observed. Some young animals can be culled prior to their use as breeding animals due to obvious defects in conformation or hair quality (Ricordeau 1981). Most dairy animals are allowed one or two lactations before they are culled for milk production.

Reproductive traits of interest include fertility, fecundity and length of the breeding season. It is especially important that the bucks are sound breeding prospects due to their greater contribution to the herd gene pool. Testicular size should be an important component of the decision to use a buck in a breeding operation. Testicular volume is correlated with sperm output. However, dairy bucks frequently are retained for the dairy characteristics of their daughters rather than their breeding soundness. Scrotal size is especially important in range animals that are expected to settle a large number of females early in a defined season. Another reason to select for scrotal size is that it is likely that, as in other species, daughters of males with large testicles reach puberty earlier than daughters of males with smaller testicles.

The Nubian dairy goat generally has a longer breeding season than dairy breeds originating in Europe. Goats are short-day (autumn) breeders, with breeding seasons generally considered to extend from late August or September to late January or February in the Northern Hemisphere. Nubians will frequently begin breeding in June and continue into March. On a worldwide basis, some breeds tend to be very seasonal breeders (Angoras) while others frequently kid almost year-round (Black Bengals) (Ricordeau 1981). In regions at high altitude far from the equator, breeding seasons may be restricted to a few months (October–December). In regions near the equator where day length varies little during the year, the breeding seasons are correlated more with rain and improved nutrition than simply with season of the year.

Table 5.1 Breed differences in litter size (adapted from Ricordeau 1981)

Breed	Country	Litter size
Anglo-Nubian	USA	2.1
	Malaya	1.43
	Israel	1.75
	Mauritius	2.29
	Mexico	1.92
Saanen	USA	1.8
	Germany	1.83
	Israel	1.95
	France	1.68
	Venezuela	1.33
	Mexico	1.68
Angora	USA	1.15
Creole	Guadeloupe	2.11
Jamnapari	India	1.11
Black Bengal	India	1.79

The heritability of litter size within a breed is low; however, this parameter can be manipulated to some extent by nutrition. There is a definite breed variation in average litter size (Ricordeau 1981) (Table 5.1). Therefore, more rapid progress in increasing fecundity may be achieved by crossbreeding with breeds that have a genetic tendency toward multiple offspring. In rangeland areas, some producers prefer single kids to twins because of the greater strength and survivability of the singles.

Management of breeding animals

Detection of oestrus

Females can best be detected in oestrus in the presence of a buck. Therefore, if oestrus does need to be identified, a male needs to be maintained in close proximity to the females. Fenceline contact with an intact male or the use of teaser animals are the most accurate methods to identify oestrous females for selective matings.

The male effect

Separation of males and females except for limited breeding seasons is a common practice. The sudden introduction of a male to females that have not been exposed to a male for at least 30 days will induce ovulation within 3 days in females if they are transitional (the male effect). Transition refers to the reproductive state in which females are not cycling, but are approaching the breeding season and so are more easily induced to cycle than during deep anoestrus. The male effect provides a loose synchronization of breeding and therefore kidding, and encourages the does to cycle and conceive early in the breeding season.

Flushing

Flushing is the technique of supplementing nutrition for several weeks prior to the breeding season. This has been shown to be economically feasible in ewes due to the increase in ovulation rate that occurs. Results are less predictable in the doe, but might be expected to be of benefit in rangeland animals on marginal planes of nutrition. If supplemental feeding of rangeland animals is not feasible, they can instead be moved to a rested pasture 2 weeks prior to introduction of the bucks. Females that are in extremely poor condition, however, will not achieve optimal ovulation rates even with flushing.

Male:female ratio

With natural service, one fertile buck per 50 does is adequate for good conception rates early in the breeding season. Bucks are capable of serving as many as 20 times per day for a limited period of time, but excessive use, especially of young bucks, may result in decreased fertility. Young bucks in their first year of breeding are best turned in with half the number of does that mature bucks are expected to handle. Bucks are very active during the breeding season and may lose weight rapidly. Therefore, they should be in good body condition when turned in with the females. If they are not in good body condition 6–8 weeks prior to the breeding season, they should be started on an increased plane of nutrition. They should also be dewormed and have their feet properly trimmed prior to the breeding season. In selenium-deficient areas, administration of selenium to bucks 6–8 weeks prior to the breeding season may be advantageous.

Timing of routine procedures

During the implementation of a breeding programme, does should not be subjected to stressful procedures. Even procedures such as deworming or foot trimming can be stressful to rangeland animals that are not used to being handled. Such procedures should be accomplished several weeks prior to the onset of breeding.

Breeding records

Breeding animals should have useful identification so that accurate breeding records can be kept. The identification method should be visible from a reasonable distance in cases where relatively large groups of females are being observed for oestrus. In addition, a teaser animal with a marking harness can be used to leave a coloured mark on the rump of does that stand to be mounted. Periodically changing the colour of the chalk in the harness allows a prediction of the time frame within which the individual does were in oestrus.

Breeding to an outside buck

Goat producers with small numbers of animals may prefer not to keep a buck. Bucks are hard on fences and have a strong odour during the breeding season. Artificial insemination (AI) can be used in these herds to reduce exposure to outside animals. If this is not possible, the does need to be taken to another location to be bred. This has inherent risks of disease transmission. Historical information on potential disease problems in the other herd should be obtained. Evidence of contagious diseases such as contagious ecthyma (soremouth), infectious keratoconjunctivitis (pink-eye) or caseous lymphadenitis (abscesses) that are not present in the doe herd should motivate the selection of an alternative breeding plan. If the outside buck is used, it is best to take the doe to the buck only when she is in oestrus and only long enough for mating to occur. Alternatively, an outside buck might be brought in and put with the does for a short period of time during the breeding season. Ideally the buck would be isolated for 30 days before being turned in with the does although this may not be practical.

Planning a breeding programme

Using the male effect

Goats will breed most successfully if they are of adequate age and size, in good body condition, and not impaired by recent parturition or heavy lactation. During the natural breeding season, most goats have not recently kidded. At this time, the main considerations would be to separate the bucks from the does at least 1 month prior to the breeding season, begin flushing the females 2 weeks prior to introduction of the males, and then introduce the males suddenly at the desired onset of the breeding season. Males can be 'introduced' using fenceline exposure although direct contact with the females may be more effective. Infertile teaser animals can be used for this purpose (see p.178). This should result in most females ovulating during the 10-day period after introduction of the males. The choice of time of the breeding season may be dictated by the type of weather that is expected 5 months later. Introduction of the males is postponed in some areas to avoid kidding during winter weather. The male effect is reduced as the breeding season progresses however, as the females will eventually begin to cycle on their own.

Short oestrous cycles

Due to lack of progesterone priming, many of the first oestrous cycles observed during the breeding season are short (4–7 days). In these cases, the first ovulation (frequently accompanied by signs of oestrus in goats) will not result in conception because the corpus luteum formed is short-lived (Chemineau 1983). With natural service and a high doe-to-buck ratio, this large percentage of infertile first breedings can needlessly tax the males. Therefore, one management technique is to use infertile teasers with the females for the first week and then turn in the desired sires. Alternatively, one group of bucks can be turned in at the beginning of the breeding season and replaced with a rested group of bucks after the length of one oestrous cycle. This technique is favoured by some Angora producers.

Because of the high proportion (up to 75%) of short cycles at the onset of the breeding season, AI might also best be postponed until the second observed oestrus.

Out-of-season breeding

Successful out-of-season breeding also requires the use of healthy animals that are of proper size and condition. Does that are less than 60 days post partum, that are nursing kids or that have recently had kids weaned, or that are lactating heavily are not good candidates for successful out-of-season breeding. Males may not be sexually active at that time of year, a factor that must be considered if natural service is to be used. If breeding males are needed, they should either be placed under lights ahead of time, or should have been continuously used since the previous breeding season. Continued use can help maintain libido in bucks during the non-breeding season, but does not prevent the seasonal decline in semen quality. Therefore, a lower female:male ratio should be considered during the non-breeding season, although I do not have data to suggest what the optimum ratio would be. When does are synchronized, there should be a buck with good libido available for approximately 10 does. If the buck has not been prepared for breeding, he may refuse to serve any does at all.

Lights

A short breeding season can be induced in goats during the natural non-breeding season by the use of lights. Goats can be exposed to 19 or 20 hour days for 2 months at which time the extra lights are turned off. This apparent decrease in day length will stimulate the goats to start cycling approximately 7–10 weeks later. With 40-W fluorescent bulbs 9 feet (2.74 m) above the floor, 1 foot (0.3 m) of bulb was needed for each 10.5 square feet (0.975 m^2) of floor space (Ashbrook 1982). Signs of oestrus during this induced breeding season may not be as strong as during the natural breeding season. The animals will cycle several times before lapsing into anoestrus again. This technique requires that the goats be kept near the lights during the hours of extra lighting for the 2-month period of time. This makes the procedure cost prohibitive for range animals.

Melatonin

The use of melatonin implants may substitute for extra lighting. Melatonin is produced by the pineal gland during hours of darkness. Exogenous melatonin signals the body that darkness is present, thus indicating that days are suddenly shorter. In sheep they are more useful to advance the breeding season than they are to induce breeding during deep anoestrus. In anoestrous dairy goats, induction of a short breeding season is most successful if extra lights are used prior to administration of melatonin. Melatonin implants have been used with success in manipulating the seasonal production of fibre in hair goats, especially cashmere goats, which produce fibre in response to decreasing day length.

Hormones

Out-of-season breeding can also be induced by use of a progestin and equine chorionic gonadotrophin (see p. 178).

Oestrus

Seasonality of breeding

Goats are stimulated to cycle approximately 7–10 weeks after perceiving a decrease in day length. Under natural conditions, days begin to shorten in the summer, resulting in a breeding season in the autumn. After days begin to lengthen in the winter, goats enter a period of anoestrus in the spring. They also experience a transitional period during the several weeks prior to each breeding season. This is a time when ovarian activity (follicular growth) begins prior to the occurrence of oestrus and ovulation. During transition, it is easier to induce oestrous activity with the male effect or hormones than it is during anoestrus. In areas near the equator, where day length is not as variable as in temperate climates, seasonality of breeding may follow rainfall and nutrition more closely than the calendar. The relative length and depth of the anoestrous and transitional periods varies with breeds. Breeds originating from northern climates tend to be more seasonal with shorter breeding seasons and deeper anoestrous periods. Breeds originating from tropical areas have more shallow anoestrous periods and so can be more effectively induced to breed out-of-season with the male effect and/or certain hormones.

Postpartum period

Goats usually breed during the autumn and kid 5 months later, in the spring. This is the anoestrous season, so the animals do not resume cyclicity post partum until the subsequent autumn. However, animals that breed out-of-season kid during the breeding season and have a postpartum period similar to that observed in cattle. In general, goats in reasonable body condition will begin oestrus cycles 30–40 days after kidding during the breeding season. Uterine involution is complete at this time (Tielgy *et al.* 1982).

Detection of oestrus

Does in oestrus will seek the male and flag their tail vigorously in response to advances by the male. More subtle signs of oestrus include vulvar hyperaemia, presence of mucus, personality changes including increased vocalization, and frequent urination. Heat detection is not reliable without the presence of a buck. Homosexual activity is not as prevalent in does as it is in cows, although it is more likely to be seen when a large number of females are in oestrus at the same time. If an intact male is not wanted with the females, teaser animals can be used. These can be androgenized castrates (150 mg of testosterone propionate given once weekly for 3 weeks will prepare a wether), vasectomized males, penile-deviated males, or intersex animals with good libido. Intact males wearing breeding aprons that cover the prepuce can also be used. Buck rags are rags that are saturated with buck odour by being rubbed on the head of a buck during the breeding season. They are kept in an airtight jar. The jar is opened and presented to the does twice daily. Does in oestrus will be unusually interested in the rag.

In situations where bucks or teaser animals run with the does, a marking harness on the male will provide a record of which females stand to be mounted. This will identify when does are bred and whether they return to oestrus.

Synchronization of oestrus

Synchronization of oestrus is useful to allow efficient use of AI and to have animals at the same stage of gestation for management purposes.

The male effect

The male effect is economical and effective for a loose synchronization. When a male is introduced to non-cycling, transitional does that have not been exposed to a male for at least 30 days, the majority of females will ovulate within 3 days. A significant proportion will ovulate again in 4–7 days at which time the mean ovulation rate is higher (Chemineau 1983). Therefore, the majority of females have a fertile oestrus during an approximately 10-day period of time.

Hormones

Prostaglandin is effective in causing luteolysis in goats with functional corpora lutea. Oestrus can be synchronized in cycling animals by the use of two injections, 11 days apart. Most goats will start showing signs of behavioural oestrus 36–60 hours after administration. Functional corpora lutea are present from approximately day 4 to day 16 of the 20-day oestrous cycle in the goat.

During the non-breeding season, oestrus is usually induced and synchronized in goats with a progestogen and equine chorionic gonadotrophin (eCG, also known as pregnant mare's serum gonadotrophin, PMSG). Progestogens can be administered by vaginal pessaries (sponges), subcutaneous ear implants, or daily injections of progesterone. They are administered for 9–15 days, with 300–600 iu of eCG being administered

48 hours prior to progestogen removal. Goats will typically be in standing oestrus starting 12–36 hours after removal of the progestogen. Oral administration of the progestogen melengestrol acetate (MGA), used to suppress oestrus in feedlot heifers, has been used successfully to synchronize oestrus in sheep (Umberger and Lewis 1992). Such a product may prove useful in goats.

Proper time to breed

Available information suggests that goats ovulate 30–36 hours after the onset of standing oestrus (Roberts 1986). Thus, goats are typically bred 12–24 hours after they are first observed in standing heat. Goats may remain in standing oestrus for 24–36 hours or even longer. Some producers rebreed does that are still in standing oestrus 24 hours after an initial breeding. Others feel this is not necessary. Generally, one breeding gives good results if the onset of oestrus was accurately determined.

Mating behaviour

Bucks have a characteristic courting behaviour in which they approach a doe toward her flank, strike with one of their front legs, flick their tongues, and vocalize. Does that are approaching oestrus will show interest without standing to be mounted. Their interactions with the buck may result in a varying amount of circling activity. Does in oestrus will readily stand still for the buck to mount and copulate. Once mounted on a female in standing heat, an experienced buck accomplishes intromission after a short series of thrusts, and ejaculates very rapidly after intromission is accomplished. Ejaculation is typically indicated by an extra vigorous, almost lunging, thrust.

Mating supervision

Hand-mating

Dairy goats are frequently mated selectively. With hand-mating, the female is kept separate from the male until she is detected to be in oestrus at which time she is introduced to the male for a single mating. Some producers reintroduce the female to the male once every 12–24 hours and allow them to rebreed if the female accepts the male. This is acceptable if the male does not have a large number of females to breed.

Pen-mating

With pen-mating, a group of does is selected to be bred to a particular buck, and the buck is allowed to run with those does during a defined breeding season. If the does are lactating and milk is being kept for human consumption, the buck may only be introduced briefly twice daily in order to reduce transmission of odour to the milk.

Pasture mating

With most meat and hair goats, pasture mating is utilized in which bucks are turned out with the females for unsupervised natural service. If possible, males should be turned out for a defined (approximately 60 day) breeding season after which they are separated from the females. With short breeding seasons it is imperative that the males be fertile when they are introduced for breeding.

Artificial insemination

Artificial insemination is commonly used in dairy goats in some developed countries. The caprine cervix, unlike that of the sheep, is structurally compatible with transcervical insemination. The technique allows the introduction of new genetic material into countries where importation of live animals is restricted. However, it is labour intensive and requires the use of drugs and/or equipment that may be prohibitively expensive in some areas.

Collection of semen

See p. 195.

Evaluation of semen

See p. 196.

Extenders

Semen may be inseminated raw, fresh extended, or extended and frozen-thawed. Semen that is to be inseminated as fresh extended or frozen semen is extended with a diluent that usually consists of skim milk or egg yolk, a natural sugar such as glucose or fructose, and a buffer such as citrate and/or Tris. When egg yolk extenders are used with buck semen, it is advisable to 'wash' the semen in order to remove the seminal plasma. Goat seminal plasma contains an enzyme that can react with lecithins in egg yolk and produce lysolecithins, which are toxic to spermatozoa. Semen is washed by adding some diluent (approximately 10 parts diluent to 1 part semen) to the semen, mixing gently, centrifuging slowly ($950 \times$ g for 15 minutes), removing the supernatant, and resuspending the spermatozoa with fresh diluent. Some feel that washing is not necessary with Angora semen if reduced concentrations of egg yolk are used (Evans and Maxwell 1987).

Insemination dose

The number of progressively motile, morphologically normal sperm that are inseminated is frequently 60–120 million cells. This means that 50 or more females can be inseminated from one good ejaculate. The volume inseminated is 0.05–0.5 ml depending on the type of system used (straws, thawed pellets, diluted fresh semen, etc.) (Evans and Maxwell 1987).

Timed insemination

Insemination of does at hormonally induced heats is best done based on detection of oestrus. Does that do not show signs of heat will have poor conception rates if inseminated. However, timed inseminations are desirable in some situations. Reasonable estimates for timed inseminations in does are 60 and 72 hours after injection of prostaglandin or 31 and 54 hours after removal of progestogens when a progestogen and eCG are being used.

Site of semen deposition

During natural service, the urethral process sprays semen around the external os of the cervix. With AI it is desirable to place the semen in the uterus to compensate for the reduced number of spermatozoa being deposited.

Insemination equipment (Figures 5.1 and 5.2)

Equipment needed for AI includes a vaginal speculum, a light source and an inseminating instrument. A variety of types of each of these have been used with success. An appropriate size for a vaginal speculum for an adult doe would be 25 mm external diameter and 20 cm in length. For doelings

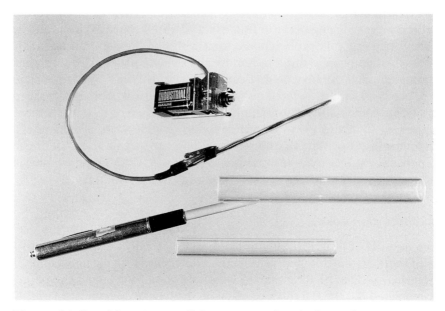

Figure 5.1 Goat AI equipment: light sources and vaginal speculae

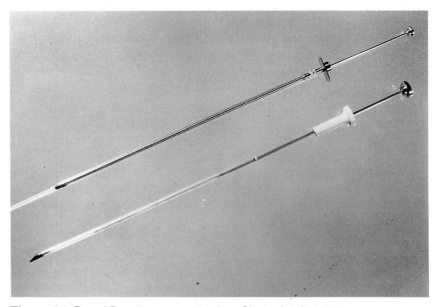

Figure 5.2 Goat AI equipment: examples of inseminating guns.

and small-breed does, a speculum 19 mm × 15 cm would be satisfactory. In some countries, goat inseminating supplies are available through commercial suppliers.

Insemination technique

The vulva of the oestrous doe should be cleaned, and the vaginal speculum inserted into the vagina with the aid of a small amount of non-spermicidal lubricant. With the aid of the light source, the external os of the cervix is visualized and the character of the cervical mucus is evaluated. Cervical mucus is clear early in standing oestrus, turns cloudy later in standing oestrus, and becomes very thick and 'cheesy' as the doe goes out of standing oestrus. The optimal time to inseminate is soon after the mucus becomes cloudy. The inseminating instrument with the semen is advanced through the speculum and visually placed in the external os of the cervix (Figure 5.3). It is manually advanced through the cervix by placing forward pressure with slight circular motions if necessary. Often the inseminating

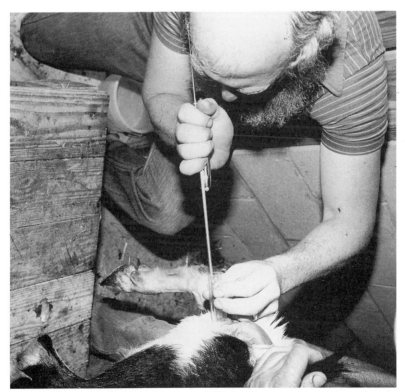

Figure 5.3 Goat AI: visual placement of AI gun in external os of cervix using vaginal speculum and light source.

gun can be heard to 'pop' through one or more of the three to five cervical rings. If after a short period of time (30 seconds to 1 minute) the instrument cannot be advanced to a point where there is no more resistance, the semen should be deposited in the cervix rather than risk trauma to the tissue. It is not uncommon to experience difficulty in achieving intrauterine insemination in maiden doelings or does of small breeds where the cervix is small and the smaller vaginal speculum may restrict visualization of the cervix.

Does being inseminated can be restrained in the standing position on an elevated platform such as a milking stand, or can be restrained with their rear ends elevated in some fashion such as over a rail.

Laparoscopic artificial insemination

Does can also be inseminated in the uterus through the use of a laparoscope in a manner similar to that used widely in sheep (laparoscopic AI). The doe is restrained in dorsal recumbency on a tilt table with her rear end elevated. A laparoscope and the insemination instrument are introduced into the abdominal cavity via two small stab incisions. The uterus is visualized with the laparoscope and the sharp end of the insemination instrument is used to puncture the uterine wall and allow deposition of the semen into the uterine lumen. Further details concerning AI are available (Evans and Maxwell 1987).

Conception rates

If does are inseminated when they are truly in oestrus by experienced operators using good quality semen, conception rates of 70% or even greater may be achieved with AI. However, novices should not unrealistically raise their expectations as conception rates of 0–40% are frequently observed with inexperienced inseminators. Goats inseminated at prostaglandin-induced heats may have slightly (approximately 10%) reduced conception rates.

Pregnancy

Early development of the conceptus

In sheep, and therefore presumably in goats, embryos enter the uterus on the third to fourth day after oestrus (Roberts 1986). They are at the 8-cell stage or later in development at this time. By 11 days after fertilization, the blastocyst is about 1 mm in diameter. Starting at 12 days the tropho-blast elongates very rapidly and by 14 days it is 10 cm long. Attachment of the chorioallantois to the endometrium is cotyledonary, beginning in the caruncular areas at about 17–20 days and being well developed by 28–30 days. The maternal caruncles are concave in shape in small rumi-nants, the opposite of what is seen in cows (Roberts 1986).

In the ewe, transuterine migration of the embryo is common, with approximately 10–20% of embryos from double ovulations on one ovary migrating to the contralateral uterine horn (Roberts 1986). Goats are presumably similar to sheep in this regard.

Estimating the stage of gestation

Approximate ages of foetuses can be determined by real-time ultrasound. Size of the uterus, placentomes, embryo, and foetal head measurements can be used to estimate the stage of gestation. The limiting factor to accurate estimation of age of the conceptus is the time required to achieve the desired view of the embryo or foetus. It can be extremely time-con-suming to obtain a precise longitudinal section of the body or head. After mid-gestation, the foetal structures are so large that only portions of them can be viewed on the screen at one time. I am not aware of published information on determination of foetal ages using real-time ultrasono-graphic evaluations of crown–nose or crown–rump measurements in goats. Experienced operators can usually estimate foetal age within 5–10 days of actual age if animals are scanned between approximately 40 and 90 days of gestation. Biparietal diameter of foetal heads has been used between days 40 and 100 of gestation to accurately determine foetal age in dairy goats (Haibel 1988). Using this method, gestational age can be calculated as $1.78 \times$ (biparietal diameter (mm) $+14.6$).

In Angora goats, foetal age can be calculated if the foetuses are available for crown–rump measurement. The foetal length in inches is divided by 0.149 and the result added to 30 to give the age in days (Shelton and Groff 1984).

Length of gestation

Breed averages for gestation length vary from 143 days for Black Bengal goats to 153 days for the Murciana breed (Ricordeau 1986). Most averages fall in the range of 146–150 days. The genotype of the foetus influences variation in gestation more than the genotype of the dam (Jainudeen and Hafez 1987). There is a tendency for does carrying female kids, does carrying multiple kids, and does kidding during the breeding season to have shorter gestations.

Nutrition during late gestation

Close attention should be paid to the nutrition of goats during the last 4–6 weeks of gestation because of their susceptibility to pregnancy toxaemia. This is especially true for females carrying multiple foetuses. Animals in confinement may be gradually introduced to 0.5–0.7 kg of a concentrate per head per day. Rangeland animals may be supplemented with a concentrate or processed feed ('range cubes') or provided a protein and energy source for self-feeding ('protein blocks'). The amount of supplementation necessary depends on the quality of the forage available.

Boosting colostral immunoglobulins

Pregnant does should be vaccinated approximately 1 month prior to expected parturition for diseases for which colostral immunity is important. These diseases include enterotoxaemia (overeating disease caused by *Clostridium perfringens*) and tetanus. Animals that have not been previously vaccinated or that have an unknown history should receive two injections of these toxoids approximately 1 month apart (or according to label directions), with the second injection being administered 1 month prior to the animal's due date. Animals that have been previously vaccinated for these diseases need only a single booster 1 month prior to their due date. This is also an appropriate time to inject does with vitamin E and selenium in deficient areas if they are not receiving adequate supplementation in their feed.

Termination of pregnancy

Because goats are dependent on the corpus luteum as a source of progesterone throughout gestation, pregnancy can be terminated at any time through the administration of prostaglandin.

Pregnancy diagnosis

Non-return to oestrus

Many producers with intensive operations use non-return to oestrus as presumptive evidence of pregnancy. Dairy goat owners may base this on failure to observe oestrus in bred females, while owners of other breeds may use a teaser animal with a marking harness to leave evidence of whether females are returning to oestrus.

Progesterone tests

A low progesterone concentration in blood or milk at one oestrous cycle's length after breeding is essentially 100% accurate as a test for non-pregnancy. An elevated concentration is only 70–80% accurate as an indication of pregnancy at this time because a corpus luteum can be present with conditions other than pregnancy. In addition, some animals that are indeed pregnant at this early stage will undergo embryonic resorption and fail to kid. Animals that were not actually in oestrus when bred, that short cycled after being bred or that are pseudopregnant might have elevated progesterone concentrations 21 days after breeding without being pregnant.

Ultrasonography

Amplitude depth, or A-mode, ultrasound is somewhat useful in the goat at approximately 60–90 days of gestation when the ratio of fluid to foetal tissue is large. With this equipment, a positive response indicates the presence of fluid which is not a cardinal sign of pregnancy. The only real advantage of this method over B-mode, or real-time, ultrasonography is cost. Real-time ultrasonography is the most rapid and accurate method of pregnancy diagnosis currently in use, but is not available in many areas due to the expense of the equipment. A linear array transducer (usually 5.0 MHz) can be used transrectally as early as 19 days after breeding with good results, but is most commonly used transabdominally 30 days after breeding. Sector scanners (3.5 or 5.0 MHz) are also widely used transabdominally as in sheep, and may be more desirable for scanning larger areas of the abdomen to count foetuses. It is necessary to clip the hair in the area to be scanned in the goat if the best picture is to be obtained. More data are available with sheep than with goats, but results are similar. Accuracy depends on the experience of the operator, body size of the females (transrectal scanning of large deep-bodied animals may miss early pregnancies), type of probe (3.5-MHz transducers penetrate deeper through tissue than do 5-MHz transducers but have poorer resolution), stage of pregnancy (pregnancies younger than 30 days are more likely to be missed), speed of scanning, and whether diagnosis of pregnancy or number of foetuses is being made. Accuracy of positive and negative pregnancy diagnosis exceeds 90% in most published reports, and exceeds 95% with most experienced operators. Accuracy of number of foetuses is less, but when predictions are restricted to singles versus multiples during the middle trimester of pregnancy accuracy can be 85% or greater (Buckrell 1988). Separation of does carrying single foetuses from those carrying multiple foetuses allows the producer to feed the animals according to their needs.

Oestrone sulphate

An elevated concentration of oestrone sulphate in blood, milk or urine is an accurate indicator of a viable foetus from 50 days after breeding to term.

Radiography

Radiographs are accurate indicators of pregnancy after 75–80 days after breeding when the foetal skeleton begins to ossify. Pregnancies can be missed by this method if animals have not been held off feed so that rumen ingesta interferes with interpretation of the radiograph. This interference can be minimized by dorsoventral positioning of the doe being radiographed.

Miscellaneous methods

Other methods of pregnancy diagnosis in goats include ballottement of the foetus (late gestation) and digital palpation of the consistency of the external os of the cervix (softer and more blunt at 30–50 days of gestation than in the non-pregnant animal). These methods require some operator experience and can provide false positives and false negatives. Recto-abdominal palpation with a Hulet rod as used in sheep is generally not recommended in goats as they resist being restrained on their backs. This can result in rectal trauma and death of the animal or abortion of the foetuses.

Prenatal losses

Compared to sheep, there is little information concerning early embryonic loss in goats. Environmental factors such as temperature and nutrition play an important role in ovulation rate and very likely in embryo survival rate (Roberts 1986). When comparing numbers of corpora lutea with numbers of foetuses, embryonic deaths in sheep have been reported to be as high as 30% with a higher rate of loss in females with three ovulations. In Angora goats, 19.9% of ova ovulated did not result in a conceptus at 25–30 days after breeding and 12.2% of embryos formed were lost prior to kidding (Shelton and Stewart 1973). Similar information is needed for the dairy goat in different environments. The discrepancy between numbers of corpora lutea and number of offspring can be due to fertilization failure, early embryonic death or abortion. Fertilization failure and early embryonic death are higher during the early part of the breeding season. Heat stress and selenium–vitamin E deficiency may also be associated with infertility/early embryonic death in small ruminants.

The Angora goat has a well-documented problem with stress abortions, which usually occur between 90 and 120 days of gestation (Shelton 1986). Other breeds of goats kept on marginal nutrition may be susceptible as well. The problem is primarily nutritional, occurring in young and/or small females, but can be exacerbated by other stresses such as shearing. Shearing of pregnant animals should be accomplished at least 2 weeks prior to the onset of the kidding season. In South Africa, habitual abortion by large Angora does has been reported to be associated with hyperadrenalism. These animals should be culled.

Infectious causes of abortion can cause significant losses in goats (see p. 204).

Parturition

Signs of impending parturition

The rate of development of the mammary glands prior to parturition varies between goats during the last few weeks of pregnancy. Some goats make the most noticeable changes in udder development during only the last few days of gestation while others show definite changes several weeks prior to kidding. The sacral ligaments relax to some extent during the last days of gestation, causing a pronounced change in the angle of the pelvis. This lowering of the caudal aspect of the pelvis results in a hollowed-out appearance of the tissue on either side of the tail. This change is most prominent during the last 12 hours prior to parturition.

Stage I of labour

Goats progress through three stages of labour. During stage I, which begins approximately 6 hours prior to parturition, the doe is restless, may decrease feed consumption, and may separate herself from other females in the herd. Uterine contractions rearrange the foetus to the birth presentation (usually front feet and head being pushed toward the cervix first) at this time. Pressure of the foetus into the dilated cervix and birth canal causes the reflex release of oxytocin. This intensifies uterine contractions and leads to rupture of the chorioallantois (the first water bag) and onset of stage II of labour and abdominal contractions (Jainudeen and Hafez 1987).

Stage II of labour and dystocia

Stage II of parturition is recognized by active labour. A doe in labour that does not deliver a kid or at least show visible signs of making progress within 30 minutes should be examined. Dystocias are not common (less than 5%) in most situations and are usually due to a large single kid in a first freshener, one front leg and/or the head being back, breech presentations, or multiple kids becoming entangled in the birth canal. Most dystocias can be corrected by elevating the doe's rear end, repelling the foetuses, and rearranging them to the normal presentation. Epidural anaesthesia will reduce straining of the doe against manual manipulations. In small females, especially in breeds such as the Pygmy, large single foetuses may necessitate caesarean sections. It is easy to apply too much force in attempting to correct malpresentations in small ruminants, especially for people with large hands. Excessive force can result in uterine rupture or torn vaginal tissue that can lead to death of the dam.

Stage III of labour and retained foetal membranes

Stage III of parturition is the passage of the foetal afterbirth. This normally occurs within 4–6 hours after delivery of the last kid. As in cattle, retention of the foetal membranes renders a doe more susceptible to uterine infection. This is more common with milk fever, dystocia, or late term abortions and stillbirths. Retained foetal membranes should not be manually removed in goats unless they fall away with almost no effort. Intrauterine medications are best administered by dilution in 250 ml of water or saline and infusion through a soft catheter. If the vagina is bruised or torn and the animal is experiencing pain, vaginal examinations and/or manipulations are contraindicated and the animal should be treated systemically.

Weak labour

Animals exhibiting weak labour may be affected by some degree of pregnancy toxaemia and/or milk fever. Treatment with calcium gluconate is advisable in these situations prior to uterine manipulations. Such animals may be prone to uterine prolapse. After delivery of the kids, oxytocin can be administered to hasten involution of the uterus.

Management of periparturient does

Dairy goats and pure-bred animals are often kept in small pens and watched closely for parturition, especially when breeding dates are known. Kids may be removed from the dams immediately after birth if disease control measures involving the feeding of heat-treated colostrum and pasteurized milk have been implemented.

Range animals may be brought up to small pastures near the producer's residence for the kidding season in order to allow monitoring and to reduce the prevalence of predation. However, breeds or herds of goats that are stressed by proximity to humans may best be left to kid relatively unattended in their usual pastures in order to prevent abandonment of newborn kids by the dams. Bonding of the dams to their newborns can be upset if females are disturbed during the kidding season. Alternatively, pregnant nannies can be brought into sheds for intensive kidding techniques similar to those used in sheep. These include the use of individual pens and the stanchioning (restraint of the head by closing two vertical poles immediately behind the head) of females that do not accept their kids until bonding is complete.

Induction of parturition

Induction of parturition is very successful in goats. It is popular with goat producers that want to schedule weekend kiddings because they have jobs away from home during the week. It is also commonly used by dairy goat producers that want to be present at kiddings so that kids can be immediately removed from their dams before they suckle colostrum. This is important to prevent the transmission of infectious agents that are spread through the colostrum. Because the species is dependent on the corpus luteum throughout gestation, prostaglandin is the drug of choice for this purpose. Retained foetal membranes are not a problem as they are in cattle. Viable kids will be produced if a goat is injected with 10–20 mg of prostaglandin $F_{2\alpha}$ after 140 days of gestation. Weak kids can best be avoided and the most predictable response obtained if the goats are at least 144 days after breeding when injected. Goats will usually kid 27–50 hours (mean 31 hours) after being injected with prostaglandin or one of its analogues.

Puerperium

Postpartum involution is poorly documented in goats. They usually kid during the non-breeding season so it is difficult to measure involution and return to cyclicity in a meaningful way. Lochia may be present up to 2 weeks post partum although the volume observed should be minimal after 7 days. Information from does kidding during the breeding season suggests that uterine involution is complete approximately 30 days post partum (Tielgy *et al.* 1982). Oestrous cycles resume approximately at this time during the breeding season. However, does nursing kids or lactating heavily may have a delayed return to cyclicity. The differences between range goats and dairy goats in this regard needs to be studied. Meat goats that kid during the breeding season are much more likely to breed back within 60 days post partum if their kids are weaned early (30 days post partum)—70% vs 24% for controls nursing kids throughout (Lawson *et al.* 1984).

Neonates

Young kids should have their navels dipped in iodine and should be watched to ensure intake of colostrum. Angora kids especially are susceptible to cold stress, particularly if the dam has been on a marginal plane of nutrition and the kids are born weak. Kid losses are commonly associated with slow parturitions and failure of kids to get up and suckle. Common causes of kid mortality are:

- predators;
- white muscle disease (selenium–vitamin E deficiency);
- colibacillosis (diarrhoea associated with *Escherichia coli*);
- coccidiosis;
- pneumonia;
- enterotoxaemia.

Most neonatal diseases can be controlled by proper vaccination programmes and environmental management. Kids should be raised in dry, well-ventilated areas if kept in confinement, and should not be overcrowded. Dams can be vaccinated for enterotoxaemia in late pregnancy to boost colostral antibodies. Pregnant does can be administered selenium–vitamin E injections to prevent a deficiency leading to white muscle disease in their offspring.

Breeding records

Good records are part of good management and should include information on occurrence of oestrus, breedings and sires used. Dairy goat producers are most likely to have information available on individual animals while producers of rangeland goats may only have a general idea of the amount of oestrous activity occurring in particular groups of animals. Availability of records allows returns to oestrus, short cycles, or other reproductive problems to be identified before the end of the breeding season. They also allow a more precise prediction of kidding.

Breeding performance

Pregnancy rates and prolificacy

Goats are a highly fertile species so that pregnancy rates well in excess of 90% can be realized. Problems usually occur due to nutritional deficiencies, intersex animals, exposure of females to an infertile male, attempts to breed subfertile females, infectious diseases, or attempts to breed out of the natural breeding season. Dairy goats very commonly produce twins or triplets, and quadruplets are not unusual. In breeds that tend to breed year round, three kid crops every two years can be achieved resulting in an average of well over three kids per doe per year (Naude and Hofmeyr 1986). First fresheners very commonly produce single kids. Multiple births are considered undesirable under some range conditions because the kids are typically smaller and weaker and have poor survivability compared to singles. However, if the pregnant females are fed properly and are in good condition when they kid, the kids will be stronger, the dams will exhibit stronger maternal behaviour, and neonatal mortality will decline.

Reproductive wastage

There are few statistics published concerning the differences between ovulation rates, fertilization rates, rates of early embryonic death and pregnancy rates in goats. Information concerning fertilization rates is available in superovulated Angora donor goats (Armstrong *et al.* 1983a, b). Approximately 88% of recovered embryos were fertilized. However, fertilization failure with embryo transfer can be associated with hormonal and other influences not present in the cycling animal. In one study of cycling Angora goats, 20% of ovulation points in bred nannies were not represented by an embryo at 25–30 days after breeding (Shelton and Stewart 1973). There can be a great deal of variation between ranches in these types of statistics, demonstrating the importance of nutrition and management in improving reproductive efficiency. The occurrence of fertilization failure or early embryonic death due to heat stress has been poorly documented. One study using real-time ultrasound in a dairy goat herd showed a pregnancy rate of 97% at 23 days after breeding but a kidding rate of only 77% (Bretzlaff *et al.* 1985). Most of the losses occurred in small, undersized doelings.

Some of the greatest documented losses occur in Angora goats where young pregnant females undergo stress abortions at 90–120 days of gestation. The prevalence of abortion varies markedly between herds depending on management and nutrition. It can be 10% or much higher in some herds, especially if young, undersized females are bred. In unsupervised range flocks, actual kidding rates and stillbirth rates may be underestimated due to lack of observation and/or predators. Stillbirths may be very high due to certain infectious diseases such as chlamydiosis, or may be high in underfed does that are weak and have slow parturitions.

Clinical examination of the male

History

The history is a most important aspect of a breeding soundness examination of a buck. If the buck is less than 1 year old, the quantity of semen is expected to be only approximately 60% that of a mature animal. The number of females the animal has been exposed to, if any, and the pregnancy status of those females should be considered. Season of year is very important also, as scrotal circumference, semen quality and frequently libido decrease during the non-breeding season. Any past illnesses, especially during the previous 2 months, should be recorded. Even transient elevations in body temperature can cause a reversible testicular degeneration that reduces semen quality 6–8 weeks later.

Physical examination

The general physical examination should include evaluation of overall body condition, feet and legs, eyes, teeth and anything else that might influence the ability of the animal to obtain adequate nutrition, seek oestrous females, and successfully copulate. The genital examination can be conducted with the animal in a standing position, restrained on its side, or sitting on its rear end. Dairy bucks usually resist being restrained on their rear ends. The testicles and epididymes should be palpated and any scrotal lesions should be noted. The spermatic cords should also be examined as well as the penis and prepuce. The penis can be manually extended by pushing on the sigmoid flexure, which is located under the scrotum in bucks sitting on their rear ends. In standing bucks or bucks lying on their sides, the penis can be exteriorized by grasping it with one hand through the prepuce in front of the scrotum, pushing it cranially, then grasping it just behind the glans through the prepuce near the preputial opening with the opposite hand, pushing the sheath caudally and then grasping it again through the sheath with the first hand, and pushing cranially. This is continued until the glans is exposed and grasped with a gauze sponge. The penis should be fully extended and any defects in the penis, prepuce, or urethral process noted. The urethral process is not necessary for fertility, so the buck need not be culled if the process is abnormally short or is missing.

Typical scrotal circumferences of fertile bucks during the breeding season tend to be somewhat less than in sheep, with values from 28 to 35 cm commonly observed. This may be because goats have not been selected for scrotal circumference. Measurements may decrease by several centimetres during the non-breeding season or during the breeding season if the animal has been used heavily for breeding just prior to the examination.

Semen collection

Semen is easily collected with an artificial vagina (AV) from tractable bucks (Figure 5.4). The use of the AV results in the most representative sample and is not stressful to the buck. However, it requires the presence of an oestrous female in most cases and is more time-consuming than electroejaculation due to the buck training required.

Electroejaculators can be successfully used in goats, but may result in

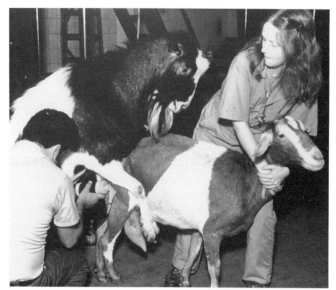

Figure 5.4 Semen collection by artificial vagina using a 'jump' doe as teaser.

ejaculates diluted by excess seminal fluids. Electroejaculators are traumatic to many bucks, and may result in rectal bleeding. Sedation may
alleviate the distress of some bucks. Xylazine at 0.05–0.1 mg/kg intramuscularly can be used but is not without risk due to its cardiovascular and
respiratory side-effects, and due to its potential to cause bloat in unfasted
animals. Alternatively, diazepam can be used at 0.8–2.0 mg/kg intramuscularly. Electroejaculator probes that can be connected to adjustable
power supplies for bulls are preferred to hand-held battery operated
models that have one power setting and are either on or off. Some probes
made for rams are uncomfortably large for many young bucks.

Semen evaluation

Gross evaluation

Semen should be collected in as small a receptacle as is practical to prevent
exposure of the small volume usually obtained to a large surface area.
Typical ejaculates are 0.5–3.0 ml in volume, depending on the age of the
buck and the frequency of collection. Semen should be kept warm (37°C)
and should only contact surfaces that are at the same temperature. Colour
and odour should be examined, with normal ejaculates having a greyish-
white to creamy colour and thick consistency. An unusual odour may

indicate that the buck has urinated (which may happen during electro-ejaculation) or that an infectious or necrotizing disease is present. Volume should also be recorded and would be expected to be smaller in young bucks, undernourished bucks, or frequently used bucks (Evans and Maxwell 1987).

Concentration

Concentration can be estimated visually by the opacity and viscosity of the sample, or more precisely by either a spectrophotometer calibrated for small ruminants or a haemocytometer. The concentration of spermatozoa in good ejaculates is $2.5-5\times10^9$/ml.

Motility

Gross motility (wave motion) should be evaluated by examining a drop of semen under low power on a microscope. A good sample will demonstrate the 'blizzard' effect due to the high concentration of buck semen. A drop of semen can then be diluted in extender or an isotonic solution such as saline and evaluated under a coverslip with higher power for the percentage of individual cells exhibiting progressive motility. This number is frequently 90% or greater during the breeding season, although numbers as low as 70% are deemed acceptable. Progressive motility may drop to 50% during the non-breeding season.

Morphology

A small drop of semen and a drop of an appropriate stain, such as eosin–nigrosin, should be gently mixed at the end of a slide and drawn out over the slide in preparation for evaluation of sperm morphology. Abnormal cells occur as in other species and include head defects, bent and otherwise abnormal midpieces, coiled tails, proximal and distal cytoplasmic droplets, and acrosomal abnormalities. The number of normal cells is commonly in excess of 90% during the breeding season in fertile bucks. A minimum acceptable figure would be 70% normal cells according to guidelines for other domestic ruminants. This may change drastically during the non-breeding season, and may explain why semen collected during the non-breeding season often does not freeze well.

Libido

Libido often is not evaluated during examinations of range animals, but should not be overlooked as an important component of male fertility.

Owners should be encouraged to observe their bucks with oestrous females. Libido can be evaluated during collection of tractable bucks with an AV, a distinct advantage of using this method of collection. Libido is seasonal in many bucks, especially those not collected or used on oestrous females continuously throughout the year. Libido can be induced during the non-breeding season in many bucks over a period of 1–2 weeks by exposing them to oestrous females, but should not be evaluated for purposes of a breeding soundness examination during this time of year.

Clinical examination of the female

History

Because of the inaccessibility of the majority of the female tract, the history is an especially important part of the examination. Documentation of interoestrus intervals, duration of heats, reaction of the female to the male or to other females in heat, breedings, fertility of the male or semen used, and AI techniques should be accomplished. Season of the year, nutrition, previous kiddings, stage of lactation and amount of milk being produced must all be considered.

Physical examination

The general physical examination includes the body condition of the animal together with an estimation of body condition during recent months. Femininity of the animal should be considered. It is important to ascertain whether the animal is polled or horned due to the association of intersexuality with the gene for polledness.

The external genital examination should include evaluation of the anogenital distance and whether the clitoris is visible without parting the lips of the vulva. These parameters can assist in a diagnosis of intersexuality (see p. 200). A vaginal speculum examination should be conducted to determine whether the vagina is complete and whether there are any membranes or adhesions present up to the level of the cervix. The presence of any discharges from the cervix or vagina should be noted. Many does resent the passing of a vaginal speculum, so the use of an endoscope may be preferable if available.

Ultrasonography

Real-time ultrasound, if available, can be used transabdominally to determine if a pregnancy, pseudopregnancy (hydrometra or mucometra) or pyometra is present. Transrectal use of a linear-array transducer may allow evaluation of ovaries, especially if follicular cysts are suspected. Transducers with 7.5 MHz capabilities are best suited for this purpose.

Surgical/autopsy examination of the reproductive tract

Because of the occurrence of intersexuality in goats, a definitive diagnosis of infertility sometimes cannot be made without examining the entire reproductive tract, especially the gonads. This may be accomplished by laparotomy in the living animal, although one gonad may need to be examined histologically for a final determination. Most intersex goats are male pseudohermaphrodites with testicular tissue in their gonads. Aberrant locations of the gonads in the inguinal region and varying degrees of maldevelopment of the internal reproductive tract may be observed. Laparotomy may also be the only way to document cystic ovaries if real-time ultrasound is not available, or to identify other conditions such as adhesions or abscesses that may involve the reproductive tract.

Infertility of individual females

Does are most commonly presented for infertility during the mid to late breeding season. The complaint is usually that the doe either has not been observed to cycle, that she has irregular cycles, or that she cycles normally but does not become pregnant despite being bred. Other common problems for which individual females may be presented include failure to observe oestrus in females that are induced with hormones, observation of abortions or a vulvar discharge, or failure of an expected kidding.

Failure to observe oestrus during the breeding season

Females may be not observed to cycle during a breeding season for several reasons:

- Anoestrus:
   Lack of male to induce cyclicity,

> Presence of night lights that prevent exposure to natural
> decrease in day length,
> Poor nutrition,
> Intersexuality.
- Missed heats:
  Poor heat detection,
  Lack of male.
- Pregnant
- Pseudopregnant with a persistent corpus luteum.

Does presented for failure to cycle should always be examined for pregnancy before significant effort is spent on other diagnostic techniques. Determination of concentrations of peripheral progesterone can be helpful in differentiating between reasons for failure to observe oestrus. Plasma/serum or milk progesterone concentrations may be determined although plasma/serum concentrations may be more reliable. With a commercially available enzyme-linked progesterone assay, determinations of whether a functional corpus luteum was present by milk progesterone levels were in agreement with determinations made by plasma progesterone levels in 79% of the samples tested in dairy goats (Bretzlaff *et al.* 1989).

A series of six progesterone tests taken every 4 days from a doe demonstrates her progesterone profile over the period of one normal caprine oestrous cycle (20 days). If a series of six progesterone tests taken every 4 days from a doe shows consistently low concentrations, then the animal is not cycling normally and cannot be pregnant or pseudopregnant. If her external genitalia appear normal so that a diagnosis of intersexuality is not obvious, her nutritional status and history of exposure to a buck should be examined. If a male has not been present, introduction of a buck will usually induce ovulation within 3 days. If the female is routinely kept in an area with night-time security lights, moving her to an area that is not lighted at night may allow her to start cycling.

Intersexuality

If the animal is polled and especially if it is known that she is the offspring of two polled parents, the intersex condition should be suspected. The gene for intersexuality is linked to the gene for polledness. The polled gene is dominant, so a polled animal can be heterozygous (one polled gene and one gene for the horned condition) or homozygous for the polled gene. Animals that are homozygous for the polled gene (one polled gene from each parent so that both parents must have had at least one polled gene and therefore were polled) are most likely to have the intersex condition.

Most intersex goats are male pseudohermaphrodites, having male gonadal tissue but having phenotypic characteristics of both sexes. Many intersex goats are phenotypically more like females than males. However, they may show a somewhat masculine appearance to the head and neck, an increased anogenital distance (≥ 3 cm), and/or a bulbous clitoris that is visible between the lips of the vulva. Vaginal examination reveals an atretic vagina in many of these animals. Intersex animals that are phenotypically more male may have small partially descended testes in the inguinal region or in a short scrotum. The urethral opening may appear in the perineal area or in the ventral midline somewhere caudal to where a normal preputial opening should be. These animals may be prone to urinary problems and/or urine scald of the rear limbs. The condition can be prevented to a large degree by breeding polled animals only to horned animals.

Pseudopregnancy

If all six progesterone tests taken every 4 days indicate elevated levels of progesterone, the doe is most likely pregnant or pseudopregnant. Pseudopregnancy is a poorly understood phenomenon in which a doe ovulates, may or may not be bred, and does not return to oestrus even though she is not pregnant. In the classical pseudopregnancy, the uterus slowly fills with fluid that is 'delivered' after approximately the length of a normal gestation (frequently referred to as a 'cloudburst'). In these cases, the condition is easily diagnosed with real-time ultrasound by observation of a fluid-filled uterus with no foetus or placentomes. In other cases, the doe may spontaneously resolve the persistent corpus luteum after a varying period of time and return to oestrus after a prolonged interoestrus interval. A haemorrhagic discharge may be observed at the vulva at this time even though the animal was not pregnant. If a pseudopregnancy is diagnosed, the treatment of choice is prostaglandin. The majority of animals will rebreed and carry a normal pregnancy if the breeding season has not passed. However, there are a few individuals in which pseudopregnancy tends to recur.

Pregnancy

If continually elevated progesterone concentrations are obtained and real-time ultrasound is not available, an oestrone sulphate test can differentiate between pregnancy and pseudopregnancy. The concentration of oestrone sulphate will be elevated 50 days after ovulation in a pregnant doe and not in a pseudopregnant doe.

Unobserved oestrus

If the six progesterone samples taken every 4 days shows the expected rise and fall of progesterone that occurs during the normal oestrous cycle, the animal is most likely cycling normally. If this is the case, the fertility of the male or of the semen used and insemination technique should be evaluated. Her reaction to the buck when progesterone levels decline should be observed also as a few does exhibit buck preferences to the point that they will not allow a non-preferred buck to serve them. If a normally cycling female that is bred by a known fertile male continually fails to conceive, diagnosis of the problem can be difficult. If the doe has never had kids, the possibility of a congenital defect of the reproductive tract exists. If the doe has had kids before, she may have had a dystocia with resultant damage to the reproductive tract and/or a chronic endometritis. In either case, a laparotomy or at least laparoscopy would be necessary to evaluate structures other than the vagina. If no anatomical or infectious problems can be discerned it would be possible to superovulate and flush the doe to document whether fertilized embryos are reaching the uterus. However, this would be cost prohibitive in most animals.

Observation of short oestrous cycles

A doe presented for irregular cycles is most commonly exhibiting short cycles, i.e. having interoestrus intervals of less than 18 days. Typically these intervals are 4–7 days in length. If daily progesterone concentrations were being determined, these 'cycles' would show a short, 1-day increase from a low to a moderately elevated concentration of progesterone, then back to a low concentration. Many goats have one short cycle at the onset of the breeding season. This is a normal phenomenon. Does that abort for any reason during the breeding season will commonly exhibit one or multiple short cycles. If enough of the breeding season remains (at least 1 month), most of these does will eventually exhibit a normal cycle once uterine involution has occurred. Does that are superovulated may also be observed to short cycle (Armstrong *et al.* 1983). If a doe exhibits short cycles under other than these circumstances, it is generally assumed that she has follicular cysts or a chronic endometritis. Cystic ovaries are poorly documented in goats due to the inaccessibility of the ovaries to palpation. With the increasing use of transrectal ultrasound in dairy goats, more information on this condition may be forthcoming. In the mean time it is generally recommended to administer one-fourth to one-half the cow dose of gonadotrophin-releasing hormone to does in which a diagnosis of cystic ovaries has been made. Chronic endometritis theoretically results in endometrial irritation and release of prostaglandin. Attempts to culture cervical discharge can be made followed by treatment with appropriate antimicrobials. If the doe is showing a rather constant sexual activity and is demonstrating unusual libido toward other does running with her, the possibility of the intersex condition should also be considered.

Failure to respond to prostaglandin

Failure of does to exhibit oestrus after being given prostaglandin can usually be explained by the doe not having a functional corpus luteum at the time of the injection.

Prolonged interoestrus intervals

Abnormally long interoestrus intervals that are not due to missed heats are generally discussed as being due to early embryonic deaths (see p. 188).

Abortion

An abortion rate of up to 5% may be considered a 'normal' occurrence but if more than one animal in a herd aborts it is recommended that aborted foetuses, foetal membranes, serum from weak newborns prior to suckling and maternal serum be submitted to a diagnostic laboratory for examination. Because goats are seasonal breeders and tend to be in a similar stage of gestation in late winter and spring, an outbreak can spread rapidly to susceptible animals and have devastating consequences. An aborting animal should be isolated immediately and the remainder of the herd removed from the area where the abortion occurred if at all possible. Uterine discharges are teeming with organisms in most cases of infectious abortion.

It is beyond the scope of this chapter to review all aspects of the aetiologies, treatments and methods of prevention of abortion in goats. Where more details are desired, the reader is directed to selected references (East 1983; Morrow 1986; Roberts 1986; Smith and Sherman 1994).

Nutrition

In rangeland areas where goats are on marginal nutrition, certain deficiencies can contribute to abortions. General malnutrition as well as vitamin A deficiency, manganese deficiency and iodine deficiency have been associated with abortions, stillbirths or birth of weak newborns (Smith 1986). Abortions in Angoras are frequently associated with low planes of nutrition, small body size and stress (Shelton 1986).

Toxic plants and chemical agents

In selected areas, toxic plants are associated with abortions and/or the birth of deformed kids. Locoweeds (*Astragalus* sp. and *Oxytropis* sp.) and broomweed (*Gutierrezia* sp.) have been associated with these problems in goats (Roberts 1986). Certain drugs, such as phenothiazine and carbon tetrachloride, should not be administered to pregnant goats.

Stress

Goats should not be subjected to stressful procedures during late gestation as stress alone can precipitate abortions. Hair goats should be shorn at least 2–3 weeks prior to onset of the kidding season for this reason.

Infectious abortion

There are a number of infectious causes of abortion in goats:

- chlamydiosis,
- toxoplasmosis,
- listeriosis,
- leptospirosis,
- Q fever (*Coxiella burnetii*),
- salmonellosis,
- mycoplasmosis,
- campylobacteriosis (rare in goats),
- brucellosis (*Brucella melitensis*, rare in the USA),
- *Sarcocystis* (protozoal parasite),
- akabane,
- foot and mouth disease,
- heartwater,
- peste des petits ruminants,
- Rift Valley fever,
- Wesselsbron disease.

The history and physical examination are extremely important in cases of abortion outbreaks in order to characterize the disease and arrive at the differential diagnosis. A number of factors aid in the selection of the most likely causative agent (Table 5.2).

The treatment and control of the various causes of abortion vary depending on the nature of the organism/cause and on the efficacy of natural immunity (Table 5.3).

Care must be taken in basing the diagnosis of an abortion on serologic

Table 5.2 Factors aiding in the differential diagnosis of abortion

Factor	Comments
Stage of gestation	Many aetiological agents associated with late-term abortions. Toxoplasmosis associated with losses throughout gestation including resorption or foetal mummification
Presence of illness	Abortion associated with stress of systemic illness in aborting females with diseases such as leptospirosis, mycoplasmosis, sarcocystis, salmonellosis, etc. Dams not seriously ill with chlamydiosis, toxoplasmosis, Q fever
Distribution of placental lesions	Non-specific with most diseases. Toxoplasmosis with pinpoint lesions in cotyledonary areas only
Identification of sources of stress	Predator attacks Severe weather
Condition of aborted offspring	Many diseases associated with birth of autolysed foetuses plus some stillbirths and live, weak newborns. Toxoplasmosis may also show birth of normal kids or mummified foetuses. Skeletal and neurological defects may implicate toxic plants or viral agents, although these are less well documented in goats than in sheep

Table 5.3 Approach to prevention and treatment of abortion

Cause	Remarks
Nutrition	Correct deficiency
Toxic plants	Restrict access to infested pasture Supplement feed so animals are not forced to graze undesirable plants
Infectious agents	Isolate aborting animals Identify vaccine (chlamydiosis) Identify treatment (tetracycline for chlamydiosis or Q fever) in outbreak Prevent exposure (hygiene; prevent cats from defecating in feed to prevent toxoplasmosis) Prevent stress (salmonellosis)

tests in the dam for toxoplasmosis, chlamydiosis or Q fever. Elevated titres can be obtained from apparently healthy animals giving birth to apparently healthy kids.

Pseudopregnancy

The failure to kid in the occasional animal that was thought to be pregnant can be due to pseudopregnancy in the goat.

Infertility of individual males

Scrotal abnormalities

Palpable abnormalities of the external genitalia should be identified. Scrotal inflammation due to mange, frostbite, chemical contamination of bedding, trauma or abscesses can adversely affect the testicles and therefore semen quality.

Testicular and epididymal abnormalities

Cryptorchidism is a heritable condition in Angora goats, probably a recessive trait with incomplete penetrance (Roberts 1986). Such animals should be culled. Other testicular abnormalities include orchitis, testicular hypoplasia or degeneration and, rarely, neoplasia (Memon 1983). These conditions are associated with an asymmetry of the testicles, abnormal size (large or small) and/or abnormal consistency. Epididymitis can also be identified by palpation of abnormally large or asymmetric epididymes. Orchitis and/or epididymitis may be associated with the occurrence of white blood cells in the ejaculate. Attempts to culture a causative organism from the semen may or may not be successful. These conditions are difficult to treat once palpable lesions are present.

With unilateral conditions, inflammation on one side may lead to a reversible degeneration of the opposite testicle. Unilateral castration may allow regeneration of the normal testicle.

Testicular degeneration may be caused by hyperthermia, whether environmental or due to an infectious process. The condition is evidenced by small, soft testicles and semen with a high percentage of abnormal cells, especially major defects such as abnormal heads, proximal droplets and coiled tails. These bucks should be retested in 60 days, as regeneration can occur.

Bucks with small testicles that have never developed to normal size have hypoplastic testicles. This is frequently associated with intersexuality (see p. 200). These animals are frequently sterile and should be culled.

An enlarged head of the epididymis may be associated with sperm granulomas in the buck, caused by accumulation of sperm in blind efferent ductules. This condition can be associated with intersexuality.

Abnormalities of the prepuce and penis

In hair goats, abnormalities of the prepuce and penis are often associated with shearing injuries. Ulcerative posthitis can affect the prepuce of goats and when healed can result in preputial strictures resulting in phimosis. This disease is associated with high dietary protein, which results in elevated levels of urea in the urine. *Corynebacterium renale* in the prepuce hydrolyse the urea to ammonia, which irritates the preputial mucosa. Affected animals should be changed to a lower protein diet and observed for preputial strictures. This condition is more common in wethers than in intact males.

Congenital abnormalities of the penis or prepuce such as hypospadias or a shortened penis may be associated with intersexuality.

Urinary calculi may lodge in the urethral process of male goats. The urethral process may slough off or be cut off to alleviate the blockage. Removal of the urethral process has not been shown to be detrimental to fertility.

Group infertility

When a large number of animals in a herd are infertile, the economic consequences can be devastating. The history and examination of the general condition of the animals are very important.

The time of year in which the problem is occurring should be considered, in addition to knowledge of whether the female animals are cycling. If the complaint is that the females are not cycling, the possibility of pregnancy must be considered first. If that is ruled out, the quality of heat detection must be determined. Progesterone tests from a representative sampling of the females should document whether the females are cycling. On a given day, 55–65% of a group of cycling does should have elevated progesterone concentrations. If this is found to be the case, yet the animals are reported not to be cycling, then an aggressive teaser animal with a marking harness should be introduced to document whether females are actually cycling or not.

If the majority of females have low progesterone, they are probably not cycling. Lack of exposure to a male or exposure to excessive lighting at night could cause this during the breeding season. Animals in poor condition and/or animals kidding during recent months could also explain this.

If females are seen to cycle, are bred and are returning to oestrus, the fertility of the buck should be investigated. If the buck appears to have good semen quality, his interaction with the does should be observed. Bucks with poor libido or young inexperienced bucks may not be serving all does in oestrus. Social interactions should also be evaluated as dominant does may prevent young or timid does from interacting with the buck. Bucks in poor body condition may not have the energy to seek does in oestrus under extensive rangeland conditions. Multisire systems may alleviate problems with individual buck infertility except in cases where dominant bucks are subfertile or infertile.

In rangeland hair goats, the pregnancy rate is often estimated by observation of udder development at shearing 2–4 weeks prior to the kidding season. If the pregnancy rate at this time is low, it is often assumed some stress abortions have occurred. However, it is difficult to make accurate diagnoses at this point in time. If there is a large discrepancy between the number predicted to be pregnant at shearing and the number of females that have kids at weaning, the difference is often attributed to predators. If this is the case, guard animals should be introduced to the herd and/or animals should be brought in for supervised kidding.

6 EQUINE FERTILITY AND INFERTILITY
S J STONEHAM BVSc, Cert. ESM, MRCVS

The non-pregnant mare
The pregnant mare
The barren mare
Early embryonic/foetal death
Abortion
Venereal diseases of stallions and mares
The stallion
Artificial insemination
Embryo transfer
Drug appendix

The non-pregnant mare

Introduction

Fillies reach puberty at about 18 months of age. The exact time will depend on nutrition and the time of year that the filly was born. Thoroughbred fillies born early in the year reach puberty during their second summer, whereas pony foals (often born later in the year) would not reach puberty until the second spring.

Fillies are not usually mated until they are 3 years old. Some Thoroughbred fillies in training do not become sexually mature until they are 3–4 years old.

Seasonality

Mares are seasonally polyoestrous long-day breeders. A long daily photoperiod during the anovulatory season (winter) will hasten the onset of the ovulatory season. Pony mares show a more marked difference between the anovulatory (anoestrus) and ovulatory season. Warmbloods and some Thoroughbreds show little seasonal variation.

In the UK the Jockey Club have imposed 1 January as the birth date of all Thoroughbred foals thereby placing those animals born later in the year at a disadvantage. The imposed breeding season for the Thoroughbred is 15 February to 15 July, some 2 months earlier than the natural breeding season. As a result considerable efforts are made by stud managers and veterinary surgeons to hasten the onset of the ovulatory season.

Considerable research has gone into this subject and current recommendations to hasten onset of the ovulatory season are as follows.

1. Housing the mares from around winter solstice (21 December) and lighting the stable using a bright white light (200–250 W). The stable should have light walls to increase reflection of the light. Neither ultraviolet or infrared light are effective.
2. A sudden increase in photoperiod to give 16 hours light and 8 hours darkness. Work by Palmer *et al.* (1982) showed that a 1-hour period of light, 9.5–10.5 hours after darkness had a similar effect.
3. It takes 8–10 weeks to hasten the change from anoestrus to ovulatory season.
4. Hastening mares into anoestrus as early as possible by reducing nutrition and decreasing temperature.
5. Providing a rising plane of nutrition including any available grass. Some people have advocated the use of hydroponic grass; however scientific data is limited.

The normal oestrous cycle

The oestrous cycle in the mare shows considerable variation in length. The dioestrous phase under progesterone influence has a fairly constant length, on average 15 days in horses and 16 days in ponies. The oestrus phase shows more marked variation, 2–11 days with an average of 5–7 days in horses. Ovulation in the mare occurs at a variable time after the onset of oestrus, therefore day 0 is taken as the day of ovulation throughout this chapter. The main endocrine changes that occur during the oestrous cycle are set out below.

Luteinizing hormone (LH)

Circulating levels are low at mid-dioestrus rising a few days before oestrus, peaking at ovulation and slowly falling to minimum levels at the next mid-dioestrus.

Follicle stimulating hormone (FSH)

FSH levels peak near ovulation and decrease to low levels 10–11 days after ovulation.

Progesterone

Progesterone is secreted by the corpus luteum; levels start to rise 24 hours after ovulation, and peak 5–7 days after ovulation. Levels are maintained until luteolysis on day 12–14, when they fall rapidly to less than 1 ng/ml during oestrus.

Oestradiol

Levels start to rise 6–8 days prior to ovulation and peak 2 days prior to ovulation. They fall to minimum levels following ovulation.

Prostaglandin $F_{2\alpha}$ (PGF_{2a})

Levels rise from day 10–14 and then rapidly fall. The presence of a viable embryo in the uterus at this stage prevents prostaglandin release.

Changes in the genital tract during the oestrous cycle

Ovarian changes

Several follicles start to develop during mid-dioestrus; one of these follicles starts to increase more rapidly and is destined to become the ovulatory follicle. During the oestrous phase of the cycle the ovulatory follicle continues to increase in size and is palpably tense. As ovulation approaches the follicle usually starts to soften and becomes wedge-shaped pointing towards the ovulation fossa. The follicle rarely ovulates until it is over 3 cm in diameter. The follicle then collapses, the ova passing into the oviduct via the ovarian bursa, which engulfs the ovulating follicle. The collapsed follicle fills with blood (corpus haemorrhagicum) which then luteinizes from the outside inwards. The other follicles undergo atresia 6–8 days prior to ovulation. Unlike the cow the corpus luteum is not palpable.

During anoestrus the ovaries are small and hard, with no palpable follicles.

Changes in the tubular genital tract

During oestrus the vulva lengthens and there is some loss of muscle tone of the vulval lips. During dioestrus the vulva appears to shorten due to increased muscular tone in the vulval lips. It is important to remember this when assessing vulval conformation.

The vagina becomes increasingly moist and hyperaemic during oestrus, with increased mucus secretion. During dioestrus the vagina is pale pink and slightly dry.

Table 6.1 Typical changes in the appearance of the cervix during the oestrous cycle

Appearance of cervix	Stage in oestrous cycle	Scoring system for cervix
Pale, dry, projecting finger-like into vagina	Dioestrus or early pregnancy	CT
Pale pink, some oedema of cervix, losing tone and falling from horizontal towards vaginal floor	Early oestrus or early dioestrus. Consider behaviour and follicular development	CR– pale
Pink, hyperaemic, glistening with marked oedema. Relaxed, lying on floor of vagina	Oestrus. Fit to cover if behaviour and follicular development appropriate	CR–pink
Pink, glistening and hyperaemic but still with some tone	Some mares, particularly maidens, show no further relaxation of cervix. Consider follicular development and behavioural signs	CR– –pink

CT, cervix tight; CR, cervix relaxed.

During oestrus the uterus loses tone and the endometrial folds become oedematous early in oestrus giving a typical 'cartwheel' appearance on ultrasound scan. During dioestrus, uterine tone increases and the uterus has a homogeneous appearance on ultrasound scan.

Table 6.1 shows the changes in appearance of the cervix during the oestrous cycle.

Behavioural changes during the oestrous cycle

Behavioural changes are routinely detected using a 'teaser'. This is usually a stallion not used for breeding; many people prefer to use a pony stallion. On some small establishments the working stallion may be used if temperamentally suitable. Both the teaser and mare are restrained using a bridle.

The mare to be teased is presented initially head to head to the teaser, separated by a solid partition ('teasing bar'). The teaser will then smell and lick the mare and her behaviour is observed. When the mare is in oestrus she will usually lift her tail and move it laterally, squat and pass frequent small quantities of urine. The clitoris is everted ('winking') and many mares will present their perineum to the teaser. These signs increase in intensity until ovulation occurs although a significant number of mares will continue to exhibit oestrous behaviour for 24–48 hours after ovulation.

During dioestrus the mare will be aggressive towards the teaser, squealing and kicking out.

It is essential to take in to account those mares that fail to exhibit oestrous behaviour to a teaser; this is particularly common in 'foal-proud' mares and maiden mares early in the breeding season.

Covering

Once it has been decided that the mare is ready to be mated she is restrained on a bridle, her tail bandaged, and perineum washed using plain warm water. She is then taken to the covering barn. Many stud farms then put large padded boots on her hind feet, apply a twitch and a quick-release leg strap to hold up a foreleg until the stallion mounts. If the stallion is particularly aggressive a leather neck cover can be used to protect the mare.

The stallion is then brought round to her left side; most stallions will rapidly mount the mare. Some aggressive, vigorous stallions require some restraint particularly with maiden and nervous mares. Care must be taken that the stallion does not enter the mare's rectum; some stallions need guiding into the vagina particularly with a mare who has had vulvoplasty. The pulsatile waves of ejaculation should be palpated on the ventral shaft of the penis. This is usually accompanied by 'tail flagging' by the stallion. Care should be taken as the stallion dismounts to avoid the mare kicking him.

Routine prebreeding examination

Veterinary examination is usually carried out early in oestrus to determine optimum time for mating, and to take necessary cervical and clitoral swabs. It is useful for the management to correlate behavioural changes with follicular development, and allows matings to be planned and reduce overuse of the stallion.

The mare should be restrained on a bridle and an attendant wearing disposable gloves should hold the tail and position the hindquarters. Many clinicians prefer the mare in stocks where possible. Adequate protective clothing should be worn and disposable full-length rectal sleeves. It is important that the examination is thorough and methodical; appropriate details should be recorded to allow maximum information to be gained from serial examinations. The following routine may be useful when a mare is first presented for examination.

1. Take a clitoral swab using a narrow-tipped swab to penetrate the clitoral sinuses and fossa. Place swab in Amies charcoal transport medium for culture.
2. Clean perineum with water and assess vulval conformation taking

into consideration stage of oestrous cycle and body condition. (If detomidine has been used to sedate the mare there will be considerable loss of vulval tone.)

3. Use a disposable speculum to examine the vagina and cervix. Note appearance of cervix and check for cervical incompetence. Take cervical swabs for cytology and bacteriology, using a plain swab for cytology and placing the swab for bacteriology in Amies transport medium. Unguarded swabs with an extension rod are adequate.

4. Carry out a rectal examination using obstetric lubricant and taking care with the relatively thin-walled rectum. Provided the mare is adequately restrained, adequate lubrication used, the examination stopped when the mare strains and care taken with manipulations, the incidence of rectal tears will be minimized. Once faeces have been cleared from the rectum the clinician should identify the cervix and the body of the uterus and then follow each horn to the ovary. Careful palpation of the ovaries will allow detection and assessment of follicles. Their approximate size and turgidity should be recorded. Corpora lutea are not palpable. Recent ovulations may be palpable as a soft, tender spot on the ovary. The routine use of ultrasound has facilitated the accurate detection of ovulation.

5. Many clinicians like to carry out ultrasound examination of the reproductive tract to allow detection of endometrial cysts, intrauterine fluid accumulations and to allow visualization of follicles (see Table 6.1.).

Information gained at this examination should be taken in conjunction with behavioural changes to determine optimal time for mating. Mating should ideally take place during the 24-hour period prior to ovulation. The follicle will frequently soften, losing its turgidity during the 24 hours prior to ovulation. It is unusual for follicles less than 3 cm to ovulate. There is no substitute for experience in predicting pending ovulation. However, serial examinations, the use of ultrasound and careful evaluation of all the information will assist the inexperienced clinician.

Examining the mare on alternate days is usually adequate; however if the information is confusing, examination on consecutive days may be helpful.

Hormone assays

Progesterone

Plasma progesterone levels may provide useful additional information on stage of the cycle, whether ovulation has occurred (levels rise within 24 hours of ovulation), and the end of the anovulatory season. During the breeding season levels below 1 ng/ml are consistent with oestrus. During the anovulatory season levels below 1 ng/ml are usual and are not accompanied by signs of oestrus.

Oestradiol

A commercial assay has recently become available. Oestradiol levels rise during oestrus and then start to fall prior to ovulation. Monitoring levels can be used to assist prediction of pending ovulation. However, experience in practice has suggested that its use is limited and rectal palpation in conjunction with ultrasound examination is more accurate at predicting ovulation.

Management of ovulation

Ovulation in the mare occurs at a variable time after the onset of oestrus. Veterinary intervention has focused on attempting to predict pending ovulation in order to minimize matings per oestrous period and for synchronization during embryo transfer. Several drugs have been used to attempt to hasten ovulation at a predictable time following their administration.

Human chorionic gonadotrophin (hCG)

Studies have shown that 3000 iu hCG (Chorulon, Intervet, UK) administered intravenously will induce ovulation of follicles over 3 cm in diameter within 24–48 hours of administration. Ideally it should be administered 24 hours prior to mating; however when natural covering is used one must be confident that no unforeseen circumstance (e.g. injury to stallion) will prevent mating in that period. Many clinicians prefer to administer hCG immediately after mating for this reason. When artificial insemination (AI) is used this is not a consideration.

Some follicles appear to be refractory to hCG and repeat dosing does not induce ovulation. Work has shown that at this dose rate fertility is not affected by hCG administration. Administration of hCG on more than three consecutive oestrous cycles may induce antibody formation in some mares with consequent loss of efficacy. These antibodies do not appear to affect the innate mechanisms triggering ovulation.

Gonadotrophin releasing hormone (GnRH)

A synthetic releasing hormone analogue, buserelin (Receptal, Hoechst Animal Health, UK), has been used in the past but work has shown it to be less effective in hastening ovulation than hCG. However it is occasionally used in mares that appear to have developed anti-hCG antibodies. The recommended dose is 0.04 mg (10 ml Receptal) intravenously 6 hours prior to mating.

Abnormalities of the oestrous cycle

Prolonged anoestrus

Signs

The ovaries are small and hard with no follicular development. Progesterone levels are persistently below 1 ng/ml.

Aetiology

The mismatch between the natural breeding season and imposed breeding season in the Thoroughbred accounts for this problem. Older mares have also been shown to come out of anoestrus later than young mares.

Treatment

See checklist for hastening the onset of the ovulatory season (p. 210). It has been shown that there may be a lag factor and events 1 year before can influence the period of anoestrus. Recently, GnRH slow-release preparations and minipumps have been used with some success; however they are not currently commercially available.

Transitional oestrus

Signs

This occurs between winter anoestrus and the normal ovulatory season; it may also occur at the end of the breeding season prior to winter anoestrus. Mares exhibit behavioural signs of oestrus for a prolonged period (10 days or more). Typically the ovaries have numerous small follicles often described as 'a bunch of grapes'. Even if one or more of the follicles enlarge they are frequently unresponsive to hCG and undergo atresia without ovulating.

Aetiology

This is a normal feature of the transition from anovulatory to ovulatory season. It causes concern to the Thoroughbred owner who wants the mare mated as early in the season as possible.

Treatment

Mares are rarely fertile at this time. Administration of exogenous progesterone to suppress follicular activity for 10 days usually results in a normal oestrus period 3–8 days after the withdrawal of exogenous progesterone. The most convenient and widely used method is oral administration of altrenogest (Regumate, Hoechst Animal Health) at a dose of 0.044 mg/kg for 10 days. This treatment is not effective in anoestrous mares.

Silent oestrus

Signs

This occurs when the mare fails to exhibit behavioural signs of oestrus despite normal follicular development and ovulation. It is most frequently seen in intensively managed mares.

Aetiology

Mares fail to exhibit signs of behavioural oestrus for several reasons: maiden mares that are inadequately teased, 'foal-proud' mares, change of environment and management, inappropriate handling.

Treatment

Careful handling and management with regular veterinary examinations is essential. It may be useful to monitor these mares using plasma progesterone levels. Most of these mares will accept the stallion at the optimal time for mating; however sedation may be necessary. Oestradiol-17β administered intramuscularly (5–10 mg) may improve behavioural signs in some cases.

Prolonged dioestrus

Signs

Failure to return to oestrus at the expected time in mares that have been diagnosed as non-pregnant, or mares that have not been mated. Plasma progesterone levels are greater than 1 ng/ml.

Aetiology

Ginther (1990) considered that periods of prolonged luteal activity can be subdivided as follows:

- development of a secondary corpus luteum during mid-dioestrus that is refractory to the luteolytic effects of prostaglandins;
- embryo loss, after maternal recognition of pregnancy, results in persistence of the primary corpus luteum;
- severe uterine pathology, e.g. pyometra, will result in reduced prostaglandin release, so failing to trigger luteolysis.

Treatment

The administration of exogenous prostaglandins is effective in inducing luteolysis in most cases. Uterine manipulation and uterine irrigation with saline solution can be used.

Lactational anoestrus

Signs

Mares go into anoestrus following the foal heat. The ovaries become small and hard, with no follicular development. Plasma progesterone levels are below 1 ng/ml.

Aetiology

Unknown but appears to be more likely to affect mares who foal early in the year.

Treatment

Treat in a similar way to those mares exhibiting prolonged seasonal anoestrus.

Failure to respond to exogenous prostaglandins

Signs

Mares fail to return to oestrus following prostaglandin administration.

Aetiology

Prostaglandin administration is a widely used method of oestrus control. However it is important to remember that prostaglandin will only induce luteolysis between days 5 and 12. Some mares appear to be refractory to prostaglandin until day 6 or 7. The onset of oestrus may be very rapid if there is a large (over 3.5 cm) follicle in the ovary. Ovulation may have occurred within 3 days of administration prior to the mare being examined. The speed of ovulation may also reduce the behavioural signs of oestrus.

Treatment

Examine the mare and take plasma progesterone levels; readminister prostaglandin when appropriate. The problem can be avoided by careful timing of administration and routine gynaecological examination at the time of administration.

The pregnant mare

Pregnancy diagnosis

Early pregnancy diagnosis in the mare has been facilitated by the widespread use of diagnostic ultrasound. The diagnosis and management of twin pregnancies has changed as a result of routine ultrasound examination. Day 0 is taken as the day of ovulation throughout this chapter.

Teasing

Most stud farms will 'tease' the mare from day 12. This can be a useful management guide, and is essential to detect mares returning to oestrus early. However mares in prolonged dioestrus or 'silent' oestrus fail to exhibit behavioural signs despite being non-pregnant.

Vaginal and rectal examination

As with any gynaecological examination the mare should be adequately restrained, many clinicians preferring stocks if available.

The cervix is examined via a speculum. In early pregnancy it is usually pale, dry and tightly closed, projecting rigidly into the vagina. However a few mares will have a moderately relaxed cervix early in pregnancy. A moist, relaxed, pink, oedematous cervix indicates return to oestrus.

In early pregnancy the ovaries are usually large and multifollicular; from day 80 they tend to be pulled craniad towards the midline by the gravid uterus.

The uterus should be carefully palpated from the tip of one horn to the opposite tip, and the body (Table 6.2). In some cases the uterus will be

Table 6.2 Typical changes in the uterus in early pregnancy

Days from ovulation	Typical findings on rectal examination
16–23	Increased tone, may be 'S' shaped, palpable 'bulge' at base of one (or both) horns from about 18 days. Pregnancy 'bulge' approximately 3–5 cm
28–35	Uterus remains turgid, bulge increasing in size. Pregnancy 'bulge' approximately 5–10 cm
42–50	Uterus becomes less turgid, bulge becoming oval and extending into both horns
60–70	Uterus become more flaccid, may be confused with bladder or a pyometra. Pregnancy extending into both horns and body of the uterus
100–200	Uterus pulled craniad and ventrally. Ovaries pulled towards midline
200 onwards	Uterus occupying large part of caudal abdomen. Foetus frequently can be palpated

'S' shaped so care must be taken to palpate the base of both horns. It is helpful to grade the tone of the uterus 16–25 days after ovulation (Table 6.3).

If there is any doubt about the diagnosis it is important to repeat the examination at a later stage or to confirm diagnosis by an alternative method.

There are some fractious mares or small ponies in which rectal examination is not safe for either the clinician or the mare. In these cases hormonal assays or, later in pregnancy, transabdominal ultrasound may be used.

Table 6.3 Scoring system used to grade uterine tone in early pregnancy diagnosis

Grade	Typical findings on rectal examination
A	Marked increase in uterine tone, often in the pelvis. May be 'S' shaped. Distinct bulge palpable. Most common in maiden and younger barren mares
B	Increased tone, no distinct bulge palpable. More common from 'foal heat' covering and in older barren mares
C	Poor tone, flaccid uterus. Typically described as 'roll of velvet'

Ultrasound examination

Most horse owners expect routine ultrasound examination. Not only does this allow earlier definitive diagnosis of pregnancy, it also allows detection of twins (see p. 226), the monitoring of the development of the foetus (Figures 6.1 and 6.2) and detection of early embryonic/foetal death.

It is important to develop a sound knowledge of developmental embryology of the horse, anatomy of the internal genitalia and familiarity with ultrasound images (Ginther 1986 and McGladdery and Rossdale 1992).

The technique is well accepted by mares accustomed to rectal examination. However for full benefit to be gained from the technique and to avoid errors being made, it is important that the correct facilities are available to the clinician.

Many clinicians prefer the mare restrained by a bridle in stocks to protect the equipment and clinician. The stocks should be situated under cover as sunlight on the screen may complicate interpretation; it will also protect the machine from rain and extreme cold. If clinicians are left-handed the ultrasound scanner should be set up on their right-hand side to allow a clear view of the screen while examining the mare. An inexperienced operator will find it helpful to have an additional attendant to operate the controls of the scanner.

It is important that ultrasound examination is thorough and methodical; with experience clinicians will develop their own technique. It may be helpful to use the following checklist for early pregnancy diagnosis by ultrasound.

1. Mare restrained adequately in appropriate location.
2. Ultrasound scanner set up and clearly visible to clinician.
3. Carry out routine visual examination of cervix and manual rectal examination to locate ovaries and uterus. Note appearance of cervix and uterine tone.
4. Evacuate all faeces from rectum.
5. Introduce probe, establish position of uterus and ovaries. Carefully sweep probe from one ovary down uterine horn and up opposite horn to the other ovary. Repeat this sweep paying particular attention to the base of each horn. Locate and scan the body of the uterus caudally towards the cervix. Remember when scanning mares less than 18 days after ovulation that the embryo may be mobile and smaller than expected if a second later ovulation has occurred.
6. Photograph findings, record position and size of the embryo. Note any other abnormalities, e.g. endometrial cysts.

The timing of ultrasound examinations is largely a matter of personal

17-day conceptus

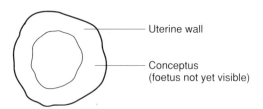
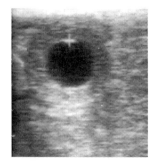

22-day conceptus

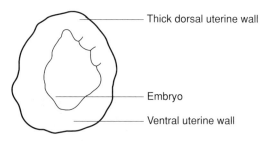
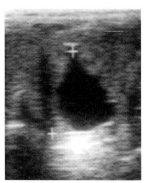

26-day conceptus

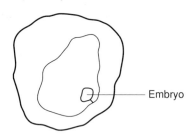
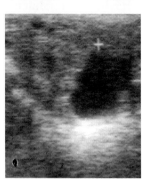

32-day conceptus

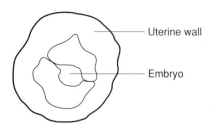
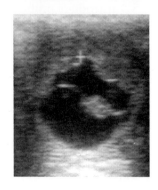

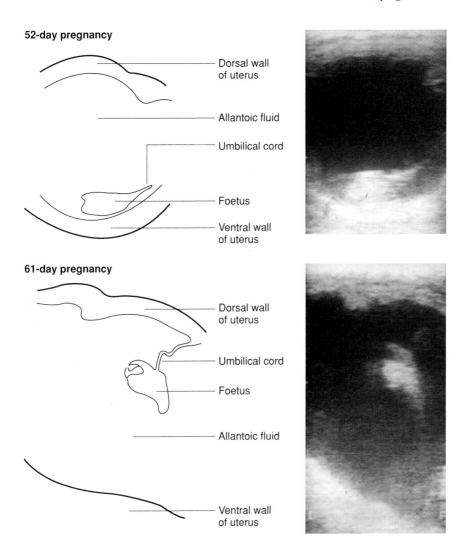

52-day pregnancy

Dorsal wall of uterus

Allantoic fluid

Umbilical cord

Foetus

Ventral wall of uterus

61-day pregnancy

Dorsal wall of uterus

Umbilical cord

Foetus

Allantoic fluid

Ventral wall of uterus

Figure 6.2 Ultrasound images and diagrams of early pregnancy (days 52–61).

preference and of the routine for the individual stud farm. It is helpful, particularly with older mares, to have a record of size and position of any endometrial cysts (Figure 6.3) prior to pregnancy diagnosis. Diagnosis of pregnancy as early as day 12 is possible; however as early embryonic loss is still high at this time it is necessary to repeat the examination a week

Figure 6.1 Ultrasound images and diagrams of early pregnancy (days 17–32).

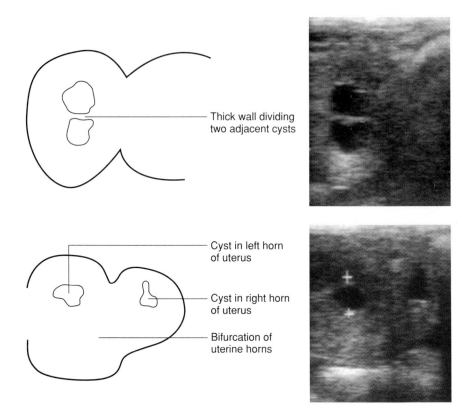

Thick wall dividing
two adjacent cysts

Cyst in left horn
of uterus

Cyst in right horn
of uterus

Bifurcation of
uterine horns

Figure 6.3 Ultrasound images and diagrams of endometrial cysts.

later. There is also an increased risk of failing to diagnose twins as there may have been a second ovulation 2 days later than the first. In my experience there are few advantages in routinely first examining the mare before day 15–17. If at this stage there is any doubt about possible twins the next examination should be at day 25–26 when a foetus and heart beat can be readily detected. If a single clear sac is detected the next examination should be carried out at about day 30 (before day 35, when endometrial cups start to form). A further examination between days 42 and 60 is usually carried out. If at any stage there is any suggestion of the pregnancy failing more frequent examinations may be carried out to monitor the situation. It is important to carry out two ultrasound examinations (one after day 25 when the foetus is visible) to reduce the risk of failing to detect twins (Figure 6.4).

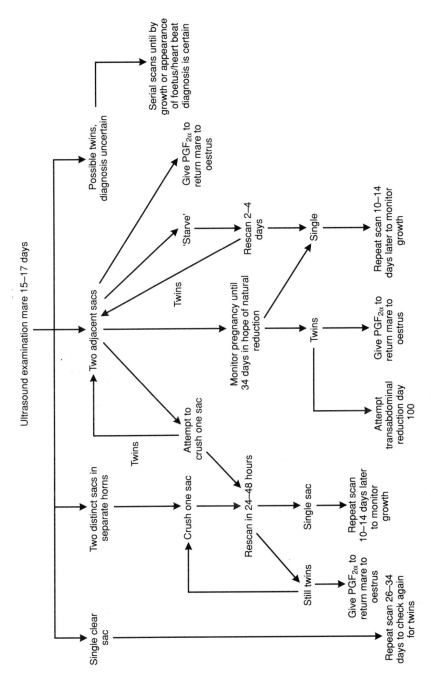

Figure 6.4 Decision plan for management of twin pregnancies.

Hormone assays

Progesterone

Progesterone cannot be used to detect pregnancy as levels may be high in dioestrus. Levels in early pregnancy are usually greater than 4 ng/ml but may also be low in some stages of pregnancy.

Equine chorionic gonadotrophin

Equine chorionic gonadotrophin (eCG; previously known as pregnant mare's serum gonadotrophin, PMSG) is produced by the endometrial cups, which are formed by foetal trophoblast cells invading maternal endometrium at day 35–38. A maternal immunological reaction about day 80 starts to destroy them. Serum levels are detectable from days 40 to 110. False positives occur when there has been foetal loss after formation of endometrial cups, as the cups will continue to produce eCG until day 110. In my experience false negatives are possible before day 45. Twins produce increased levels of eCG.

Oestrogen

Oestrogen produced by the foeto-placental unit, in particular the foetal gonads, can be detected from day 90 onwards. The plasma levels peak at day 210. It is a useful test after day 90, and confirms a viable foetus. Urinary oestrogens can be used from day 120, although this test has been superseded by testing for circulating oestrogens.

The management of twin pregnancies

The routine use of ultrasound for early pregnancy diagnosis has substantially increased the detection of twin pregnancies (Figure 6.5) and allows appropriate steps to be taken to prevent the mare carrying twins to term. Nearly all twin conceptions result from a double ovulation.

There is a marked variation in the incidence of double ovulations. Ginther (1986) reports a 20–25% incidence in Thoroughbred and draft mares as opposed to 10% in ponies. In my experience a few individual mares appear to be predisposed to double ovulations. The twin conception rate in Thoroughbred mares is reported to be 7–10%.

Even with the use of ultrasound to monitor ovulation, many double ovulations are not detected. This is likely to occur when the ovulations are adjacent or asynchronous (there may be 24–48 hours between ovulations).

Ginther (1989a, b) has reported the incidence of natural reduction of twins in Standardbreds. The highest incidence of natural reduction occurs

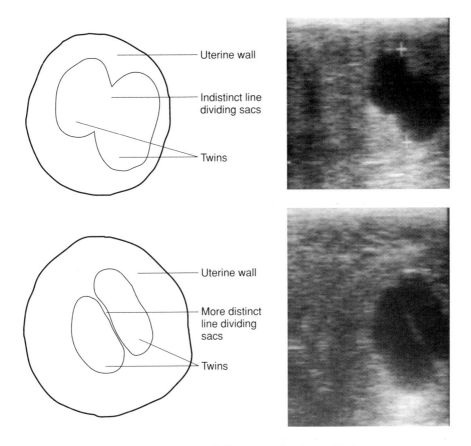

Figure 6.5 Ultrasound images and diagrams of twins at 17 days.

in unilateral twins of disparate size, and it is likely to occur before day 20. Reduction of twins of the same size is less probable but if it does occur it is more likely to be after day 20.

Mares should be mated during those periods of oestrus with twin follicles as there appears to be an enhanced conception rate. Twin follicles or twin ovulations should always be recorded to ensure that these mares are carefully scanned at an early stage.

Before any steps are taken to reduce twins one must be certain of the diagnosis. In mares with endometrial cysts it is possible to mistake an endometrial cyst for a 15–24-day conceptus. If there is any doubt the examination should be repeated before any action is taken. Serial examinations will allow growth to be monitored and by day 23–24 the foetus becomes visible, and at day 25–26 the appearance of a heart beat will be diagnostic.

The accepted method of reducing twin embryos to a singleton is by manual crushing of one embryo between forefinger and thumb per rectum or compressing the embryo between the scanner probe and the pelvis. Obviously this is easier when the twins are bilateral. When the twins are adjacent it is very difficult to exert sufficient pressure on one embryo without damaging the other. If the embryo is still mobile it may prove more difficult to crush; however this feature can allow unilateral twins to be separated prior to crushing. If crushing is difficult it is usually worth leaving it and repeating the procedure 24–48 hours later because changes in uterine tone can facilitate crushing.

The use of anti-prostaglandins to aid survival of the remaining embryo has been suggested. Recent studies, and experience in practice, indicate no difference in survival of the pregnancy after reduction with or without their use.

There are clinical reports of the use of a limited period of reduced food intake to reduce twins early in pregnancy. The mare is kept stabled on non-edible bedding and minimal rations for 2–4 days.

When twin pregnancies are diagnosed it is essential that the options are fully discussed with the owner. If the clinician takes no action to reduce the twins or terminate the pregnancy, it may be advisable to put this in writing. Likewise if the mare returns home from stud the implications of the situation must be fully reported.

Rantanen and Kincaid (1988) report the use of a transabdominal ultrasound-guided needle to inject potassium chloride into the heart of one foetus. This procedure can be performed from day 100. As many clinicians are not familiar with transabdominal ultrasound, success is dependent on the experience of the operator.

Main events of normal pregnancy in the mare

Fertilization occurs in the oviduct, with only fertilized ova passing into the uterus. Unfertilized ova remain in the oviducts where they degenerate. The embryo reaches the uterus at day 5–6, then migrates freely around the uterus. It is thought that as the embryo migrates around the uterus it releases an antiluteolytic factor about day 14. Increasing uterine tone at day 15–16 results in fixation of the embryo, usually at the base of one of the horns. By day 36, cells from the chorionic girdle migrate and invade the maternal endometrium, clumping together to form endometrial cups. The endometrial cups secrete eCG, which has FSH and LH like activity. A maternal immunological reaction results in maternal leucocytes invading and encapsulating the cups. By day 120 minimal quantities of eCG are produced.

During the first 90 days of pregnancy the ovaries are multifollicular.

Ovulations occur about days 35–40 resulting in the formation of secondary corpora lutea. By day 120 the placenta plays a primary role in progesterone secretion.

During the second half of pregnancy the ovaries become inactive. The follicular activity in the first half of pregnancy may account for some mares exhibiting signs of behavioural oestrus during early pregnancy. Mares showing behavioural signs of oestrus should be examined to confirm the pregnancy. From day 70 onwards there is a sharp rise in oestrogens, which originate from the foeto-placental unit. In parallel with this rise there is a marked growth and then regression in size of the foetal gonads.

Abnormalities during pregnancy

Pregnancy is usually uneventful in the mare. When problems occur they cause concern. Colic is a relatively common complication and it is essential to differentiate gastrointestinal problems from those associated with pregnancy (Table 6.4). A careful clinical examination including vaginal and rectal examination should indicate whether the gastrointestinal or reproductive tract is involved.

Premature lactation, often described as 'running milk', may be idiopathic or due to some abnormality in the placenta or foetus. Careful examination of the mare including milk samples for electrolyte analysis, plasma for progesterone levels and transabdominal ultrasonography can be used to detect any abnormality. A complication arising from premature lactation is loss of all colostrum prior to parturition. The foal is entirely dependent on antibodies ingested in colostrum for passively derived immunity. Failure of passive transfer of maternal immunity can be avoided in these cases if the colostrum is milked and tested for IgG levels. If IgG levels are greater than 70 g/l the colostrum should be frozen until the foal is born. It is then thawed and fed to the foal prior to the foal suckling the mare. If IgG levels are inadequate donor colostrum must be used.

Cervical pole placentitis may present as a vaginal discharge during pregnancy. Vaginoscopic and rectal examination should be carried out if a mare has a significant vaginal discharge. Transabdominal ultrasonography can be used to monitor foetal health. Discharge swabs should be cultured for bacteria and fungi. Treatment with systemic antibiotics and vaginal douches is frequently unrewarding. If the mare carries the foal to term it is likely to be infected and should be considered 'high risk' for developing septicaemia.

Gestation length

The average length of gestation for a Thoroughbred mare is 330–340 days.

Table 6.4 Differential diagnosis of gynaecological abdominal pain in late gestation

Condition	Occurrence during gestation	Diagnostic features	Treatment
Foetal hypermotility	Last third	Mild signs of pain, excessive foetal movements. More common in maiden and old mares. Common condition	Spasmolytics are usually adequate. If signs persist check foetal health
Uterine dorsoretroflexion	Last third	Moderate to severe signs of colic. Foetus is palpable just cranial to anus; marked pain response when palpated. Uncommon	Smooth muscle relaxants, e.g. clenbuterol or isoxuprine, should be given. Repeated administration may be necessary
Uterine torsion	Late pregnancy or at parturition	Chronic colic of varying intensity. Foetus is not palpable. Careful palpation of crossed broad ligaments indicates the direction of torsion. Vaginal examination is unrewarding as rarely involved in the mare. Uncommon	Surgical correction is necessary without delay
Hydrops allantois	Last third	Acute, excessive abdominal distension, with signs of low-grade colic. On rectal examination excessively distended flabby uterus and foetus not palpable. The condition is progressive	Manual rupture of the allantochorion after using warm water douches to relax cervix. Drain half of allantoic fluid. Administer oxytocin drip to contract splanchnic vasculature. Then drain remaining fluid from the uterus and deliver foal, which is frequently deformed

However there is a wide variation and in my experience normal mature foals can be produced from 310 to 365 days. In pony mares gestation is frequently shorter than Thoroughbreds. Mares that foal early in the year (January/February) often carry foals 10–14 days longer. Gestations over 350 days tend to cause concern, although provided mare and foetus are healthy there is no indication to induce parturition. It has been suggested that prolonged gestation may be due to an embryonic/foetal diapause earlier in pregnancy. Foetal oversize is not usually a problem in prolonged gestation in the mare.

Signs of imminent parturition

During the final month of pregnancy the mammary glands develop, increasing in size and tone. Early in this process the swelling of the glands increases overnight and tends to diminish with exercise during the day. As parturition becomes imminent (usually 24–48 hours prior to foaling) wax develops at the end of the teats, known as 'waxing up'. Marked changes occur in the mammary secretions close to term. The following electrolyte changes in mammary secretions indicate parturition will probably occur within 24 hours:

- calcium >10 mmol/l,
- sodium <30 mmol/l,
- potassium >30 mmol/l,
- magnesium >10 mmol/l.

A rapid strip test method to assess mammary secretions can be used to predict foaling (Cash *et al.* 1985). The test utilizes strips used to assess water hardness.

There is marked relaxation and lengthening of the vulva and relaxation of the cervix. Relaxation of the cervix is accompanied by loss of the cervical plug, which may be seen as a sticky discharge on the perineum or tail. There is also relaxation of the sacroiliac and sacrosciatic ligaments but this tends to be less obvious than in the cow.

Normal parturition

First-stage labour

The mare starts to show signs of restlessness and discomfort—sweating, pawing, walking the box and getting up and down repeatedly. The foetus changes from a flexed to an extended posture and from a ventral to a dorsal position. This is due in part to myometrial contractions and in part to reflex foetal movements. The length of this stage shows marked individual variation from a few hours to several days. Thoroughbred mares are particularly prone to 'false alarms'. There are some mares who exhibit very few external signs of first-stage labour.

Second-stage labour

The start of second-stage labour is marked by rupture of the placenta and loss of allantoic fluid (similar in appearance to urine). Most mares lie down and abdominal straining becomes appreciable. The amnion should appear at the vulva lips within a few minutes of the rupture of the placenta. The foal should be in anterior presentation, in a dorsal position with an extended posture with one foot slightly in advance. A check should be made that this is the case. Once the head has been delivered, straining continues forcefully until the hips are delivered when efforts will cease. If undisturbed the mare will lie quietly in sternal position for up to half an hour. The foal is usually born with the amnion intact, and unless rapidly broken by the foal struggling should be quickly cleared from the nose and mouth. If the mare has had a Caslick's operation, episiotomy is usually performed by the stud groom early in second-stage labour. Second stage is rapid (average 20 minutes).

Third-stage labour

The umbilical cord remains intact until either the mare stands or the foal struggles to its feet. The umbilical cord stump on the foal should be dressed with iodine. The placenta usually is expelled within 1 hour. The mare frequently exhibits signs of pain, rolling, sweating and ignoring the foal.

The foal should show reflex sucking movements within 10–15 minutes of birth, stand within 2 hours and suck within 4 hours. Anything outside these times should be considered abnormal.

Induction of parturition

Conditions that compromise either the mare or the foal are the usual indication for induction of parturition in this country. In the USA it is used routinely to facilitate management. It is a straightforward procedure provided certain guidelines are followed. Complications most frequently occur when parturition is induced prior to term; these include premature/dysmature foals and traumatic injury to the mare due to inadequate relaxation of the birth canal. The following is a checklist of criteria for induction of parturition:

1. gestation over 340 days,
2. relaxation and lengthening of vulva,
3. relaxation of the cervix,
4. relaxation of pelvic ligaments,
5. adequate mammary development,
6. 'mature' mammary secretion on electrolyte analysis.

Methods of induction of parturition

Oxytocin

Oxytocin is considered by many clinicians to be the drug of choice. All the above criteria should be met as it will induce parturition in preterm mares. There is considerable variation in dose rate and route. Recent studies have indicated that 2.5–5.0 iu of oxytocin diluted in 10–20 ml of sterile water given as an intravenous bolus is most likely to provide a successful outcome. It can be repeated after 30 minutes if the initial dose does not initiate parturition. This method is unlikely to hyperstimulate the myometrium but can induce premature placental separation or malpresentations. Parturition usually is complete within 1.5–2 hours of administration.

Prostaglandins

Fluprostenol can be used to induce parturition. It is unlikely to initiate parturition unless the foetus is ready for birth. Fluprostenol (250 μg) given intramuscularly is likely to initiate parturition within 0.5–3 hours; 1000 μg may be required in larger mares.

Dystocia

Dystocias are reported to occur in 1% of deliveries. Dystocia in the mare requires immediate attention if mare and foal are to be saved. The foal has a very limited period in which it will survive in cases of dystocia, this period lasting no longer than an hour and in many cases considerably less. Dystocia occurs most commonly as a result of a deformity of the foal, e.g. severe carpal flexion, incomplete turning of the foal from a ventral flexed to a dorsal extended position, or maternal abnormality, e.g. previous pelvic fracture, twins or a dead foal.

The mare should be restrained with an additional attendant to hold the tail and position the hindquarters. It is easier to evaluate the situation with the mare standing; however in some cases the mare will not stand for the examination to be completed. Walking the mare will usually reduce abdominal straining. It is essential to use plenty of lubrication. In cases when abdominal straining hinders examination and manipulations, epidural anaesthesia should be used. It is essential to check that the foal is alive, not deformed and in anterior presentation.

The principles of correcting dystocia are similar to other large animals, although in the mare embryotomy should only be considered as a last resort. The mare's birth canal is readily damaged and recent advances in surgical techniques have resulted in acceptable fertility rates following caesarean section under general anaesthesia. However the speed with which surgery is carried out influences the final outcome. General anaesthesia and raising the hindquarters may allow correction of the dystocia without the need for caesarean section. If embryotomy is to be performed it should be carried out under sedation and epidural anaesthesia with the administration of smooth muscle relaxants. Great care must be taken of the cervix as damage will adversely affect future fertility.

Common problems associated with parturition and dystocia

Premature placental separation

A red velvety sac of allantochorion is presented at the vulval lips. There is failure of the allantochorion to rupture at the cervical star prior to placental separation. The allantochorion should be manually ruptured without delay. It is a condition when it is essential to give appropriate advice by telephone in order to save the foal. Delivery is then usually uneventful.

Failure of the mare to lie down during second-stage labour

This complication is usually due to the environment in which the mare is foaling or due to a musculoskeletal problem. When the mare is obviously going to remain standing, gentle traction may be necessary as abdominal straining is not as effective. The foal should also be supported during birth. Continually disturbing the mare, using bright lights or having attendants in close proximity are frequently contributing factors.

Foetal oversize

This is a relatively uncommon complication, more frequently reported in maiden mares. Inadequate relaxation of the birth canal may cause an apparent oversize; in these cases there may have been premature intervention. Usually plentiful lubrication and coordinated traction will result in rapid delivery.

Postural abnormalities

Postural problems of the limbs or of the head and neck are the most common cause of dystocia. Carpal flexion will readily become impacted in the birth canal. The foetus should be repelled and the limb extended. Where there is a flexural deformity of the carpus and the limb cannot be adequately extended to allow vaginal delivery, caesarean section should be undertaken. In cases of flexion or lateral deviation of the head, the foetus should again be repelled to allow correction. The application of colour-coded foaling ropes is often helpful. In cases of wry neck vaginal delivery is rarely possible.

Abnormalities of presentation

These are uncommon in the mare. Posterior presentations should be delivered as rapidly as possible with gentle traction. However, if it is a breech presentation with limbs extended cranially caesarean section should be considered. Tranverse presentation is extremely rare and exceedingly difficult to correct; again caesarean section should be considered.

Abnormalities of position

These usually occur due to incomplete rotation of the foal. They can usually be corrected by twisting and traction.

Once manipulation and reposition is complete, manual traction may be applied with care. When traction is applied the birth canal must be adequately relaxed and plentiful lubrication used; colour-coded ropes on legs and head are helpful. Traction should coincide with abdominal straining and be in a downward curving arc. It should again be reiterated that if vaginal delivery is proving very difficult caesarean section should be considered before there has been significant damage to the mare, and while the foal is still viable.

Postpartum complications

Several complications can arise in the postpartum period and affect future fertility or threaten life.

Retained placenta

The most commonly encountered complication is a retained placenta. There is some controversy as to the time interval that is considered abnormal. In the Thoroughbred, intervention usually takes place after 6–8 hours. It is usual that either the complete placenta or the non-pregnant horn is retained. In some cases manual removal is easily accomplished. However, if the retained placenta does not separate readily, manual removal should not be attempted as microvillous retention and uterine haemorrhage may occur.

An oxytocin drip, 30–100 iu in 500 ml sterile saline, administered intravenously over about half an hour usually results in expulsion of the placenta within 1 hour. Some clinicians prefer to administer 30–50 iu of oxytocin intramuscularly. If the placenta has not been expelled the treatment may be repeated. Flunixin meglumine should be administered for its anti-endotoxic and anti-inflammatory effects. Systemic antibiotics and intrauterine large-volume flushing may be indicated in cases of prolonged retention.

Perineal injury

Perineal injury is relatively common, particularly when foaling is unattended. Injuries range from first-degree tear of the dorsal commissure (easily repaired using Caslick's operation) to third-degree tears involving rectovaginal tears that require extensive specialized standing surgery to salvage the mare for breeding. Second- and third-degree tears that are not suitable for immediate repair should be kept clean. Topical and systemic antibiotics may be required in some cases. When there has been severe perineal bruising, non-steroidal anti-inflammatory drugs (NSAIDs), e.g. phenylbutazone, should be administered.

Cervical injury

Cervical lacerations are most commonly associated with dystocia or incomplete relaxation of the birth canal. They should initially be treated daily with topical antibiotic ointments and digital manipulation to prevent adhesion formation. Full thickness tears require surgical repair and, despite surgery, carry a poor prognosis for further breeding.

Haemorrhage

Haemorrhage from the uterine artery is a serious life-threatening complication. It most commonly presents as a severe colic in older mares in the immediate postpartum period. However, I have seen fatal haemorrhage in a primiparous mare and also in a mare initially presented 48 hours after parturition. Veterinary intervention appears to have little effect on the final outcome. If the haemorrhage is contained within the broad ligament the mare is likely to survive; rupture of the broad ligament almost always results in fatal intra-abdominal haemorrhage. Efforts should be concentrated on controlling the pain with analgesics and mild sedation. The use of fluid therapy remains controversial. The use of hypertonic saline, followed up with isotonic therapy has been reported. However, the increase in blood pressure and dilution of clotting factors may be undesirable.

Uterine rupture

Uterine rupture may occur during dystocia. The severity of clinical signs is dependent on the position and size of the tear. Mares with large tears in the uterus rapidly show signs of shock and die. Small or incomplete tears may not be noticed until the mare presents with signs of peritonitis. Surgical repair and abdominal lavage should be considered. Broad-spectrum antibiotic therapy should be instituted without delay.

Uterine prolapse

Prolapse of the uterus is uncommon due to the cranial attachment of the broad ligament. Incidence in Thoroughbreds is lower than in Standardbreds. Dystocia and placental retention may predispose to prolapse. Sedation and epidural anaesthesia should be administered. The uterus should be supported, carefully cleaned with a dilute iodine solution, checked for tears and replaced. Systemic antibiotics and NSAIDs should be administered.

Toxaemic metritis/laminitis

This may be seen as a complication of retained placenta, dystocia or severe uterine contamination. It is a serious condition due to rapid onset and progress that, unless treated aggressively, may be fatal.

Diagnosis

This condition usually occurs in the immediate postpartum period. The mare becomes inappetent, depressed and pyrexic and may exhibit signs of laminitis. The uterus contains a large volume (several gallons in severe cases) of fetid brown fluid.

Treatment

The fluid should be drained from the uterus. This is most readily done by placing two sterile stomach tubes through the fully open cervix into the uterus. One tube is attached to a hand pump and a dilute warm solution of povidone-iodine gently pumped into the uterus. The other tube is used as an egress tube, the fluid flowing out under gravity. The procedure should be continued until the egress fluid is clear. If it proves difficult to remove all of the fluid, a drip containing 50 iu of oxytocin in 500 ml of sterile saline may be helpful. The mare should be given broad-spectrum systemic antibiotics and NSAIDs. It may be necessary to repeat the uterine lavage for several days. The mare should also be treated for laminitis.

Foal heat

A foaling mare will come into season 5–10 days after parturition; this is known as the 'foal heat'. Controversy exists over mating mares in this heat period. The advantage of conception at this time is that the mare will foal earlier the following year. Studies indicate that although this oestrous cycle is as fertile as any other, early embryonic death occurs more frequently.

The mare should not be mated if:

1. the uterus has not contracted satisfactorily after foaling,
2. there is any fluid accumulation in the uterus,
3. there is significant bruising or damage to the cervix,
4. the perineum has not healed adequately after any damage,
5. cervical cytology and bacteriology results are abnormal,
6. the mare is pooling urine in the vagina at the optimum time for mating.

If the owners are keen to mate the mare during foal heat she should receive adequate exercise in the postpartum period and be examined when she first comes into season so treatment may be carried out prior to mating. Each individual case should be assessed to allow mares to be rested if mating might adversely affect future fertility.

The barren mare

The breeding industry requires maximum reproductive efficiency from mares; consequently any mare that fails to conceive is a cause for concern. Considerable research efforts have been put into investigating the pathogenesis of the various aspects of subfertility and infertility in the mare.

Mares are expected to produce one foal a year, and most Thoroughbred owners do not like to have foals born after the beginning of May. This, coupled with the long gestation period in the mare, provides a limited number of heat periods when it is desirable for the mare to conceive.

- A barren mare is considered to be a mare that is not pregnant at the end of the covering season either because she has failed to conceive or has not been mated.
- An infertile mare is a mare who is incapable of conceiving and carrying a pregnancy to term.
- A subfertile mare has a reduced fertility rate when mated by a normal healthy stallion.

Uterine defence mechanisms

At natural mating the stallion ejaculates through the relaxed cervix directly into the mare's uterus. This inevitably results in intrauterine contamination with bacteria and foreign material. The repeated insult of mating and pregnancy results in a clearly demonstrated linear decline in fertility with age (Jeffcott *et al.* 1982).

It is important to understand the normal defence mechanisms of the reproductive tract in the mare when considering a barren mare.

1. The vulva provides the first line of defence. When this seal is incompetent it allows air and bacteria into the genital tract producing infection and inflammation (pneumovagina). During dioestrus and pregnancy the muscular, tubular structure of the cervix provides an effective seal; however any damage that may occur at foaling or, rarely, at mating will impair its function. At mating both these seals are breached.
2. Uterine defence mechanisms are of paramount importance in the normal elimination of infection that occurs at mating. The mechanical defences involve smooth muscle and mucociliary clearance. There is also a cellular and humoral component, with an influx during oestrus of neutrophils and serum proteins, including immunoglobulins and complement. These mechanisms rapidly clear the contamination that occurs at mating leaving a suitable environment for the embryo when it enters the uterus 5–6 days after ovulation.

Investigation of the barren mare (Figure 6.6)

Mares are usually presented for investigation either after the end of the breeding season when they have failed to conceive or in the latter part of the breeding season after several unsuccessful matings. Examination must be thorough and methodical to allow accurate diagnosis, prognosis and treatment to be given.

It is important to take a careful history including previous breeding record, fertility of the stallion used, history of venereal infection and management practices on the stud farm. A checklist for recording the history of the subfertile mare is shown below.

1. Has the mare had any foals?
2. Have there been any problems at parturition?
3. Has the mare a history of early embryonic/foetal death or abortion?
4. Is the mare in good health and condition?
5. Have there been any fertility problems with the stallion used?
6. Is there any history of venereal disease on the stud farm?
7. Has the mare been intensively managed (more important with non-Thoroughbred mares): How many heat periods was she mated on? How many times was she mated per heat period? Were follicular development and ovulation monitored?

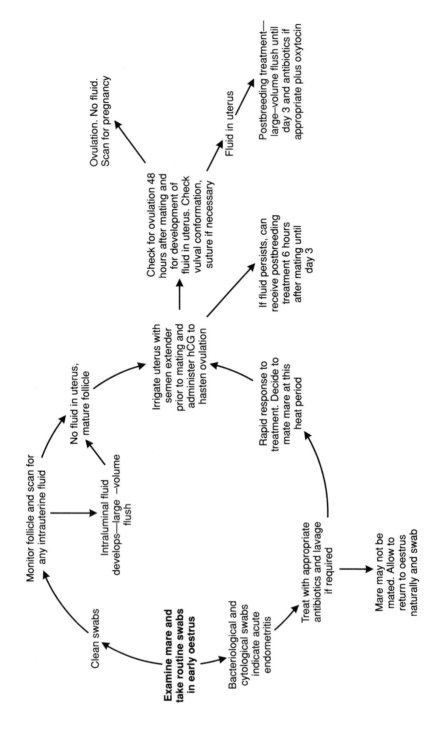

Figure 6.6 Decision plan for management of the subfertile mare.

If there is any doubt of the mare's state of health a full clinical examination should be carried out.

Gynaecological examination

The mare should be prepared for gynaecological examination as previously described. The vulval conformation should be assessed as to whether there is a predisposition to pneumovagina. The position of the dorsal commissure of the vulva in relation to the pelvic brim and angle of declination of the vulva is assessed (Pascoe 1979). The efficacy of any previous vulval surgery should be determined. Occasionally there are small holes in a previously stitched vulva, which will require debridement and restitching to complete the seal, or there may have been wound breakdown.

If the vulval seal is inadequate and there has been no previous attempts to correct it, Caslick's operation should be performed once investigation and any intrauterine treatment is complete. If there have been previous unsuccessful attempts to correct poor vulval conformation it may be necessary to consider Pouret's operation (Pouret 1982).

Vaginal examination

The vagina and cervix should be examined using a speculum. In mares where the cervix has been pulled cranially and ventrally there may be urine pooling in the cranial vagina, which in some cases will partially submerge the cervix producing a severe cervicitis, vaginitis and endometritis. In these cases efforts should be made to reduce the size and increase the tone of the uterus. The condition is most commonly seen in older mares with delayed uterine involution at the foal heat. Increasing the exercise routine is also helpful in reducing urine pooling.

The cervix should be carefully examined both visually and digitally. Any defect in the muscular integrity of the cervix, adhesion or scarring will result in inadequate closure and infertility. Mucosal defects will usually heal with topical antibiotic ointments and digital manipulation to prevent adhesion formation. Defects in the cervix are usually wedge-shaped, being widest caudally. Surgical repair is difficult due to limited exposure and having to work 'down a tunnel'. Even if the surgery is undertaken, prognosis must be guarded for future breeding.

Bacteriological and cytological swabs

Endometrial swabs should be taken for bacteriological and cytological examination when the mare is in oestrus. A clitoral swab should also be taken. The samples should be screened for aerobic, microaerophilic and anaerobic bacteria (Ricketts et al. 1993).

Table 6.5 Standard system for interpreting endometrial smears

	No cells seen	+/-	1+	2+	3+
Epithelial cells	No epithelial cells	Epithelial cells present			
Interpretation	*Inadequate smear*	*Good smear*			
Polymorphs (PMNs)		<1%	1-5%	5-30%	over 30%
Interpretation	*No PMNs seen in normal healthy mare*	*Often foal heat or 1st oestrus of year*	*Endometritis*		

Endometrial cytology has been shown to be useful in interpreting bacteriological results, and as a rapid test can provide early information on acute endometritis. Wingfield Digby (1978) describes the technique using Pollack's Trichrome stain, which gives excellent nuclear detail. Alternatively, Testsimplets (Boehringer Corporation) prestained slides may be used. These are simple to use and require no specialized equipment. The slides should be examined under a good laboratory microscope. The slide should then be scored using the standard system shown in Table 6.5. Vaginal cells indicate a vaginal sample, while erythrocytes may be seen during the foal heat.

Endometrial and clitoral swabs are screened for the following venereal pathogens: *Taylorella equigenitalis, Klebsiella pneumoniae* (capsule types 1, 2 and 5), *Pseudomonas aeruginosa*. These are described on p. 255–8.

Opportunist pathogens that can produce acute endometritis include:

Streptococcus zooepidemicus (ß-haemolytic),
Staphylococcus aureus (coagulase positive),
Haemolytic *Escherichia coli,*
Enterobacter aerogenes,
Proteus spp.,
Klebsiella pneumoniae (capsule types 7 and 68),
Bacteroides fragilis (commonly isolated anaerobe, other anaerobes may be significant),
Candida spp.,
Mucor spp.

Rectal examination

A rectal examination should then be undertaken with evaluation of the size and position of the uterus and any palpable abnormalities noted. The size and follicular activity of the ovaries should be assessed. Ultrasound examination of the uterus and ovaries should be undertaken.

Endometrial biopsy

In most cases it is appropriate to take an endometrial biopsy. Before the procedure is carried out it is essential to confirm the mare is not pregnant. Histological findings are most readily interpreted when the sample is taken during dioestrus. Basket-jawed biopsy forceps are required to take an adequate sample.

1. Mare prepared for examination as before.
2. Confirm non-pregnancy.
3. Remove faeces from rectum.
4. Clean perineum and wear clean gloves.
5. Guard closed jaws of biopsy punch in left hand and introduce into vagina.
6. Use forefinger to pass through the cervix and slide biopsy punch alongside finger.
7. Gently, with a finger, ease cervix caudally along the biopsy punch ensuring that it is through the cervix.
8. Remove hand from vagina and palpate end of biopsy punch per rectum.
9. Carefully manipulate end of punch into uterine body/horn, open jaws of punch and (per rectum) ensure contact of endometrium with biopsy punch.
10. Close biopsy punch and sharply withdraw.
11. Place sample in Bouin's fixative and take swab for bacteriological examination from inside biopsy punch.

It is essential to ensure that the biopsy punch is positioned correctly as samples of bladder and cervix have been submitted unintentionally. Rarely some endometrial haemorrhage may occur; the risk is reduced if the biopsy is taken during dioestrus.

Detailed discussion of histological changes is beyond the scope of this chapter but is well described in the literature (Kenny 1978; Van Camp 1988; Ricketts 1989). Common findings and recommended treatments are discussed below.

Acute endometritis

Polymorphonuclear leucocytes are seen migrating through luminal epithelium into stratum compactum. Eosinophils are seen in association with pneumovagina. These signs are usually associated with bacterial infections and treatment with intrauterine infusions of appropriate antibiotics selected with the aid of sensitivity testing is recommended. A combination of 5 Mu of crystalline penicillin, 1 g neomycin, 40 000 iu polymyxin B and 600 mg furaltadone dissolved in 100 ml of warm sterile water administered once daily into the uterus for 3–5 days has proved successful in practice.

Chronic infiltrative endometritis

Plasma cells and mononuclear cells are seen, which indicate immunological response to antigenic challenge. There is no specific therapy.

Chronic degenerative endometritis

Degenerative changes in the glands of the endometrium with formation of 'gland nests', groups of dilated glands of inactive appearance surrounded by layers of fibrous tissue. Occasionally lymphatic lacunae may be seen. The condition is progressive and develops as a result of repeated challenge at mating and repeated pregnancy. The age of the mare must be taken into consideration when judging whether the degree of change is excessive. I have used treatment with large-volume 'hot' saline uterine flushes with some success. Various treatments have been advocated: endometrial curettage (Ricketts 1989), chemical curettage (Bracher et al. 1991) and dimethyl sulphoxide (DMSO) and antibiotic solutions (Ley et al. 1989).

Endometrial hyperplasia

Glandular hyperplasia, normally seen in the immediate postpartum period (usually resolving 10–14 days post partum), may persist for several weeks or be seen following pregnancy loss. Treatment with an oxytocin drip (50 iu oxytocin in 500 ml sterile saline) given intravenously is usually effective. This can be used in combination with warm large-volume lavage in refractory cases.

Endometrial hypoplasia

Underdevelopment of glandular structure of the endometrium associated with immaturity, ovarian or chromosomal abnormality.

Endometrial atrophy

This may be seen as a temporary feature in deep winter anoestrus. In the ovulatory season it may be a result of senility or occasionally secondary to severe acute endometritis with Pseudomonas aeruginosa infection. There is no treatment, and the mare should be retired from breeding.

Hysteroscopy

The videoendoscope has made hysteroscopy a more widely available technique. However as the equipment is costly it is usually performed at specialist centres. The technique allows visualization of endometrial cysts, neoplasms, adhesions and fluid accumulations. Specific biopsy samples can be taken. The advent of the laser (via a channel in the videoendoscope) has facilitated treatment of some conditions, particularly adhesions and large endometrial cysts (Bracher and Allen 1992 and Bracher *et al.* 1992).

Specific conditions

Pyometra

A pyometra is defined as the accumulation of excessive amounts of abnormal fluids in the uterus that may be sterile or contain bacteria or fungi. The cervix may be closed or adhesions may be present producing physical obstruction to drainage of fluids through the cervix. If the cervix is relaxed there may be a vaginal discharge. Oestrous cycles may be short due to recurrent inflammatory stimulus resulting in premature prostaglandin release and luteolysis. If endometrial damage is severe there may be a failure of prostaglandin release and prolonged dioestrus.

Diagnosis

The condition is diagnosed on rectal examination as a large uterus with a characteristic 'doughy' feel. Ultrasound shows a large fluid-filled uterus containing 'scintillating' hyperechoic particles.

Swabs should be taken for bacterial and fungal culture. The histological appearance of an endometrial biopsy typically shows severe acute endometritis imposed on advanced chronic infiltrative and degenerative endometritis. In advanced cases there may be endometrial atrophy.

The prognosis for these cases must be very poor; many cases are refractory to intensive therapy. In riding mares ovariohysterectomy may be considered.

Treatment

Large-volume uterine lavage to physically flush the fluid from the uterus plus intrauterine antibiotics for a period of 5–7 days is the recommended treatment. Dilute hydrogen peroxide may be added to the flushing fluid in the early stages. If the mare is in prolonged dioestrus prostaglandin should be administered. When the mare comes into season the cervix will relax and this will facilitate drainage of the fluids.

Fungal endometritis

Candida and *Aspergillus* are the most commonly isolated fungi. Fungal infection is most frequently associated with intensive management systems. Tissue invasion occurs when there is a failure of defence mechanisms or extensive antibiotic use.

Diagnosis

Fungal infections may initially be picked up on routine bacteriological and cytological examinations. Endometrial biopsy indicates the degree of tissue invasion.

Treatment

Treatment involves uterine lavage. Dilute povidone-iodine preparations have been used but may produce severe inflammatory reactions; alternatively 2% hydrogen peroxide or natamycin can be used. The use of human preparations, e.g. clotrimazole, have produced some encouraging results in my experience.

Endometrial neoplasia

Endometrial neoplasia is rare. Leiomyomas and fibroleiomyomas are most commonly seen. These are firm masses up to about 5 cm diameter often located in the caudal uterine body. They are usually benign and do not appear to affect fertility unless they interfere with cervical function or become large and pedunculated.

Diagnosis

The tumour is palpable as a firm mass on rectal examination, may be visible on ultrasound and can be confirmed histologically from a biopsy sample.

Treatment

Leiomyomas can be removed surgically.

Ovarian haematoma

Haematomata occur at ovulation and can be up to 50 cm in diameter. The ovum is unaffected and can be fertilized.

Diagnosis

The ovary is large on rectal examination. The enlargement is sudden and will gradually start to decrease in size over several weeks. It can be differentiated from a granulosa cell tumour by ultrasound, on which the ovary has a diffuse echogenic mottled appearance.

Treatment

None is required unless the ovary becomes very large, when it can produce signs of colic.

Ovarian neoplasia

The most common neoplasm is a granulosa–theca cell tumour. Teratomas, which contain misplaced embryonic structures, are also seen; they can be removed surgically. The contralateral ovary functions normally.

Granulosa–Theca cell tumours

Diagnosis

Diagnosis is based on palpation of a firm, persistently enlarged ovary. A granulosa cell tumour has a multiloculated honeycombed appearance on ultrasonic examination (White and Allen 1985; Hinrichs and Hunt 1990). The contralateral ovary is small and inactive. The mare may exhibit stallion-like behaviour, be nymphomaniacal or anoestrous. The mare will be infertile until the tumour is removed, although the tumour may develop during pregnancy.

Treatment

Surgical removal of the ovary is the treatment of choice. The contralateral ovary may take several months to start functioning again.

Chromosomal abnormality

The normal chromosome number in the horse is 64. The most commonly reported abnormality is 63, XO where one X chromosome is missing; 63,XO/64,XX mosaic, 64,XY sex-reversed males have also been reported (Long 1988). The incidence of abnormality is unknown.

Diagnosis

Mares that are 63,XO usually present as barren maidens. On rectal examination the ovaries are often tiny, hard and inactive. The cervix is pale and gaping. They may exhibit erratic oestrous behaviour. These fillies are usually infertile. Diagnosis is confirmed on chromosomal analysis from a heparinized blood sample.

Non-specific treatments for mares 'susceptible' to persistent endometritis

There is a group of subfertile middle-aged mares who present a challenge to the clinician. Following full investigation they appear 'susceptible' to repeated episodes of acute endometritis following mating. These mares require intensive treatment to assist conception.

Pneumovagina must be adequately corrected in these mares and any cervical problems treated. Intrauterine treatment should be carried out during oestrus as immune function is enhanced in the oestrogen-dominated uterus.

If there is any fluid in the uterus it should be flushed with warm sterile saline until the flush fluid is clear. Flushing is readily performed using a 28 or 30 French gauge Foley-type embryo flushing catheter. When the cuff is inflated it forms a tight seal in the cervix. One litre bags of intravenous saline can usually be fitted directly into the catheter and the fluid squeezed in; if the seals are good the fluid then drains back out into the bag. If fluid retrieval is poor the uterus can be gently massaged per rectum, or a low dose of oxytocin administered.

Large-volume uterine lavage removes fluid, bacteria and debris from the uterus, stimulates uterine contractility and increases opsonin and neutrophil concentrations in the uterus.

Lavage can be used prior to mating and again 4–6 hours after mating until 3 days after ovulation to optimize the uterine environment for the embryo. Oxytocin may be used to stimulate physical clearance of accumulated fluid.

When bacteria have been cultured from the uterine swabs, appropriate antibiotics should be administered in 100 ml of sterile water.

Homologous plasma (100 ml) has been used to increase opsonins and immunoglobulin concentrations (Asbury 1984); although scientific evaluation has produced equivocal results in practice it appears to be a useful adjunct to therapy.

Kenny *et al.* (1975) suggested a minimal contamination breeding system. This system advocates the use of semen extender, which is placed in the uterus approximately 1 hour prior to mating. The semen extender recommended has the following composition:

Dried low-fat skimmed milk	2.5 g
Gelatin	0.5 g
Glucose	5.0 g
Crystalline penicillin	300 mg
Crystalline streptomycin	300 mg

This can be made up in individual sachets and stored at 4 °C and then dissolved in 100 ml of sterile water, and heated to 37 °C prior to use.

Early embryonic/foetal death

Early pregnancy loss is a major factor in subfertility and gestation failure. Estimates of loss rate have shown considerable variation, dependent on method and time of pregnancy diagnosis. Most studies agree on an average loss of 10% of pregnancies after day 18.

Widely recognized types of loss are:

- early pregnancy loss: prior to day 150,
- embryonic death: prior to day 40,
- early foetal death: between days 40 and 100,
- abortion: beyond day 150.

A large recent study based on manual pregnancy diagnosis from day 18 reported that the highest pregnancy loss was in mares with a foal at foot, particularly when implantation occurred on the side of the previous pregnancy. Maiden mares had the lowest pregnancy loss rate (Gilbert and Marlow 1992).

Detection of early pregnancy loss

The use of diagnostic ultrasound has increased the ability to detect pending embryonic loss. Through observations in practice and in experimental studies the following changes on ultrasound may indicate a failing pregnancy:

1. irregular shape of vesicle—may be due to changes in uterine tone;
2. undersized vesicle—vesicles more than 2 SD below normal are more likely to be lost;
3. intraluminal uterine fluid;

4. prolonged mobile phase;
5. failure to detect an embryo after day 25;
6. loss of heart beat or failure to detect a heart beat after day 26;
7. oedematous appearance of endometrial folds.

If any of the above changes are detected the mare should be more closely monitored, using ultrasound more frequently and monitoring growth carefully. Once pregnancy loss has been confirmed the mare should be returned to oestrus using prostaglandins. The formation of the endometrial cups at about day 36 marks an important point because once they have formed the mare can rarely be returned to fertile oestrus prior to day 100. To eliminate this risk, frequent assessments should be carried out to allow a rational decision to be made if the pregnancy is failing. In my experience, if the pregnancy fails shortly after day 36, eCG levels should be checked as in some cases when the pregnancy is failing, development of endometrial cups may be delayed.

Early foetal death (EFD) may go undetected for some time as the mare will not return to oestrus until after day 100, and routine examinations are less frequent at this stage in pregnancy. Mares with a history of EFD should be examined more frequently in this period, using ultrasound to monitor foetal development rather than standard manual examinations. However in most cases of EFD, particularly in Thoroughbreds with a short breeding season, it is not possible to return the mare to a fertile oestrus prior to the end of the breeding season.

Causes of early embryonic and early foetal loss

Many causes have been suggested.

1. Low plasma progesterone is the explanation used by many owners; however scientific studies indicate that this is rarely the case. Levels below 4 ng/ml for more than two consecutive days are likely to result in pregnancy loss. Obviously once the pregnancy starts to fail, levels will fall as a secondary effect and exogenous supplementation is unlikely to save the pregnancy. In cases with true low levels of progesterone, supplementation is most readily administered orally as Regumate, started when pregnancy is first diagnosed and continued without interruption until day 120. Withdrawal should be gradual over a 3-week period.
2. Ageing gametes have been shown to increase pregnancy loss. Mating should be timed as close to ovulation as possible because semen can remain viable in the mare's reproductive tract for up to 72 hours.

3. Subfertile mares have been shown to have a pregnancy loss rate of up to 80% from fertilization to day 50, the majority of this being prior to day 14. Both periglandular fibrosis and endometritis have been shown to increase loss rates significantly.
4. Age. Loss rates increase with age of the mare; rates are lowest in maiden mares.
5. Maternal stress. Severe dietary restriction particularly between days 25 and 31 has been shown to be a factor. Likewise long-distance travel and surgical intervention may contribute.
6. Chromosomal defect of the embryo (increased by inbreeding).
7. Some studies indicate that loss rates are higher when foaling mares conceive from a foal heat mating. My experience would tend to substantiate this.

Treatment

Treatment should involve returning the mare to oestrus, carrying out full gynaecological examination and trying to identify any contributory factors.

Prophylaxis

A checklist for the treatment of mares with a history of early pregnancy loss is shown below.

1. Full gynaecological examination and routine swabbing.
2. Assess vulval conformation: is Caslick's operation necessary?
3. Take an endometrial biopsy if appropriate.
4. Treat any genital abnormality detected.
5. Use minimum contamination breeding techniques.
6. Time mating as close to ovulation as possible using daily ultrasound examination if necessary.
7. Minimize stress to mare, avoid long journeys prior to day 40 and ensure adequate nutrition.
8. Increase frequency of pregnancy examinations to once or twice weekly.

Abortion

Abortion is defined as expulsion of the foetus between 150 and 300 days. The signs of abortion are similar to those of birth, and may be confused with colic. There is a wide variation in premonitory signs: some mares carrying twins or with placentitis will show mammary development and 'run milk'; others (e.g. EHV-1 abortions) are sudden with no premonitory signs. Placental retention is more common following abortion.

Abortion is due either to death of the foetus or to abnormality in the foeto-placental unit. The causes can be infectious or non-infectious.

Infectious causes

Equine herpes virus 1

Equine herpes virus 1 (EHV-1) abortion is a major concern to the mare owner. Due to the infectious nature of EHV-1 any abortion should be treated as an EHV-1 abortion. The respiratory form of the disease is prevalent in youngstock. For this reason care should be taken to separate youngstock and horses out of training from pregnant mares.

Two strains of EHV-1 occur: type 1 is commonly known as the abortion strain and type 2 as the respiratory strain. However type 1 can cause respiratory disease or neurological signs.

EHV-1 abortions usually occur between 5 and 11 months of gestation. The foetus may be found within the membranes and there are rarely any premonitory signs. The foetus is usually fresh and the placenta may be oedematous. The foetus and membranes contain large amounts of virus so should be handled with care. Attendants should wear protective clothing when handling the mare. The bedding should be burnt. If the abortion occurs in the paddock it should be considered contaminated for at least 1 month. The mare can be considered non-infectious after 1 month, although it is advisable to return her to a group of barren mares.

The typical post-mortem findings in an EHV-1 infected foetus include:

- increased serosal fluids, often amber coloured,
- tiny white spots (pinhead sized) beneath the liver capsule,
- marked perirenal oedema,
- pneumonic lungs.

Pathognomonic histological findings are intranuclear inclusion bodies (Cowdray type A) in hepatocytes surrounded by an area of focal necrosis. Similar inclusion bodies are found in the bronchiolar epithelium.

A killed EHV-1 vaccine in an oil adjuvant is commercially available (Pneumabort-K). It should be administered in the fifth, seventh and ninth months of pregnancy. Although the level of immunity raised is relatively poor, vaccination is thought to reduce the incidence of abortion storms but individual abortions in the face of heavy challenge may not be prevented.

Equine arteritis virus

Equine arteritis virus has recently been recorded in the UK, is widespread in the non-Thoroughbred population in Europe and outbreaks have occurred in Kentucky. The increasing international movement of breeding stock and the reduction of health controls in the European Community make introduction of the virus into this country increasingly likely.

Equine arteritis virus is a togavirus that produces systemic signs involving panvasculitis. Abortion rates are high following infection in naive animals.

Bacterial infections

Bacterial infections are usually chronic, involving the cervical pole of the placenta. Abortion can occur from 5 months to term. The foetus is frequently growth retarded, and may show signs of septicaemia. It is usually autolysed. The affected area of the placenta is thickened and necrotic and may have a greyish exudate. The organism may be cultured from the foetus, placenta or cervical discharges.

Fungal infections

The pathology is usually confined to the placenta, with a large area covered with a brown sticky exudate. Fungal hyphae can be identified by microscopy. There may be necrotic plaques on the amnion. The foetus is usually very small for dates and emaciated. The abortion often occurs at about 10 months.

The mare will frequently show premonitory signs including mammary development, running milk and a vulval discharge with either bacterial or fungal placentitis.

Non-infectious causes

1. Twinning. The increased use of ultrasound for early pregnancy diagnosis has substantially reduced the incidence.
2. Abnormality of the umbilical cord. The cord may be severely twisted occluding the blood supply to the foetus. In some cases the cord may be very long.
3. Uterine body pregnancy with shrivelled placental horns.
4. Foetal developmental abnormality, e.g. CNS or organ malformations.
5. Maternal stress or disease, e.g. colic, surgery.
6. Iatrogenic administration of drugs that can cause abortion.

Checklist for action following an abortion

1. Consider abortion to be due to EHV-1 until proved otherwise.
2. Put the mare into strict isolation in a stable; attendants to wear protective clothing and use foot dips.
3. Check mare has expelled complete placenta and undertake gynaecological examination to check for damage, e.g. perineal or cervical injury.
4. Submit foetus and membranes to laboratory for investigation, or carry out gross post mortem and submit samples to appropriate laboratory (Table 6.6).
5. If mare aborted in a paddock, isolate direct in-contact animals and keep as a group. Avoid any stress to these animals.
6. Stop movement of animals on or off the stud until EHV-1 eliminated.
7. Burn all bedding from aborting mare, and use iodophor disinfectants.

If EHV-1 is subsequently confirmed:

8. Inform Breeders Association, neighbours and owners of any animals that have recently left the premises.
9. Maintain strict isolation until 30 days after last confirmed case.
10. Keep in-contact mares in small fixed groups and minimize overcrowding and stress.
11. Leave paddock for minimum of 1 month if EHV-1 confirmed, then use for barren or maiden mares.
12. Take serum samples from in-contact mares and other animals on the stud and monitor antibody titres.

Table 6.6 Samples required for detection of EHV-1 from an aborted foetus

Test	Sample	Fixative
Virus isolation	Liver, lung and thymus	Viral transport medium
Histology: H&E stain	Liver and lung	10% formalin
Histology: rapid	Liver and lung	Carnoy's solution
Histology: F.A.T	Liver and lung	Unfixed

Venereal diseases of stallions and mares

The Horse Racing Betting Levy Board code of common practice for control of contagious equine metritis (CEM) established in 1980 in Thoroughbreds in the UK has considerably reduced the incidence of bacterial venereal diseases. The CEM outbreak in 1977 encouraged the development of preventative measures on stud farms, which has also contributed to the decline of these diseases.

Bacterial diseases

There are three bacterial venereal infections in horses in the UK: *Taylorella equigenitalis* (CEM), *Klebsiella pneumoniae* and *Pseudomonas aeruginosa*.

The stallion acts as a passive carrier of disease, harbouring the organisms in the penile and preputial smegma. Clinical signs are rarely seen although ascending urinary tract infection has been reported as an uncommon complication of *Ps. aeruginosa* and *K. pneumoniae* infections. The normal commensal organisms provide protection against overgrowth of pathogenic bacteria. The practice of washing the penis and prepuce with water or mild antiseptics disturbs the normal flora and encourages overgrowth of pathogenic bacteria.

These infections may be acquired congenitally or before going to stud, so all potential stallions should be swabbed before taking up stud duties and the first few mares mated should be monitored.

Mares may present with a vaginal discharge and inflammation of the cervix and vagina, or a group of mares covered by a particular stallion may return to oestrus earlier than expected. Mares can act as carriers, these individuals having clitoral infection with no endometrial involvement. At natural mating, the clitoris is everted and pathogenic bacteria contaminate the stallion. The clinical signs vary with the type of infection. The signs with CEM are striking and severe.

Following treatment affected animals must have three negative swabs of the prepuce/penis, urethra, urethral fossa, and pre-ejaculatory fluid before the treatment is considered to be effective. There should be a 7-day interval between swabs; however there has been a change in the 1992 code of practice for CEM allowing swabs of stallions to be taken at 2-day intervals during the breeding season. The mares mated by a treated stallion should be monitored, particularly in cases of *Pseudomonas* infection. Likewise the stallion and any mares mated subsequently should be monitored after a treated mare has been covered.

Taylorella equigenitalis

The organism has not recently been isolated from Thoroughbreds in the UK but cases have occurred in non-Thoroughbreds in Europe. It is most commonly isolated from the clitoral sinuses in the mare or the urethral fossa in the stallion. Both streptomycin-sensitive and resistant strains have been isolated. The organism has a wide range of sensitivity.

Treatment of mares

Mares with a clitoral infection usually respond to a 7–10 day course of cleaning the clitoris with a 4% w/v chlorhexidine solution, followed by packing the sinuses and fossae with 0.2% nitrofurazone ointment. Any smegma must be removed prior to treatment. A small syringe with a narrow nozzle may be useful to ensure adequate treatment of the sinuses. However, this treatment may produce local irritation. Intrauterine treatment with an appropriate antibiotic, e.g. penicillin, should be used for endometrial infections; systemic antibiotics may also be used. Clitoral treatment should be carried out for 2–3 days prior to undertaking intra-uterine treatment. In resistant cases of clitoral infection sinusectomy or clitorectomy may be considered.

Treatment of stallions

Parenteral antibiotics are inappropriate as there is no invasion of tissues. Treatment should involve thorough removal of smegma and topical application of appropriate antibiotics. If the stallion is manageable he should be teased by a mare to achieve an erection and then the shaft of the penis and prepuce thoroughly cleansed using a dilute chlorhexidine solution and then dressed topically with nitrofurazone ointment. If the stallion is difficult to handle acepromazine (ACP) at a low dose may be required; however the owner must be warned of the potential risks of using ACP in breeding stallions. Attention must be paid to the degree of irritation caused to the penile skin as there can be a severe inflammatory response to any of these agents.

Klebsiella pneumoniae

Capsule typing allows differentiation of true venereal forms of K. pneumoniae. Capsule types 1 and 5 are the most commonly occurring in the UK; type 2 is also considered to be pathogenic.

Treatment is similar to that for CEM, although Klebsiella is a more resistant organism and difficult to treat effectively. It may require prolonged treatment with topical and systemic antibiotics. Sensitivity testing should be carried out to determine appropriate antibiotics; aminoglycosides, particularly gentamicin and amikacin, are useful. Care must be taken regarding toxicity if aminoglycosides are used systemically; they may also cause local irritation. Following the course of treatment, a bacterial broth made of normal commensal organisms should be applied to encourage establishment of normal protective flora.

Clitoral infections usually resolve satisfactorily, but if there is persistence of the organism following extensive treatment clitorectomy may be considered.

Kenny and Cummings (1990) report on the use of dilute sodium hypochlorite to treat *Klebsiella* infections in stallions. The treatment involves cleaning the penis and then rinsing it with dilute sodium hypochlorite solution once daily for 2 weeks. The solution is made up by adding 40 ml of 5.25% sodium hypochlorite (bleach) to 1 gallon (4.5 litres) of water.

Pseudomonas aeruginosa

Pseudomonas aeruginosa is the most difficult pathogenic bacterium to treat successfully. Pathogenic and non-pathogenic strains cannot be differentiated in the laboratory. The organism may also recur after a negative swab. Sensitivity testing must be carried out prior to treatment. Aminoglycosides, particularly gentamicin and amikacin, may be useful.

Treatment of mares

Clitoral infections can be treated with topical application of 0.5% silver nitrate solution, which acts as a desiccant, prior to application of an appropriate antibiotic cream. Some clinicians prefer the use of povidone-iodine as a cleansing agent. Silver nitrate solutions may be irritant after repeated applications. Clitorectomy may be considered in persistent cases. When there is an endometrial infection clitoral treatment should precede intrauterine treatment by 2 or 3 days. Application of bacterial broth containing normal flora may be a useful adjunct to therapy. In persistent cases continued contamination from urine or faeces should be considered. Following treatment an additional precaution of applying silver nitrate and gentamicin cream to the clitoris prior to mating may be useful.

Treatment of stallions

The penis and prepuce should be thoroughly cleansed using povidone-iodine solution, followed by the application of 0.5% silver nitrate solution and appropriate antibiotic cream. Treatment should be carried out daily for a minimum of 1 week. Care must be taken with regard to any local inflammatory reaction. Application of bacterial broth containing normal commensal flora following treatment may be useful.

Kenny and Cummings (1990) report that *Pseudomonas* rarely survives in acid conditions, so they suggest rinsing the cleansed penis with a dilute solution of hydrochloric acid once daily for 2 weeks. The solution is made up of 10 ml of concentrated hydrochloric acid in 1 gallon (4.5 litres) of water. The concentration may be reduced in 2-ml steps if there is a marked inflammatory response.

Viral diseases

Equine herpes virus 3 (coital exanthema)

Equine herpes virus 3 (EHV-3) is a relatively common infection. It presents as small vesicles on the vulval lips or shaft of the penis. The vesicles rupture to form ulcers, which take 10–20 days to heal, frequently leaving the affected area unpigmented. The incubation period is 7–10 days. Systemic signs are rare but pyrexia and depression have been reported.

Treatment in both mares and stallions involves sexual rest, and topical application of antibiotic ointment to prevent secondary bacterial infection of the ulcers. EHV-3 infection does not depress fertility.

Recrudescence may occur as with other herpes virus infections. Recurrence may be spontaneous or triggered by stress.

Equine arteritis virus

Equine arteritis virus (EAV) is a togavirus that produces a panvasculitis. Infection may occur either via the respiratory or venereal route. Severity of clinical signs depends on the pathogenicity of the strain and previous exposure of the population. In populations where EAV is endemic clinical signs may be minimal. Clinical signs include anorexia, depression, lacrimation and severe conjunctivitis, nasal discharge and generalized oedema; in the stallion this may included marked oedema of the scrotum and sheath. Abortion can occur due to death of the foetus or more commonly due to endometrial lesions. Signs usually develop within 14 days of infection. Diagnosis should be confirmed by virus isolation, virus neutralization and enzyme-linked immunosorbent assay (ELISA) tests. Treatment involves isolation, rest, nursing and control of bacterial secondary infections. All in-contact animals should be identified and isolated.

The carrier state has not been reported in mares. Approximately 30%

of infected stallions can become chronic carriers, persistently shedding the virus in the sperm-rich fraction of semen. Chronic carriers are only infective via the venereal route. Extending, freezing or chilling semen has no effect on reducing infectivity. Equine arteritis virus can be transmitted in semen used for AI.

A vaccine is available in the USA that has been shown to prevent the development of the carrier state in stallions but produces high virus neutralization titres, which may prove problematical if the horse is to be exported.

The stallion

Anatomy and physiology

The testes are maintained at 35 °C; any rise in temperature will affect sperm quality, the effects being seen 10–40 days later. The testes descend into the scrotum between 300 days' gestation to 10 days of age. They can remain in the inguinal canal for several months.

The epididymis is a single convoluted tubule with the head at the cranial pole, the body running dorsolaterally along the testis and the tail attached by a fibrous ligament to the caudal pole of the testis.

The penis is a haemodynamic musculocavernous structure. It consists of the root, body and glans, which is the enlarged end that may form a seal with the cervix at ejaculation, allowing the semen to be deposited directly into the uterus. The prepuce protects the non-erect penis.

The accessory sex glands are listed below.

- The ampullae are the distal portion of the deferent ducts that converge over the neck of the bladder.
- The vesicular glands open into the pelvic urethra and produce the gel fraction of the ejaculate.
- The prostate gland, lying about a hand's breadth from the anus, is a bi-lobed structure connected by an isthmus over the pelvic urethra.
- The bulbourethral glands lie dorsolateral to the pelvic urethra at the ischial arch. They produce pre-ejaculatory fluid.

Gonadal function is under neuroendocrine control, the hypothalamus acting as the primary regulator. The hypothalamus integrates neural input with hormonal output: in response to neural input GnRH is released that in turn acts on the anterior pituitary, which produces LH and FSH; LH acts on the Leydig cells in the testes stimulating testosterone production, which stimulates spermatogenesis; FSH acts on the Sertoli cells in the testes.

Spermatogenesis occurs in the convoluted part of the seminiferous tubules and takes approximately 57 days. Transport along the tubules takes 7–10 days.

Seasonality and puberty

The stallion is a seasonal long-day breeder, with an endogenous circannual rhythm. There are seasonal fluctuations in FSH, LH and testosterone, peak levels occurring in May, June and July.

Puberty occurs at 1–2 years of age and testicular size continues to increase until the stallion is 7 years old. Degenerative changes may be observed in the testes from 15 years of age, although some stallions will maintain good fertility into their early twenties.

Fertility evaluation of the stallion

A stallion may be presented for fertility evaluation prior to purchase, to investigate apparent subfertility or to maximize efficiency in an AI programme. The only accurate assessment of fertility is the pregnancy rate achieved in mares mated. No single criterion correlates accurately with fertility, but a combination of physical examination, behavioural observation and semen evaluation acts as a guide and will highlight any problem involved in subfertility.

Physical examination

This should include a general clinical examination, paying particular attention to musculoskeletal problems such as laminitis, lameness or back pain that may have a significant effect on mating behaviour and fertility. Musculoskeletal pain may account for poor mounting behaviour, instability on the mare or failure to ejaculate.

A checklist for recording the history in fertility evaluation of the stallion is given below.

1. Previous use, e.g. horses in training are usually punished for exhibiting sexual behaviour.
2. Frequency of mating, e.g. has there been a marked increase in number of mares mated?
3. Previous injuries or disease.

4. Previous medication, e.g. anabolic steroids can have a marked negative feedback on endogenous hormone production.
5. Patterns of mating behaviour.
6. Management changes.
7. Are there previous fertility figures available for comparison?

An examination of the external genitalia should be undertaken. It is a matter of personal preference whether this is undertaken before or after observation of mating behaviour. Often the stallion may be more amenable to handling after mating; the testes are often well descended and easier to palpate thoroughly. Swabs of the prepuce/penis, urethra, urethral fossa and pre- ejaculatory fluid should be taken for aerobic and microaerophilic culture. These swabs should be taken when the stallion has an erection while teasing a mare at teasing boards. It is important to have an experienced handler restraining the horse; with some stallions the sight of the mare may be adequate to allow the swabs to be taken. At this time a visual examination of the erect penis can be made, noting any ulcerated areas, signs of trauma or neoplasia.

If the stallion is used to natural mating he should be taken to the normal covering area and presented with a quiet oestrous mare. The stallion's behaviour towards the mare, number of attempts to mount, thrusting and ejaculation should be noted. It is also useful at this time to note the practices of the handlers, one of whom should palpate and count the pulsatile waves of ejaculation on the ventral shaft of the penis. There are normally six to nine pulsatile waves.

If the stallion will use an artificial vagina (AV), a semen sample may be taken rather than let the stallion cover the mare. If the stallion is unused to the AV, it is more useful to observe natural mating behaviour before collecting a semen sample.

The external genitalia should be palpated. The consistency of the testes should be noted. They are normally firm and smooth and slip easily within the scrotum. Soft, spongy testes indicate hypoplasia or atrophy; hard fibrous testes suggest degenerative change. The tail of the epididymis can be palpated at the caudal pole of the testes. If the stallion is amenable the body of the epididymis can be palpated along the dorsolateral aspect of the testis. Testicular rotation of 180° can occur; this may be temporary or permanent and does not appear to affect fertility. Testicular dimensions should be measured using calipers; in a mature stallion each testis is about 8–10 cm long, 5–6 cm wide and 4–6 cm high. Pickett et al. (1981) report that total scrotal width is the parameter most closely correlated to daily sperm output. They consider a total width of less than 8 cm to be abnormal, and the average measurement to be greater than 10 cm.

A rectal examination should be undertaken with the stallion adequately restrained or sedated to evaluate the accessory sex glands and inguinal canal. Ultrasound examination with a 7.5 MHz linear array rectal probe allows evaluation of the accessory sex glands (Weber and Woods 1992).

Semen collection

A semen sample should be collected for evaluation. Ideally an AV should be used to collect two ejaculates 1 hour apart. The stallion should have a period of several days sexual rest prior to collection. This is not always possible when evaluation is undertaken during the breeding season.

Some stallions, particularly those used to natural covering are reluctant to use an AV. In these circumstances it may be preferable to perform a somewhat limited analysis in order to reassure the client that the stallion is ejaculating live, progressively motile sperm. This can be done by collecting a dismount sample into a warmed container, or by aspirating semen from a mare immediately after natural cover.

A more complete ejaculate can be collected using a 'condom'. McDonnell and Love (1990) suggest two alternative methods for semen collection, either using a rectal glove attached to the erect penis before natural cover, which allows the semen to run into the fingers of the glove, or by attaching a plastic bag to the mid-shaft of the penis and manually stimulating the stallion using warm towels at 45–50 °C to compress the glans and base of the penis.

The type of AV used is a question of personal preference on the part of the stallion and clinician. The most commonly used types are listed below.

- The Colorado is large and has a rigid outer casing. It contains a large volume of water, which has good heat retention, but also makes it heavy
- The Nishikawa is lightweight, easy to clean and assemble. The main disadvantage is water leakage so the handler should wear waterproof clothing!
- The Missouri is lightweight and flexible with a watertight seal.

It is essential that the AV is correctly prepared to maintain an internal temperature of 45–50 °C and adequate pressure. The lubricants used must be non-spermicidal. The collection area must be safe, easily cleaned with a secure footing. Collection techniques vary considerably, but whichever method is used the AV should mimic the position of the mare's vagina and should be held firmly as the stallion thrusts; the temperature and pressure of the AV should stimulate ejaculation.

Once collected the semen must be handled with care; all equipment must be prewarmed and free from chemicals. The gel fraction should be filtered off and the volume of the ejaculate measured. The semen should be milky to creamy white in colour, odourless with no blood or urine contamination or clots visible. The pH should be between 7.3 and 7.6.

Semen evaluation

Volume

Volume of the gel-free ejaculate is usually between 15 and 100 ml. The volume can be reduced by 40% in December, January and February. The second ejaculate is usually a smaller volume than the first. Volume does not appear to be an important factor in fertility. It has been suggested that large volumes, in excess of 100 ml, may stimulate uterine motility and so reduce fertility.

Motility

A sample of semen should be placed on a warmed microscope slide and percentage motility and percentage progressive motility estimated. These measurements are subjective and when sperm density is high extending the semen will reduce agglutination. Total motility is usually between 60 and 80% and progressive motility should be between 40 and 70%, with little variation between the first and second ejaculates. Initial motility is an important characteristic of semen.

Motility should be observed on a prewarmed slide at 5, 10, 30 and 60 minutes after collection. Raw semen should be kept in an airtight container at 22 °C and observed hourly until there is no motility. The extended semen, kept at 4 °C, should be observed at 6 hours and 24 hours. The reduction in motility should be slow during the first half an hour and declines to about 10% by 6 hours. However conditions are not the same as in the mare's genital tract, and poor longevity *in vitro* does not preclude good fertility.

Several slides should be smeared with semen for eosin–nigrosin and haematoxylin staining. A portion of semen should be diluted 1:1 with formal citrate and returned to the laboratory for further evaluation.

Concentration

The semen is diluted 1:100 or 1:200 with formal citrate or buffered formal saline. The dilution must be accurate. The concentration of spermatozoa is then measured using a spectrophotometer or a haemocytometer; it can vary between 50 and 700×10^6/ml.

Morphology

Slides are usually stained with eosin–nigrosin for live/dead counts and assessment of sperm morphology. Two slides should be examined and 100 sperm per slide checked for abnormalities. Less than 10% of one particular abnormality is considered to be within normal limits. The relationship between morphology and fertility is less clear in the stallion than in farm animals.

Evaluation of findings

The total number of progressively motile morphologically normal sperm per ejaculate can be calculated using the following method:

concentration × volume × % progressively motile × % morphologically normal

This is the most meaningful figure when assessing potential fertility. There is considerable monthly variation. Kenny *et al.* (1983) suggest that for a stallion to cover 40 mares in a breeding season this figure for the second ejaculate should be approximately:

February	1.7×10^9
April	1.8×10^9
June	2.2×10^9
August	1.7×10^9
October	1.2×10^9
December	1.0×10^9

Care should be taken when attempting to predict fertility on the basis of any of these findings. Season, age, management, number of mares covered and handling of the semen should all be taken into account. Any obvious variation in the findings merits full evaluation. It may allow recommendations regarding the management of the stallion to be made. The single most reliable figure is the number of mares the stallion gets in foal.

Subfertility in the stallion

Infertility in the stallion is uncommon and is due to a sperm-free ejaculate, ejaculation of only dead sperm or inability to mate in naturally bred stallions. Subfertility is difficult to define as numerous variables are involved: number of mares mated, management system, time of year and fertility of the mares mated.

Abnormalities detected in the preceding examination may reveal specific problems or a more vague subfertility. In the latter situation, careful management of mares, timing mating as close to ovulation as possible, spacing matings carefully to reduce the frequency of matings and good stallion management will maximize fertility.

There are many specific conditions that will be detected during the preceding examination that have an adverse affect on fertility. The non-specific problems usually require management changes for both the stallion and mares to maximize fertility.

Specific conditions

Traumatic injuries to penis and prepuce

These injuries are usually a result of trauma at mating, e.g. a kick from the mare, an incorrectly prepared or used AV, or accidental injury, e.g. from a fence, or stable door if the stallion is teasing over it.

Signs

Initially there is marked oedema and haemorrhage. Lesions involving the prepuce tend to produce generalized reaction whereas those involving the penis produce a more restricted reaction.

Treatment

Treatment should be directed towards limiting and then rapidly reducing the swelling. Cold hosing, subsequent massage and alternate hot and cold therapy are useful. Incorporating the penis in an abdominal bandage will support it and help return of fluids from damaged tissues. Depending on the extent and depth of the injury topical and systemic antibiotics should be administered. Non-steroidal anti-inflammatory drugs and analgesics, e.g. phenylbutazone, should be given. Until the injury has resolved satis-factorily the stallion should have a period of complete sexual rest.

Penile paralysis (priapism)

Signs

This can be the result of neurological damage or the use of phenothiazine tranquillizers, e.g. ACP. There is a partial erection with filling of the corpus cavernosum rather than oedema.

Treatment

The penis should be supported with an abdominal bandage or padded plastic guttering, and alternate hot and cold therapy applied. In severe cases amputation may be necessary following reduction of acute inflammation.

Penile neoplasms

Signs

Neoplasms usually interfere with intromission and may result in haemospermia. Squamous cell carcinoma is most commonly seen; it affects the non-pigmented skin and may be locally invasive. Metastasis to the local lymph node has been reported though infrequently. Melanomas, sarcoids, haemangiomas and fibropapillomas have been reported. Diagnosis can be confirmed by biopsy.

Treatment

Small lesions may be removed cryosurgically; others require surgical removal or amputation of the penis (Howarth *et al.* 1991). Stallions with fibropapillomas should not be mated during the infectious period.

Urethral trauma

This may be due to urethral calculi, improper catheterization, endoscopy or tight stallion rings.

Signs

Inflammation is marked and if trauma is severe a stricture may form.

Treatment

Topical application of 1% silver nitrate solution following removal of the cause is the treatment of choice.

Trauma to testicles and epididymis

Signs

A kick is the most common traumatic injury to the scrotum. It produces scrotal oedema and pain, often increasing testicular temperature that in turn damages the sperm. It rarely results in testicular swelling.

Treatment

Cold water therapy is important in the acute phase; analgesics and NSAIDs should be administered.

Orchitis

Signs

Acute orchitis can be due to infection, e.g. strangles, or trauma. The scrotum and testes become painful, hot and swollen. Early initiation of therapy is essential to prevent chronic orchitis. Chronic orchitis presents as firm nodular small testes. Semen analysis reveals a low sperm density with large numbers of abnormal spermatozoa.

Treatment

In the acute stage cold water therapy, analgesics, systemic antibiotics and NSAIDs are essential. In cases where there is marked swelling and dependent oedema, support for the scrotum is helpful. In cases where one testis is severely affected and the other apparently normal, early unilateral castration may preserve the unaffected testis. If this decision is delayed unduly the second testis may develop orchitis. When testicular temperature is raised for more than a few hours sperm quality will decrease. Raised temperature for 48 hours will produce considerable reduction in sperm motility 1–5 days later. The most significant changes will be seen 25–40 days after the insult.

Epididymal obstruction can occur following an episode of orchitis. Usually extreme sexual excitement will unblock the duct. The stallion should then be used frequently to prevent recurrence.

Zang *et al.* (1990) reports on the development of anti-sperm antibodies following an episode of traumatic orchitis.

Testicular torsion

Signs

Acute 360° torsion is uncommon. It presents as an acute, severe colic in a younger stallion. Clinical examination will reveal the cause of the severe pain. Sedation may be required to complete the examination.

Torsion of 180° may be detected on routine examination. The tail of the epididymis is at the cranial end of the scrotum. The torsion may be temporary or permanent. It does not appear to affect fertility or libido.

Treatment

Torsion of 360° requires early surgical intervention. Torsion of 180° requires no treatment.

Testicular neoplasia

Signs

Seminomas (most common), lipomas, Sertoli cell tumours, interstitial cell tumours and teratomas are seen in the older stallion. Tumours are usually unilateral and present as painful firm swellings that result in testicular degeneration and reduced sperm numbers.

Treatment

Unilateral castration is the treatment of choice. Local lymph nodes should be checked for evidence of metastasis.

Cryptorchidism

One or two testes can be retained anywhere along their path of descent in the foetus. After the first few weeks of life an abdominal testis can no longer pass through the inguinal canal. Testes retained in the inguinal canal can descend; they are usually palpable and descend as the animal matures. A testis may be permanently retained in the inguinal canal in which case it is usually small and misshapen. Abdominal testes can be either completely retained, i.e. testes and epididymis within abdominal cavity, or partially retained when the vaginal process and epididymal tail pass through the inguinal ring.

Signs

Diagnosis is made on palpation. Animals who have had little handling may require sedation to allow adequate palpation of the inguinal region.

Diagnosis can be confirmed in animals over 3 years of age by measurement of plasma oestrone sulphate levels. Cryptorchids have levels in excess of 400 pg/ml, whereas geldings have levels less than 100 pg/ml. Donkeys and animals under 3 years old do not produce significant levels of oestrone sulphate; in these animals a testosterone stimulation test can be carried out. A resting sample is taken then 6,000 iu hCG is administered intravenously and a further sample taken 30–120 minutes later. Testosterone levels are measured in both samples and a significant rise following hCG infection suggest that functional testicular tissue has been stimulated. The normal range for testosterone levels in an entire male is 5.0–30 nmol/L, in cryptorchids 0.3–4.3 nmol/L and in "false rigs" (geldings) 0.15–0.3 nmol/L.

Treatment

Testes in the inguinal canal can easily be removed under general anaesthesia; those in the abdominal cavity require an exploratory laparotomy.

Haemospermia

Signs

Blood contamination of semen reduces fertility proportional to the degree of contamination. Contamination can be constant or intermittent. Blood causes sperm agglutination and reduces progressive motility.

Treatment

The source of haemorrhage should be located. It may be urethral, penile or from the internal genitalia. Urethral endoscopy may be necessary to locate and treat the lesion. Treatment is dependent on the nature of the lesion, but is likely to include topical antibiotics (after appropriate sensitivity testing); occasionally topical corticosteroids or 1% silver nitrate solution are necessary. The stallion should have a period of sexual rest until the lesion has resolved satisfactorily.

Urospermia

Signs

Semen is yellow to amber in colour with a distinct urine odour. The pH is raised and urea levels are greater than 5 mmol/l. There is low motility. Fertility is reduced by the effect of the urine on sperm and on the mare's endometrium. The problem may be intermittent.

Treatment

The cause is unknown, but urination frequently occurs towards the end of ejaculation. The stallion can be used for AI as semen collection can be modified to collect the early part of the ejaculate. For natural mating the stallion should be encouraged to urinate prior to mating.

Ejaculation problems

Unless the stud routinely palpates the pulses of ejaculation the staff may be unaware of a problem. Behavioural changes are frequently associated with failure to ejaculate. The stallion may exhibit excessive libido and restless fidgety behaviour. There may be more than 10 pelvic thrusts, and the stallion becomes increasingly frustrated and can be aggressive. Diagnosis is confirmed at the time of semen collection.

Mounting and thrusting difficulties are frequently associated with musculoskeletal problems causing pain or weakness. Aortic–iliac thrombosis, which compromises hindlimb circulation, can cause these problems.

Treatment

Management changes may be enough to overcome the problem. The stallion should reach a stage of maximal sexual arousal before being allowed to mount the mare and stimulus to the penis should be maximal. Any musculoskeletal pain should be alleviated with phenylbutazone and the footing of the covering area should be secure.

The use of various drugs to stimulate ejaculation in the stallion has been reported (Klug 1987). Adrenergic α-agonists and β–antagonists can be used to stimulate smooth muscle contracture: L-norepinephrine at a dose of 0.01 mg/kg is administered intramuscularly 15 minutes before mating, followed 5 minutes later by 0.015 mg/kg carazolol. Diazepam at a dose of 0.05 mg/kg up to a total dose of 20 mg administered by slow intravenous injection 5–7 minutes before mating will help some horses. GnRH has been used to increase testosterone levels in horses with poor libido; 50 µg given intramuscularly 2 hours and 1 hour before breeding has been recommended. In my experience results may be disappointing. Xylazine will induce ejaculation without mating in 25–30% of stallions; 0.66 mg/kg should be administered intramuscularly and the horse then left undisturbed.

Retraining has an important role to play in many disorders involving poor libido, behavioural and ejaculatory problems. Discussion is beyond the scope of this chapter and readers are recommended to consult McDonnell (1992a,b).

Artificial insemination

Artificial insemination has been used successfully in the horse for most of this century in Europe. An increasing number of breed societies accept AI, although it is not yet acceptable in Thoroughbreds. Artificial insemination has several advantages over natural mating:

1. it increases the number of mares that can be inseminated by the stallion and reduces the load on the stallion, as a single ejaculate can be collected and split to inseminate several mares;
2. it reduces the risk of injury to the mare or stallion;
3. it increases hygiene, control of venereal disease and reduces bacterial contamination of the mare at mating.

However there are also several disadvantages that must be carefully explained to the client before embarking on an AI programme:

1. it requires a high level of skilled veterinary attention to achieve fertility levels comparable to natural mating;
2. as a result of this, costs are higher than natural mating;
3. the stallion must be trained for semen collection.

Artificial insemination can be undertaken using fresh, chilled or frozen semen. Conception rates are highest with fresh semen and lowest with frozen semen. Fresh semen used on the stud farm where it is collected is the simplest system and high conception rates are readily attainable. It is useful to use this system to familiarize staff with procedures before setting up a more extensive AI programme.

Chilled semen is extended, cooled to 4°C and can be stored for 24–48 hours. This allows transportation in specialized containers, e.g. Equitainers (Hamilton-Thorn Research Ltd, Danvers, MA, USA). Conception rates can be similar to those achieved with fresh semen provided management is good.

Frozen semen can be maintained in liquid nitrogen at –196°C for long periods. Frozen semen is least well accepted by breed societies but allows international trade in semen provided strict import regulations are followed. A programme of test-freezing and inseminations is necessary to determine whether a stallion's semen is suitable for freezing. Due to reduced conception rates this is not a suitable alternative for subfertile mares. To achieve acceptable conception rates with frozen semen it is important to select fertile, young mares who are cycling regularly. Insemination should be carried out within 12 hours of ovulation.

The stallion used should be swabbed for equine venereal diseases, have his markings taken and blood typed and registered with the breed society before being used for AI.

Semen collection

The stallion should be trained to use an AV, either with a quiet mare or with a dummy mare. It is essential that the semen is handled with the greatest care to maximize conception rates. There should be a special collection area with an adjacent well-equipped laboratory for semen evaluation and processing. Each stallion should have separate collection equipment with his own AV, disposable or sterilizable liners for the AV, and separate collection receptacles.

After collection, the gel fraction should be rapidly removed using a filter, and the semen evaluated for volume, motility and sperm concentration. The semen can then be diluted using semen extender (see below) and divided into insemination doses of $250–500 \times 10^6$ progressively motile sperm. A semen extender suitable for semen maintained at room temperature or chilled has the following composition:

D-glucose	4.9 g
Powdered low-fat milk	2.4 g
Crystalline penicillin	150 iu
Streptomycin sulphate	150 mg

Made up to 100 ml with sterile deionized water.

Semen to be used fresh can be stored at room temperature for 2 hours. Semen to be used chilled should be cooled carefully at a rate of 0.3°C/minute to 4–6°C and stored or transported in a special thermostatically controlled container, e.g. a Hamilton-Thorn 'Equitainer'. These containers should be sealed and labelled appropriately. Semen to be frozen requires dilution, centrifugation and resuspension in a special freezing extender. Special packaging and labelling equipment is required. Liquid nitrogen is needed for freezing and long-term storage.

Preparation of the mare

It is important to discuss fully with the owner of the mare the requirements and likely costs of using AI. Owners of single mares often think AI is going to be cheaper than sending the mare to stud!

All equipment used must be sterile and prewarmed; all syringes should have plastic rather than rubber plungers. Lubricants used must be non-spermicidal. The semen should be protected from air, sun and temperature fluctuations.

The mare should be swabbed and examined as for natural mating. The mare should have her markings recorded. Insemination should be carried out in the 12 hours preceding ovulation, or immediately after ovulation. To hasten ovulation 3000 iu hCG can be administered 12 hours before, or at the time of, insemination. The mare should be prepared as for a gynaecological examination. Particular attention should be paid to cleaning the perineum. There is no need to warm the semen as the mare will act as an incubator. The insemination catheter should be guided with a sterile gloved hand through the cervix into the body of the uterus where the semen should be gently expelled.

Either before or immediately after insemination a sample of semen should be examined on a prewarmed microscope slide. A few minutes should be allowed for the temperature to equilibrate. The semen should be assessed for motility and density.

The mare should be examined 12–24 hours later to check for ovulation. If ovulation has not occurred, insemination should be repeated. The mare should be examined 15–17 days later to detect pregnancy.

Embryo transfer

Introduction

Embryo transfer was first successfully carried out in the horse in 1972. Since then it has been increasingly used by certain sections of the horse breeding industry. It has been used to obtain foals from performance mares allowing them to continue competing, to increase production from quality mares and to obtain foals from subfertile mares. The techniques for embryo collection and transfer are now well established. However, before embarking on such techniques the high production costs and regulations of breed societies must be discussed with the owners.

The high cost of maintaining suitable recipients, and of intensive specialized veterinary input is a major limiting factor. The absence of an effective commercial method of superovulating mares limits the maximum number of embryos obtained per breeding season to six to eight. The variable length of oestrus and unpredictability of the timing of ovulation necessitate two possible recipient mares for each transfer attempt.

Donor and recipient selection

The donor and recipient mares should be kept at the same premises and closely monitored for one or two cycles prior to the transfer. If fresh semen is to be used it is easier if the stallion is also at the same premises. It is usual practice to have two possible recipient mares available at each attempt.

Ideally the donor mare should be a genetically superior, proven, broodmare cycling regularly. Older subfertile mares show a significant depression in embryo recovery rates; mares with a history of repeated abortion or early embryonic death are better candidates than those with a history of recurrent endometritis. The mare should have a full gynaecological examination including an endometrial biopsy to assess suitability, and be carefully monitored through one or two heat periods prior to insemination.

The selection of the recipient mare is crucial to success. The recipient should be 3–10 years old, in good health and condition, and either a maiden mare or a mare of good breeding history. The recipient should be a similar size to the donor. A full gynaecological examination, including endometrial biopsy, should be undertaken. Only those mares cycling regularly with no gynaecological abnormalities should be used. Mares that do not become pregnant following two transfer attempts should be removed from the programme.

Synchronizing donor and recipient mares

Recent studies have shown that recipient mares should ovulate either 1 day before to 2 days after the donor mare. Mares that ovulate soon after the donor are most suitable.

Both mares should be cycling regularly; transitional oestrus should not be used. Methods for synchronizing donor and recipient are detailed in Table 6.7.

The donor mare should be teased and examined both manually and by ultrasound. Insemination should be carried out on the day before or on

Table 6.7 Different methods of synchronizing oestrus in donor and recipient mares

	Day	Mare	Treatment
Method 1	0–10	Donor	12.5 ml Regumate
	11	Donor	Inject PGF$_{2\alpha}$
	1–11	Recipients	12.5 ml Regumate
	12	Recipient	Inject PGF$_{2\alpha}$
Method 2	0–10	Donor	Inject 150 mg progesterone in oil and 10 mg oestradiol-17β
	1–11	Recipients	Inject 150 mg progesterone in oil and 10 mg oestradiol-17β
Method 3	6–12 after ovulation	Donor	Inject PGF$_{2\alpha}$
	1 day later	Recipients (6–12 days post ovulation)	Inject PGF$_{2\alpha}$

Day 0, start of programme; PGF$_{2\alpha}$, prostaglandin F$_{2\alpha}$.

the day of ovulation. The recipient mares should be examined until ovulation is detected.

Embryo recovery

All equipment used for recovery and transfer must be sterile, and if ethylene oxide is used the equipment must be allowed to air for 48 hours. Syringes must not have a rubber plunger.

Embryo recovery is carried out on day 7. The mare should be restrained in stocks, tail bandaged and the perineum cleaned. A 28 or 30 French gauge silicone embryo flushing two-way catheter is used. The catheter is inserted through the cervix and the cuff fully inflated. The catheter is withdrawn until it lodges in the internal os of the cervix, forming a tight seal. One litre of prewarmed (32–35°C) Dulbecco's phosphate buffered saline (DPBS) with 1% foetal calf serum is infused into the uterus under gravity; it is then allowed to drain out via a 75-μm filter cup. A minimum of 20 ml of fluid should be maintained in the filter cup. Some operators advocate a 3-minute wait before draining the fluid from the uterus. The process is repeated twice, and 90% of the fluid should be recovered. The uterus may be gently massaged per rectum to assist recovery. The recovered fluid should be clear and uncontaminated. Excessive massage of the uterus will result in contamination by blood. The catheter is then removed and any fluid in the catheter drained into the filter cup. The fluid from the filter cup is poured into a Petri dish and examined under × 10 magnification. Once the embryo has been located a fire-polished pipette attached to a 1-ml syringe is used to move the embryo to the culture medium (DPBS with 10% foetal calf serum). The embryo is then maintained at room temperature until transfer. This should take place within 2 hours of collection. The embryo recovery rate from healthy donor mares by an experienced operator is about 75% (Squires 1993).

Several factors influence recovery rate:

1. Day 9 embryo recovery rate is highest but these embryos are less viable so day 7 is optimal.
2. Semen quality and treatment. Fresh raw semen is reported to have the highest embryo recovery rates (Squires 1993).
3. Donor fertility. Older subfertile mares have considerably lower embryo recovery rates.

The donor mare should then be given prostaglandin to return her to oestrus. This will eliminate any contamination introduced at collection and allow another attempt at embryo collection to be made.

Transfer

Several studies have shown higher pregnancy rates following surgical as opposed to non-surgical embryo transfer. Obviously experience of the operator is a significant factor particularly with non-surgical transfer. Lower pregnancy rates following non-surgical transfer are thought to be due to breaching the cervical seal and contaminating the progesterone-dominated uterus, thereby increasing the risk of endometritis.

Surgical transfer may be carried out through a midline laparotomy. The embryo is transferred into the tip of the uterine horn on the same side as ovulation has occurred. The embryo is transferred using a fire-polished pipette in a minimal quantity of culture medium. This method has several disadvantages:

1. the risk involved in general anaesthesia,
2. the high cost of a laparotomy,
3. a midline surgical wound.

Alternatively, and increasingly used, a standing flank incision can be made. The mare is sedated and restrained in stocks. The paralumbar fossa is prepared surgically and a line block instituted. The area is then prepared aseptically. A grid incision is made, the tip of the uterine horn exteriorized and the embryo transferred using a fire-polished pipette into a relatively avascular area of the uterus. The wound is then closed routinely.

For non-surgical transfer the mare is restrained in stocks, the tail bandaged and perineum thoroughly cleaned. A 10-ml syringe is attached to an insemination pipette. A volume of air (4 ml) is drawn into the syringe; then small amounts (0.5 ml) of medium from the dish containing the embryo are drawn into the syringe in the following order: medium, air, medium with embryo, air, medium, air. A rectal glove and sterile surgical gloves are worn. The catheter is then carefully threaded through the cervix, using a finger to cannulate the cervix and the contents of the syringe expressed into the uterus. Experienced operators are now obtaining similar pregnancy rates to surgical transfer.

Whichever method of transfer is used, the mare is examined for pregnancy with ultrasound 6–8 days after transfer (13–15 days from ovulation). Follow-up ultrasound examinations are carried out at days 20, 35 and 60 if the mare is pregnant. If the mare is not pregnant one further attempt can be made.

Embryo culture and freezing

A suitable culture system has been devised to allow storage of embryos for 12–24 hours to enable transport of the embryo prior to transfer. Ham's

F10 plus CO_2 at 5°C was found to produce satisfactory pregnancy rates. Squires (1993) reports that fertility rates for cooled, transported embryos are similar to those for fresh embryos. Storage for longer than 24 hours appeared to depress fertility.

Bovine embryos have been successfully frozen, thawed and transferred. However results from attempts with equine embryos have had limited success, with low pregnancy rates. More studies are required before a commercial method of embryo freezing is available.

Recent work has been reported on successful *in vitro* fertilization, and immature oocyte manipulation. This is an area currently being intensely investigated and may prove the most effective way forward with older infertile mares.

Drug appendix

Trade name	Active ingredient	Manufacturer	Dose
Regumate	Altrenogest	Hoechst Animal Health	0.044 mg/kg (1 ml/50 kg) orally
Chorulon	Chorionic gonadotrophin	Intervet UK Ltd	1500–3000 iu intravenously
Receptal	Buserelin	Hoechst Animal Health	10 ml intravenously
Estrumate	Cloprostenol sodium	Pitman-Moore Ltd	0.5–2 ml intramuscularly
Lutalyse	Dinoprost	UpJohn Ltd	5 mg (1 ml) intramuscularly
Oestradiol benzoate	Oestradiol benzoate	Intervet Ltd	5–10 mg intramuscularly
Utrin	Neomycin sulphate 1 g, furaltadone hydrochloride 600 mg, polymyxin B sulphate 40 000 iu	Univet Ltd	3 g dissolved in 100 ml sterile water for intrauterine irrigation
Ovalyse	Fertirelin	UpJohn Ltd	2 ml intramuscularly
Oxytocin-S	Synthetic oxytocin	Intervet Ltd	5–40 iu (see text) intramuscularly or diluted intravenously

CHAPTER

7 PIG BREEDING AND INFERTILITY
M J Meredith MA, BSc, BVetMed, PhD, MRCVS

Reproductive physiology
Management of breeding
Planning a breeding programme
Breeding performance
Breeding problems
Specific diseases

Reproductive physiology

Puberty

The earliest indication of reproductive activity in gilts is the appearance of macroscopic antral follicles on the surface of their ovaries from about 80 days of age. These increase in number until about 110 days. Ovulation can be induced in prepubertal gilts by means of equine chorionic gonadotrophin (eCG; formerly known as PMSG) either alone, or in combination with human chorionic gonadotrophin (hCG).

The most important stimulus initiating puberty is contact with a boar, provided that the gilts have reached a responsive age (150–170 days) and a reasonable liveweight. Continuous contact with a boar is not necessary; 15 minutes per day appears to be sufficient. It is unimportant whether gilts are exposed to a boar before reaching the responsive age. The boar effect can be augmented by relocating gilts to a new pen at the time of boar exposure. Direct physical contact is more effective than contact through a gate or fence. The main mechanism of the boar effect is olfactory (salivary and urinary pheromones), but sound, sight and touch play subsidiary roles. Young boars are less able to stimulate ovarian activity than boars of 11 months or older.

Gilts loose-housed in groups tend to reach puberty earlier than gilts in individual stalls, tethers or small groups (three pigs). However, crowded group housing can inhibit ovarian activity.

As far as climatic environment is concerned, moderately low temperatures do not adversely affect puberty, provided that growth rate is not affected. Prolonged high temperatures can delay puberty.

Genetic influence on pubertal age is important—breed, strain, sire and dam effects have all been reported. Heterosis markedly advances puberty. Miniature pigs and Meishan gilts show earlier puberty than commercial pigs. In a recent trial, where gilts were loose-housed and exposed daily to a boar, Meishan gilts attained puberty (first oestrus) at 118 ± 3 days of age and crossbred white commercial gilts reached puberty at 217 ± 3 days.

Seasonal effects on puberty have been widely reported, but the findings are inconsistent, probably reflecting interacting variables such as temperature, wind speed and photoperiod. Typically, puberty may be delayed during the summer. Increasing photoperiod can hasten puberty and 6 or less hours of light per day can delay puberty. In a recent experiment in controlled environment rooms, the percentage of gilts reaching puberty by 225 days was reduced from 54% to 3% by exposure to a summer photoperiod (Paterson and Pearce 1990). However, this effect was overridden by the presence of a boar. During summer and autumn, pigs have higher levels of the hormone melatonin. In pigs, nocturnal increases in melatonin are more likely if light intensity is high during the day. Melatonin can be increased even further by feed restriction to 60% of *ad libitum* for 3 weeks; it has been suggested that seasonal effects on puberty can be overridden by high levels of feeding (Love *et al.* 1993).

In the boar, puberty is defined as the time at which viable spermatozoa appear in the ejaculate. This is typically at about 5 months of age (age being the most important factor), although spermatozoa can be detected in the epididymis (the site of sperm maturation) about 1 month earlier. Development of full sexual capacity may take a further 2–4 weeks. Miniature boars can reach puberty about 1 month earlier.

Oestrus and ovulation

Oestrus (commonly referred to as 'coming in heat') is the period of time in which a female will voluntarily copulate, given a conducive environment. Pro-oestrus is the period of increasing oestrogen influence preceding oestrus and arising from follicular development. It lasts a few days and is particularly noticeable (because of vulval swelling) in gilts. Prepubertal gilts show episodes of follicular growth and external pro-oestrus signs that do not culminate in oestrus or ovulation.

Oestrous behaviour is stimulated by high oestrogen levels (initially from ovarian follicles developing in pro-oestrus) acting on the hypothalamus, but there is a delay in this behavioural response. Oestrogen concentrations actually fall during oestrus. Oestrus is probably terminated by a combination of falling oestrogen plus the postovulatory rise in progesterone, which inhibits oestrous behaviour. 'Split oestrus' is the phenomenon where a pig

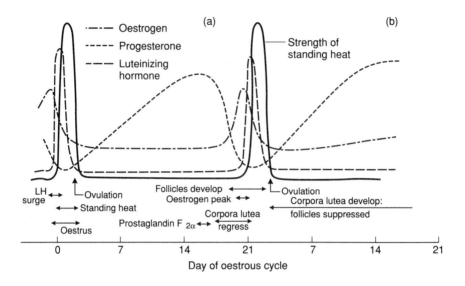

Figure 7.1 Relative changes in the blood concentrations of hormones of the oestrous cycle (a) in the absence of pregnancy and (b) in the presence of pregnancy (from Whittemore 1993).

goes out of oestrus for a day or two but then oestrus recurs; it has been linked with disturbances in ovulation.

The oestrous cycle is the period from the beginning of one oestrous period to the next (Figure 7.1). In unmated pigs, oestrus recurs at a mean interval of 21 days. Cycle lengths are normally distributed around this mean with 95% being in the range 18–24 days. After mating, most non-pregnant pigs return to oestrus at 18–24 days (regular return). There is also a second, more minor, peak of sows returning at 25–30 days due to loss of early embryos.

Oestrous cycles begin at puberty, but are usually absent during pregnancy and lactation. Some sows exhibit anovulatory oestrus 3–7 days after farrowing, but this is due to oestrogens produced by the foetuses and placentae in late pregnancy. However, some pigs will cycle during lactation under conditions of multiple suckling, *ad libitum* feeding and exposure to a boar.

Ovulation starts at 36–44 hours after onset of oestrus (range 0–96 hours) and lasts for 1–3 hours (range 0.5–7 hours) (Flowers and Esbenade 1993). Thus, there is great variation. Most follicles (68–95%) ovulate early in the ovulatory period, but the residue take longer. Coitus can advance and shorten the process of ovulation. Slightly more ovulations occur from the left ovary compared with the right. In the Meishan breed, ovulation occurs later in oestrus and is shorter in duration.

Table 7.1 Mean ovulation rates (from Christenson 1993)

	At puberty	Age (days)				
		220(G)	280(G)	417(S)	608(S)	735(S)
Meishan	12.3	16.7	16.5	18.1	20.1	24.6
White crossbred	12.7	12.7	13.9	15.2	17.1	16.6

G, gilts; S, sows.

In a recent trial the number of ovulations (corpora lutea) increased markedly (mean increase 4.3) from the first (pubertal) oestrus to the sixth oestrus in Meishan gilts, but only increased slightly (1.2) from the first to fourth oestrus in white crossbred gilts (Christenson 1993) (Table 7.1).

Mating and conception

In the brief 'courtship' preceding mating, the boar gives a characteristic series of grunts, quaintly referred to as his 'courting song'! He noses her flanks and vulva vigorously and champs at the jaws, producing frothy saliva containing a pheromone that excites the sow to show what has been termed the 'mating reflex' of rigid immobility. Repeated short protrusions of his spiral-tipped fibroelastic penis occur as mounting is attempted. Intromission is accompanied by repeated pelvic thrusting, followed by a quiescent phase during which ejaculatory waves of contraction can be palpated at the root of the penis, below the anus. Copulation lasts 1–10 minutes.

Fertilization occurs in the ampullary (middle) segment of the uterine tube (oviduct) and requires spermatozoa to be already present at the time of ovulation. The sperms are 'stored' at the utero-tubal junctions after insemination and progressively escape from there to ascend the tubes. This seems to be part of the mechanism to avoid deleterious fertilization of an egg by more than one sperm (polyspermy).

Pregnancy

The mean duration of pregnancy is 114 ± 1.5 days. This predicts that 99% of sows will farrow in the period 110–119 days (first day of oestrus is day 0).

Maintenance

In the first 10 days of pregnancy, transplanted embryos only survive if there is close synchrony between their age and the days since ovulation of the recipient uterus. How progesterone influences the uterine environment at this time is not well understood, but this is a period of marked endometrial development. After day 10, the uterus synthesizes and secretes significant quantities of a variety of proteins as components of the nutritive uterine secretion known as 'histotrophe' or 'uterine milk'. Embryo survival and development are very dependent on this secretion because the diffuse epitheliochorial placenta of the pig does not allow the intimate contact between foetal and maternal capillaries that would facilitate transfer of large molecules. One of the best known of the histotrophe proteins is uteroferrin, which is secreted by the uterine glands, beginning in the attachment period, increasing markedly after day 30 and peaking at day 60. As the name suggests, uteroferrin is known to function in iron transport to the conceptus. Retinol-binding protein (RBP) is detectable from day 12 and is believed to supply vitamin A to the conceptus. Other uterine protein secretions have antibacterial, immune or development-regulating functions. In addition to secreting proteins, the endometrial epithelium takes up some plasma constituents and releases them into the uterine lumen.

Porcine pregnancies are dependent on progesterone produced by the corpora lutea for maintenance and normal development. The developing embryos must produce a 'signal' (oestrogen is believed to be a component of this) at day 11–12 (day 0 is first day of oestrus) to prevent the regression of corpora lutea (luteolysis), which would start at day 12 in a non-pregnant female. It is also essential that viable embryos are present in both horns of the uterus at this time to prevent release of luteolytic quantities of prostaglandin $F_{2\alpha}$ ($PGF_{2\alpha}$) from unoccupied uterine horn.

Corpora lutea appear to function autonomously for the first 2 weeks of pregnancy, but subsequently (days 14–50) require luteinizing hormone (LH) as a luteotrophin. In the last half of pregnancy, prolactin appears to be an important luteotrophin (Dusza and Tilton 1990). A second phase (days 14–18) of embryonic oestrogen stimulation seems to be necessary for uterine arterial vasodilatation and luteal maintenance beyond day 25 of pregnancy.

Pregnancy is very resistant to adverse nutritional influences: prolonged periods of starvation do not cause embryo death or pregnancy failure.

Porcine corpora lutea were the source from which the hormone relaxin was first discovered in 1930. They are particularly rich in relaxin during pregnancy, in fact the most concentrated biological source known. In early pregnancy, relaxin promotes uterine growth and expansion. In later pregnancy it suppresses uterine contractions and is necessary for normal udder tissue development.

As farrowing approaches, relaxin acts on the oestrogen-primed connective tissue of the cervix to promote softening and dilatation. In this process, the collagen fibrils disperse and become more chaotically orientated, with an increase in the interfibrillar matrix. Prostaglandin $F_{2\alpha}$ causes luteolysis and therefore a fall in ovarian progesterone output. Ovarian progesterone is essential for maintenance of pregnancy during late gestation in the pig and goat.

Conceptus development (Table 7.2)

Fertilization occurs in the ampullary–isthmic junction of the oviduct (uterine tube). Cleavage begins about 15 hours after ovulation with the 2-cell stage lasting 6–8 hours (14 hours *in vitro*) and the 4-cell stage 20–27 hours. Up to the 2-cell stage, embryos are dependent on maternally derived mRNA to direct development. Embryos (mainly 4-cell) or unfertilized ova enter the uterus at about 48 hours after ovulation, probably due to rising progesterone concentrations.

In the period after hatching and before attachment, blastocysts migrate from the cranial extremities of the uterine horns, to spread throughout the uterus. At this time they secrete oestrogen, which appears to be important to the distribution process, modulation of uterine secretions and uterine attachment. Embryos also secrete prostaglandins and proteins, including the antiviral protein interferon, which probably reduces maternal immune response to the conceptuses.

After day 11 blastocysts elongate to form filamentous structures up to 100 cm in length. Attachment is quite superficial, so the term 'implantation' is not appropriate in the pig. It commences on day 13, in the region of the embryonic disc, and continues to progress until at least day 26.

Embryos can be sexed by immunofluorescent detection of the HY antigen on male embryos. This is possible from the 8-cell to early blastocyst stage, with an accuracy of 81%. In miniature pigs, the swine leucocyte antigen (SLA) gene has been shown to influence the rate of embryo development. This may be one of the factors accounting for the considerable variation in rate of blastocyst development in pigs.

Compared with the Yorkshire breed, embryos (of either breed) growing in dams of the Meishan breed appear to have lower growth rates and oestrogen secretion up to day 12 of gestation. This may account for their higher survival rate (Ford and Youngs 1993).

Foetuses can be aged conveniently from the 'crown of head to anus' dimension. They should be in a natural (slightly curved) posture when this is done. From 26 days onwards a simple age estimate can be made with the following formula (Marrable 1971)

Age (days) $=$ 3 × crown/anus length (cm)+20

Table 7.2 Development of porcine conceptuses

Days after ovulation	Developmental stage	Events
1	2-cell	Cell division begins
2	4-cell	Enters uterus. Begins to produce mRNA
3	8–16 cell morula	Compaction and blastulation (differentiation of inner and outer cells) begins. Sexing by HY antigen becomes possible
4	32-cell	Blastocyst formed
6–7	Hatching	Hatching from zona pellucida of 0.2 mm blastocyst
7–12	Free blastocyst	Blastocyst expands to 10 mm sphere. Migration and spacing of embryos around uterus
9–14		Separate formation of embryo and placenta (primitive streak, gastrulation and neurulation)
10–12	Spherical blastocyst	Blastocyst expands from 4 to 10 mm, produces oestrogen, which stimulates endometrial secretory activity. Maternal recognition of pregnancy
12–13	Elongation	Conceptus lengthens (up to 50 cm) in response to uterine secretions? Much variation in size. Secretion of interferons
13–14		Blastocyst begins to attach to uterus by loose contact between uterine and trophoblast membranes. Knob-like microscopic proliferations of the uterine epithelium anchor it to the mesometrial side of the uterus. Increased uterine blood flow. First somites form
16–17		Front leg buds form
17–18		Interdigitation of uterine and trophoblastic microvilli begins. Hind leg buds form
20–21		Pigmentation of eyes. Genital tubercle and olfactory pits present
28		External genitalia and mammary glands differentiate
30–33		Four digits become apparent on each foot
35–36	Foetal period begins	End of embryo period, organ and limb formation completed—looks like a pig. Onset of calcification of skeleton. Palate fuses, limbs project beyond belly
44		Scrotum/labia present
60–75		Teeth can be felt. Claws apparent
90–100		Bristles appear on skin
105–115		Testicles in scrotum

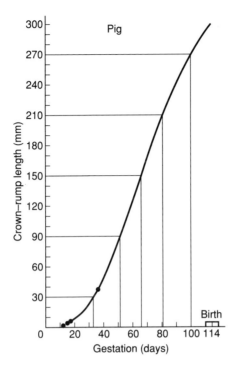

Figure 7.2 Foetal growth curve.

More accurate ageing can be done from a foetal growth curve (Figure 7.2). Degenerate foetuses may require a radiograph for determination of ossification centres or long bone dimensions.

Prenatal losses

Losses of potential offspring vary greatly from one sow to another and from one pig herd to another, but some general biological trends are apparent. In western breeds of pigs, the overall prenatal loss of potential offspring is estimated to be 30–40% of ovulated eggs.

The proportion of unfertilized eggs is quite low (<10%). Most of the prenatal loss occurs between days 12 and 18 of pregnancy, a particularly crucial stage for nourishment, development, and uterine spacing and attachment of pig embryos. This loss is particularly insidious because the tiny dead embryos quickly degenerate and are rarely seen. If the entire litter is lost, this will be obvious by return to oestrus or failure to farrow, but mostly prenatal losses involve only a few embryos per litter and there is no sign that this is occurring.

In pubertal gilts, high embryo losses have been found before day 10 of gestation, but in general most (20–30%) of porcine embryos die between days 10 and 25, particularly between days 12 and 18; losses are greater in sows than gilts, and higher with higher ovulation rates. These high losses are largely unexplained but there is much interest in the theory that asynchronous development of the embryos in a litter is an important factor, i.e. that less-developed embryos succumb when more advanced embryos trigger changes in the uterine environment. A particularly crucial period for this is day 10–12 of pregnancy, when the larger embryos produce oestrogen, provoking a marked secretory response from the endometrium. At this stage of gestation, it is quite possible to find a mixture of small spherical and expanded elongate blastocysts in the same uterus. However, this asynchrony is also seen in Meishan dams, which have a very high embryo survival rate (Ford and Youngs 1993). Lower oestrogen production by embryos in Meishan dams may result in more gradual changes in the uterine environment during a critical period of embryo development.

When deaths occur in the foetal period, the piglets are much larger, with a calcifying skeleton that cannot degenerate without trace, so losses are more likely to receive attention. The foetuses have to be aborted, or delivered with their viable littermates at farrowing time. In rare cases, e.g. some viral infections, the whole litter dies *in utero*, without bacterial infection. In this event, the dead foetuses can remain in the uterus almost indefinitely.

Parturition (farrowing)

Initiation

The initiation of parturition involves a complex interaction of hormonal changes culminating in increasing uterine muscle contractions (Figure 7.3). The key to these complex changes seems to be the foetuses, because parturition will not occur at the normal time if they are all dead. Possibly as a result of increasing distress as they outgrow the capacity of the uterus to support them and certainly in part due to their maturation process, the foetuses produce increasing quantities of corticosteroids and oestrogens. These act on the uterus, stimulating myometrial contractility and also stimulating it to induce regression of the corpora lutea, which have been critical in maintaining the state of pregnancy.

First-stage labour

The first stage of labour lasts 4–12 hours and is characterized by the dilatation of the cervix and development of significant uterine contrac-

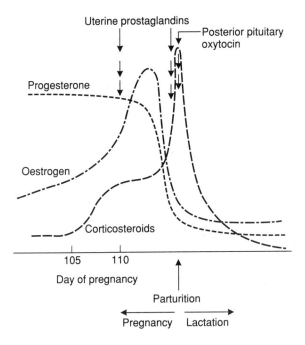

Figure 7.3 Hormonal activities involved in parturition.

tions, which begin to transport piglets down from their uterine locations. Pressure of foetal parts on the birth canal (cervix and cranial vagina) initiates Ferguson's reflex in which nerve ending stimulation stimulates the hypothalamus to initiate oxytocin release from the posterior pituitary gland. Oxytocin stimulates uterine contractions (both directly and also by causing release of uterine $PGF_{2\alpha}$), which lead to further stimulation of nerve endings—a positive feedback mechanism. The progress of this oxytocin release is apparent by the increased milk flow obtained when the teats are milked—an initial drop of milk becomes a jet of milk.

There is, as yet, no maternal straining, but the sow's rectal temperature rises by about 1°C and she shows increasing discomfort, manifested as grunting and champing of the jaws and twitching of the flanks. In a group situation, the sow will separate and take diminishing interest in food and activity. At the same time, she is restless and engages in nest-making. If there is straw available, she will move this around in her mouth. In situations of little or no bedding, she can only paw the ground as if gathering imaginary bedding materials under her.

Physiologically this is an important stage in which the birth canal is prepared (shortening and dilatation of the cervix), separation of the foetal and maternal parts of the placenta begins, and the first foetus is delivered to the pelvic inlet ready for birth. Quite often, the appearance of a blood-stained fluid discharge at the vulva signifies that the chorioallantois of the first piglet's placenta has ruptured and the second stage is about to begin.

Second-stage labour

This is the stage of actual delivery of the litter. It can take less than an hour, but more usually lasts 2–3 hours. The commencement of second stage is signalled by the onset of abdominal contractions (straining) as pressure of foetal parts onto the pelvic wall initiates the pelvic reflex. Pressure on the placenta and umbilical cord during this second stage produces increasing distress for the piglet being delivered, as blood oxygen levels fall and carbon dioxide rises.

In this stage, the sow lies on her side, moving her legs during straining. Swishing of her tail often precedes expulsion of a piglet. The feet or snout of a piglet may appear first; 25–45% of piglets are born in posterior (backwards) presentation. In the delivery process, foetuses come randomly from each uterine horn and they can occasionally overtake one another. The umbilical cord of the piglets is long and remains unruptured, until the newborn piglet moves, in 60–70% of cases. The interval between birth of each piglet ranges from 1 minute to half an hour in healthy farrowings. Some afterbirths may pass out during the second stage, particularly in cases of dystocia, but most are expelled in the third stage.

Third-stage labour

This is the stage of expulsion of the remaining foetal parts (allantochoria or 'afterbirth') of the placentae. In the pig, the allantochoria of adjacent piglets are usually fused and most or all of the afterbirth is passed together about 4 hours (range 0.5–12 hours) after completion of farrowing. Uterine contractions continue in the third stage, though much reduced. They aid placental degeneration and separation. The uterine surface of the afterbirth is velvety and reddish-purple in appearance, while the foetal surface is shiny and smooth. White calcium-containing plaques are sometimes seen in the membranes; they are apparently quite normal.

Fourth stage (puerperium)

The puerperium is the phase when the genital tract returns to normal size ('involution') and function after farrowing and the bacterial contamination, which commonly occurs, is eliminated. Continuing, though reducing, uterine muscle activity is vital in these processes. Most of the recovery is completed in the first 5 days after farrowing and it is usual for some discharge from the vulva ('lochia') to occur at this time. Full uterine recovery, sufficient for good fertility, takes about 3 weeks.

Lactation and weaning

A periparturient rise in prolactin concentrations is believed to be important in the initiation of lactation. Suckling stimulates release of prolactin and oxytocin. Besides reproductive effects, these hormones promote utilization of maternal energy and protein reserves to support milk production. Prolactin concentrations gradually decline as lactation progresses, probably due to the progressive decrease in suckling frequency. Prolactin (and possibly oxytocin) are thought to be important factors contributing to the lactational anoestrus that commonly occurs in the pig (Dusza and Tilton 1990), but the precise mechanisms resulting in lactational anoestrus are not clear; endogenous opioid peptides and possibly ovarian inhibin may also be involved. During lactation gonadotrophin releasing hormone (GnRH) synthesis is inhibited (probably due to neuroendocrine reflexes arising from suckling) and secretion of follicle stimulating hormone (FSH) and LH is usually suppressed during lactation although there is some progressive increase with time. Suckling produces increases in oxytocin, prolactin, progesterone and corticosteroids. After weaning, both basal and pulsatile LH levels rise while prolactin declines dramatically. Oestrus typically occurs 4–7 days after weaning.

Management of breeding

Gilts

Gilts are not mated at puberty, because ovulation rate is poor. In some circumstances, delaying mating has been known to increase litter size by half to one pig per oestrous cycle and it is common practice to delay breeding until gilts are about 220 days old for this reason. However, with modern high-quality feeds and prolific strains of crossbred pigs, it seems that there is little advantage in waiting longer than the second oestrus, provided that the gilts are in good condition.

Some herds use a vasectomized boar to stimulate and detect the initial heats of gilts. This can also have the advantage that they are accustomed to mating before fertile service is undertaken. Unfortunately the vasectomized boars have to be replaced frequently because they become too large.

In most instances gilts will be replacing sows that are about to be culled and it is advantageous to synchronize their heat with the expected heats of the batch of sows they will farrow with. This can be achieved with the oral synthetic progestagen, altrenogest (Regumate, Roussel-Uclaf, France), which is added to the feed daily for 18 days. The cost per gilt treated is approximately £7.

Gilts come into oestrus at approximately 6 days after cessation of altrenogest. Altrenogest simplifies oestrus detection, facilitates planning of artificial insemination (AI), allows synchronization of batch farrowing groups and avoidance of weekend matings. It also means that a much smaller 'pool' of replacement gilts is necessary to replace sows as they are culled, because they can be induced into oestrus as required.

Detection of oestrus ('heat')

Missing the occurrence of 'heat' is a common reason for unnecessary loss of breeding time. The definitive test of oestrus is to expose a female to a keen and desirable male in a conducive environment and see if copulation occurs (copulation refers to the full process of mounting, intromission and ejaculation). However, this ideal test is not always possible, e.g. when AI is being used or where females have to be moved elsewhere for service (mating). In some situations, it is necessary to use the following specific tests for evidence of oestrus:

- response to mounting attempts by boar, or
- response to a 'riding test'.

In each case, a positive response is manifested by immobility and rigidity and a negative response by vocalization and attempts to escape.

The 'riding test' (Figure 7.4) begins with a 'back pressure test', i.e. hands placed gently, but with increasing pressure, on the sow's loins. If the sow stands still for this, the stockperson's weight is then gradually transferred onto the sow's back, in the sitting position. Many sows require some male stimulation to give a positive result to this test, so negative results are not reliable unless a boar (preferably) or aerosol spray of boar odour are present. Skilful supplementary use of the 'back pressure' and 'riding' tests by the stockperson can do much to increase the accuracy of testing for oestrus with a boar.

Testing pigs for heat with a boar is very expensive in time. This cost can

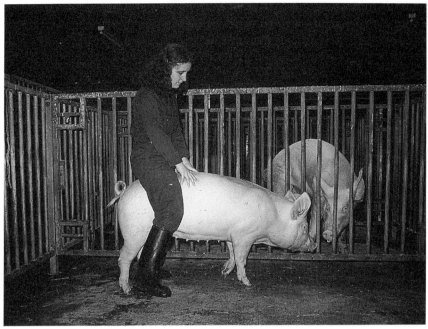

Figure 7.4 Riding test in presence of boar.

Errors in oestrus detection using a boar

Incorrect diagnosis of 'in oestrus' (rare)

'Rape' occurs because female is too ill to resist or cannot escape, e.g. because of stall or mating crate

Incorrect diagnosis of 'not in oestrus'

- boar libido poor (does not 'court' female and attempt mating)
- female (usually virgin gilt) has pain during mating
- female does not like a particular boar (uncommon)
- female distracted by pain or fear (e.g. of stockperson)
- stockperson not ensuring *every* sow in group contacts boar
- stockperson not ensuring *every* sow mounted or back pressure tested

---

Sources of oestrus detection problems

Oestrus not expected

- Poor identification of sows
- Poor breeding records
- Not predicting oestrus from date of weaning/previous service

Not testing each day with boar

- Undue reliance on human observations
- Boar not kept near sows
- Staff overworked
- Lack of libido in boar

Unsuitable housing

- Poor lighting
- Restricted movement of sows (tethers/stalls)
- Female group size too large (more than about 20)
- Stocking density too great
- Slippery floors

Inhibition of oestrous behaviour

- Food present
- Humans too close (where pigs afraid of humans)
- Dominant sows too close
- Distracting sounds and smells

Staff lack skill or care

- Insufficient training, experience, aptitude or motivation
- Not using boar mounting or riding test on every pig
- Not testing each day that heat might occur
- Lack of special attention to nervous or subordinate females
- Rough handling of pigs
- Not detecting lack of libido in boar
- Not detecting illness or lameness in females or boar

be reduced by focusing on the times when heat is likely to occur, i.e. from 3 days after weaning, 17–25 days after an unmated heat and 17–30 days after a mating. Time and effort can also be saved by preliminary human selection of females showing signs indicative of oestrus or of approaching oestrus (pro-oestrus). Skilled pig breeders mark pigs in pro-oestrus or record their details in a notebook or on a displayed record card so that they can be checked carefully with a boar over the next few days.

Signs of pro-oestrus:

- Vulval swelling/reddening (especially in gilt)
- Restlessness, especially at night
- Cloudy, watery vulval discharge (trace)
- Attractive to male (but boars may mount non-oestrous sows)
- Attempts to get to a male ('boar seeking')
- Standing immobile to 'back pressure' by human hands

Signs of oestrus:

- 'Pricking' of ears (more subtle movement in lop-eared pigs)
- Characteristic 'earthy' grunt or 'growl'
- Standing immobile to
    mounting by boar,
    'riding' test,
    mounting by females (not common)
- Mounting evidence: reddening or abrasions in loin area

Loose-housing of females is the most suitable situation for sows to display signs of heat and show the clearest response to an oestrus test. Designs that allow the females to display 'boar-seeking' behaviour are particularly effective and can save much time in detection.

Oestrus detection: could there be a problem?

- Are some gilts >240 days old without being served?
- Is it taking >3 weeks to serve some weaned sows?
- Are >10% sows served only once in the heat period?
- Are pigs returning at 36–48 or 54–72 days after service?
- Are >2% sows 'not-in-pig' (failure to farrow or return to heat)?

Boars

Before using them for breeding, it is advisable to subject newly acquired boars to a thorough health and performance check. A significant proportion of young boars are unfit for breeding, the commonest reasons being poor semen quality and lack of libido. As with all introduced breeding stock, they should also undergo a quarantine period of at least 3 weeks' isolation followed by a microbial/managemental acclimatization period of at least 3 weeks in which they contact cull sows from the herd they are about to join. This can avoid some expensive disruption of the breeding programme.

Modern strains of young boars, which have been performance tested, tend to be too lean and may require some building up of backfat for their working life. They must also have plenty of exercise to prevent locomotor system problems. Twice-daily feeding is recommended and commercial sow diets contain an adequate balance of nutrients. Yorkshire boars on 25 MJ metabolizable energy (ME)/day produced 26% fewer spermatozoa than boars on 47 MJ ME/day (Colenbrander and Kemp 1990).

Boars are commonly vaccinated against erysipelas and porcine parvovirus. In enzootic areas or particular risk situations they might also be vaccinated against Aujeszky's disease, leptospirosis or influenza. Regular treatment for ectoparasites and endoparasites is also important.

Prevention and prompt treatment for locomotor problems is a high priority because they feature prominently as reasons for low libido and culling of boars.

Boars are usually friendly and safe to handle, if treated well, but it must always be borne in mind that they are potentially dangerous. Their razor-sharp tusks are powered by a highly muscular neck with the result that deep wounds can be instantly gouged into pigs or people with an upwards and sidewards thrust. The particularly dangerous times are when another boar (or even the smell of one on pig or human) or a female in heat are around. A pig board should always be used when working with boars and protruding tusks must be cut short. Lots of good contact with people and pigs are important when a boar is growing and when in quarantine.

First use of a boar can begin as early as 7 months. Initial services should be closely supervised and on gilts or small sows that are standing firmly. These matings should be followed up by a proven boar to ensure good farrowing rate and litter size. In the first few months a boar can be used up to twice per week. Farrowing rate and litter size tend to improve up to about 18 months of age (Pearson 1988). Mature boars can be used up to twice per day and five times per week. If a boar is not used for 2 weeks or more, it would be advisable to cover his initial services with another boar or AI. After illness, boars should be well rested and any services within 6 weeks may need to be covered.

Conception

In most countries, conception is still mainly achieved by natural mating, but usage of AI is steadily increasing. In skilled hands and good husbandry conditions AI with semen less than 48 hours old can give similar fertility to natural mating and there are many advantages to using it (Tables 7.3–7.5). There are recent reports that using AI (in the same oestrous period) to follow an initial natural mating gives better farrowing rate and litter size than do entirely natural matings or entirely AI. This may be because AI can be less stressful, but an initial natural mating has advantages for oestrus detection and for stimulation by the penis and seminal fluid components (Flowers and Esbenade 1993). This combined approach is becoming more widespread; however, as with all mixed sire matings, it is more difficult to monitor boar fertility in this situation. One way around this is to use a vasectomized boar for the initial mating.

Table 7.3 Labour time per pig for breeding tasks (from Flowers and Esbenade 1993)

Task	Average time (min)
Natural service: oestrus detection	9.7
Natural service: mating supervision	12.3
AI: oestrus detection	9.2
AI: collection of semen	11.3
AI: semen processing	6.7
AI: insemination	3.4
AI: equipment cleaning	3.1

Table 7.4 Labour time (minutes per sow) for breeding (from Flowers and Esbenade 1993)

	No. of sows bred per day							
	1	2	3	4	5	6	7	8
Natural service	23	24	25	24	23	24	23	23
AI	35*	26	22	20*	19*	18*	18*	17*

*, Significant difference $P\,0.05$.

Table 7.5 Comparison of service protocols (from Flowers and Esbenade 1993)

Day 1:	NS	NS	NS (a.m.+p.m.)
Day 2:	NS	AI	NS
Farrowing rate (%)	88.5	93.2	89.4
Born alive/litter	10.2	10.3	10.5
Labour/sow (min)	35.6[a]	24.6[b]	50.4[c]
Ejaculates/sow	2.0	1.1	3.0
Pigs produced per labour hour	15.2[a]	23.5[b]	11.2[a]
Pigs produced per ejaculate	4.5[a]	8.7[b]	3.1[a]

Values are means. Those in same row with different superscripts (a, b or c) are significantly different ($P<0.05$). AI, artificial insemination; NS, natural service.

Natural mating

Matings may be carried out in the sow's pen, the boar's pen or in a special mating pen. Better matings have been obtained in a special octagonal mating pen than in a small boar's pen, apparently because of improved sexual behaviour of the boar (Hemsworth et al. 1989). The advantage of using a sow's pen, if suitable, is that it avoids the difficulty of moving a sow in heat. Mating pens need to be at least 3×2.6 m, with bedding of straw, wood shavings, sawdust or sand to avoid slipping. Projections that might produce injury, such as feeders or drinkers, must be avoided. Also avoid, if possible, the presence of other pigs and high environmental temperatures.

Mating sows twice during oestrus gives better pregnancy rate and litter size than a single mating. A third mating, when sows are in heat long enough, can improve litter size even further. The optimum time for mating can vary in individual cases from 12 to 40 hours from onset of oestrus. This has led to recommendations that detection of oestrus should be carried out twice daily. In practice many herds only detect oestrus once daily without any obvious detrimental effect on fertility and with considerable saving in labour. With twice-daily detection there is a danger of doing the job less conscientiously than when it is only done once per day. After the initial service sows should be remated at 24-hour intervals (after natural mating the spermatozoa retain their fertilizing capacity for at least 24 hours).

Using two or more boars to serve a sow in the same oestrous period has increased litter size, in some trials, by about half a pig per litter. This is sometimes termed heterospermic (cf. homospermic) insemination. The disadvantages are that this precludes monitoring of the fertility of individual boars, plus there is a greater risk of spreading disease venereally.

Supervision of matings ('hand mating') produces better fertility than just allowing the boar to run with the females. The pigs can be given assistance with alignment, mounting and intromission. Good mating facilities and supervision will ensure that ejaculation is fully completed. A sack placed on the sow's back before the boar mounts will avoid injury by the boar's claws and ensure the sow is not averse to a subsequent mounting. Inexperienced boars may try to mount the head of a female, risking a nasty bite to their working equipment!

Ideally a boar should be slightly larger than the female he is to mate. If there is a marked discrepancy in size, problems with intromission are likely. The penis may pass into the rectum or over the back, side or between the legs of the female. Human assistance, grasping the shaft and not the spiral tip of the penis, is required to guide the penis into the vagina in these situations.

Artificial insemination

Due to the absence of a boar and the shorter effective life of AI sperms in the sow, success with AI is very dependent on good detection of oestrus and accurate timing of insemination. Other important factors are listed below.

Disease control

Because of the potential for spreading disease, most countries control the usage of AI in pigs, primarily by requiring registration and inspection of boar studs and the keeping of records of semen distribution. These statutory requirements often include specific checks of stud boars for epidemic diseases. In addition, AI studs may undertake their own checks that particular diseases are absent from their boars. It is difficult to test the semen itself for pathogens because of enzymes that interfere with diagnostic tests, so serological tests on boars are mainly employed in checking for specific diseases.

Microorganisms known to enter pig semen include:

- adenovirus,
- *Brucella suis,*
- foot-and-mouth disease,
- Japanese B encephalitis,
- leptospirosis,
- *Mycoplasma* and *Ureaplasma* spp.,

- porcine parvovirus,
- porcine reproductive and respiratory syndrome virus,
- pseudorabies (Aujeszky's disease),
- reovirus.

Although not known to be transmitted by semen, precautions are usually taken to ensure that the following diseases are also absent from boar studs:

- classical swine fever (hog cholera),
- swine vesicular disease,
- African swine fever.

Apart from microorganisms that can enter the boar's genital tract, semen can easily become contaminated with infected urine or blood, so theoretically there is potential for spreading many diseases. To some extent the disease risk is reduced by adding antibiotics, e.g. penicillin and streptomycin, lincomycin, gentamicin, kanamycin, neomycin, spectinomycin, to semen, but their role is more to extend storage life by inhibiting microbial multiplication rather than eliminate disease risks. In the European Union, addition of antibiotics is required, by Directive 90/429/EEC, for intracommunity trade in semen. Spread of leptospirosis via semen can be prevented by treatment with 500 iu/ml streptomycin for at least 45 minutes at a minimum of 15°C.

Semen collection

On-farm semen collection can be undertaken by getting the boar to mount a sow in oestrus or a cull sow with inactive ovaries that has been induced into oestrus with oestrogen injection. The penis is deflected before intromission. For boar stud purposes, contact with a female is inconvenient and an unacceptable disease risk. These boars need to be conditioned (trained) to arousal by a 'dummy sow' mounting frame. Training is easier if the boar has no experience of natural mating. Electroejaculation does not give a good enough ejaculate and there is grave concern about the distress it can cause to a boar.

Once arousal (possibly aided by massage of the penis within the sheath) has produced protrusion of the penis, ejaculation is stimulated by contacting the spiral ridges of the penis tip with a latex-gloved hand. It is important not to grip the penis too tightly.

For AI purposes, semen is commonly collected from boars one to three times per week, depending on age, individual performance and demand. Boars with high sperm concentration may show improved semen quality if ejaculated more than once per week.

Semen quality

A typical insemination dose of semen contains 3 (range 2–5)×10^9 spermatozoa of which at least 70% should show progressive motility. After 48 hours of storage (at room temperature) more than 60% sperms should still show progressive motility.

Monitoring of microorganisms in the AI processing laboratory and in the semen produced is vital if fertility and storage life are to be maximized. Seminal components from healthy boars do not usually contain bacteria, but during ejaculation and collection the semen usually becomes contaminated with bacteria from the boar's prepuce, diverticulum, skin and the collection environment. Contamination is reduced if the initial spurts of semen are not collected. Common contaminants, even after addition of antibiotics, are staphylococci, streptococci, *Pseudomonas* spp. and yeasts. Further contamination can occur during processing of ejaculates.

Insemination and fertility

Optimum fertility is obtained when semen is used within 24 hours of collection, but with modern long-life diluents semen doses can be stored at room temperature for 2–5 days prior to use. However, over this period a 5–10% drop in farrowing rate and a decrease in litter size of up to one pig can be expected (Table 7.6).

Single inseminations can give acceptable performance in pigs with a short oestrous period but, if they are still in oestrus the next day, it is advisable to give a second insemination (Table 7.7). Pigs should never be inseminated when not in oestrus, because there is a serious risk of inducing endometritis (Meredith 1991).

A variety of disposable catheters are now available for pigs and, under farm conditions, are preferable to the traditional rubber catheter, which had to be carefully cleaned, sterilized and dried after each use. Pigs, particularly gilts, are sometimes injured by careless insertion of a catheter. It is important to have the pig very still, and insert the catheter carefully,

Table 7.6 Comparative fertility of natural mating and artificial insemination (AI) (from Colenbrander *et al.* 1993)

	Natural mating	AI: semen storage time (hours)		
		<12	18–26	26–36
No. of sows	1529	8853	1419	1337
Farrowing rate (%)	87.3	87.8	88.4	85.8
Litter size	11.3	11.7	11.7	11.1

Table 7.7 Effect of timing and frequency of inseminations (gilts) (from Flowers and Esbenade 1993)

	n	Farrowing rate (%)	Pigs born alive/ litter
Gilts in oestrus for 1 day			
a.m. day 1	35	87.4	8.5
p.m. day 2	36	85.3	8.3
a.m. day 1+p.m. day 1	25	88.2	8.7
Gilts in oestrus for 2 days			
p.m. day 1	65	72.3	8.0
a.m. day 2	68	74.3	8.0
a.m. day 1+a.m. day 2	80	86.4	8.6
p.m. day 1+a.m. day 2	84	85.7	8.7
a.m. day 1+p.m. day 1+a.m. day 2	67	87.5	8.9
p.m. day 1+a.m. day 2+p.m. day 2	72	86.5	8.8
a.m. day 1+p.m. day 1+a.m. day 2+p.m. day 2	78	88.7	9.2

Insemination protocol: a.m., 07.00–09.30; p.m., 15.00–17.30.

following the top wall of the vagina so that the urethral diverticulum is not entered.

There have been reports that semen doses containing sperms from more than one boar (mixed sire semen) produce improved farrowing rate and litter size; however recent and extensive Danish experience revealed no advantage (Colenbrander *et al.* 1993). However, production of mixed ejaculate doses in the AI laboratory is quicker and cheaper.

Pregnancy

Feeding

It is important that sows are in good condition at the time of service, so that high feed intake and weight gain during pregnancy can be avoided— these are known to lead to greater weight loss in lactation and delayed postweaning oestrus.

There has been much controversy about possible detrimental effects of high feed levels in early pregnancy. In some circumstances it seems that high feed levels in the first 2 weeks after mating can increase embryo losses. Increased feed or protein at this time can lower plasma progesterone and this is associated with lower embryo survival rates (Einarsson and Rojkit-tikhun 1993). It has been suggested that this may arise from increased clearance of progesterone under conditions of increased blood flow to the liver.

Feeding strategies for pregnant sows have been reviewed (Cole 1990). Target weight gains during pregnancy are 25 kg for sows and 45 kg for gilts. Sows kept on straw can eat about 0.5 kg/day (digestible energy (DE) about 0.5 MJ/kg dry matter). A target backfat thickness (P2) for gilts at parturition is 20 mm; backfat should never be allowed to fall below 13 mm for gilts or 10 mm for sows (improved hybrids). Within reason, feeding practices are unlikely to have much influence on the development of conceptuses except in the last few weeks of gestation when extra energy intake can be beneficial for birthweights. Insufficient energy intakes in late pregnancy (less than about 30 MJ DE/day) can lead to mobilization of the dam's fat reserves.

Management

The first 35 days of pregnancy are the embryo period when organs and limbs are developing. This is a time when the piglets are very vulnerable to damage by chemicals, so all drugs and pesticides should be avoided or used with great care at this time. In the period from 10 to 18 days after the first mating, the developing embryos are especially susceptible to any stress of their mother. This is a time when moving, mixing, handling, changing feed or any other disturbance should be rigorously avoided if breeding performance is to be maximized.

Pregnancy diagnosis

Non-return to oestrus is the most widely used indication of pregnancy. In herds with good performance this can be the most cost-effective technique (Meredith 1989). Where fertility is lower, for individual problem sows or for 'peace of mind' purposes, a variety of ultrasonic pregnancy testers are widely used (Meredith and Maddock 1995). A-mode (amplitude-depth) instruments are the cheapest and simplest to use, but very prone to false-positive errors. Doppler instruments are now more popular, but require skill for good results and negatives have to be rechecked. The cost-effectiveness of using them routinely is often doubtful.

Rectal palpation can be cheap and highly accurate, but it requires training and in some countries could only be undertaken by a veterinarian. It is very useful in the investigation of infertility problems, because other clinical information is obtained. The technique for the future is undoubtedly real-time ultrasound scanning, but the high cost of the instruments limits usage at present.

Farrowing

Induction of farrowing

The applications of farrowing induction are listed below.

1. Convenient timing:
   (a) minimizing night, weekend or holiday period work,
   (b) supervision of farrowing is easier and cheaper.
2. Stillbirth and preweaning mortality reduction:
   (a) improved attention to dystocia,
   (b) improved care of litter,
   (c) improved colostrum intake.
3. Financial efficiency improvement:
   (a) less time per litter in expensive farrowing accommodation,
   (b) gestation length 2 days less = 1% increase in litters/sow/year.
4. Postpartum sow illness and mastitis reduction:
   (a) improved attention to dystocia,
   (b) hygiene: sow less time in farrowing pen before birth.
5. Induced birth desirable:
   (a) sow disease/injury in late pregnancy,
   (b) dam is immature in size,
   (c) farrowing is overdue,
   (d) litter is dead (mummified),
   (e) piglets born exceed teats, induce gilt to farrow early.
6. Weaner health/performance improvement:
   (a) variation in weaner age reduced by farrowing synchronization,
   (b) variation in weaning weight reduced by better litter care.

The risks of induced farrowing are shown in Table 7.8.

Induction of farrowing is now widely practised, using an intramuscular injection of $PGF_{2\alpha}$ or a synthetic analogue. Pharmaceutical companies differ in their recommendations regarding how early the injection can be given. Some advise against injecting sows more than 2 days early (which precludes treating sows due to farrow on Sunday); most advise against injection more than 3 days early. Premature birth does risk low viability of piglets, so accurate service records and careful calculation of expected farrowing dates are vital. Some of the sows induced would of course have naturally farrowed later than their 'due' date. Experience shows that average pregnancy length can differ between herds, so it is important that each herd analyses its own experience of average farrowing time for untreated sows.

Prostaglandins can produce a variety of side-effects in some sows:

Table 7.8 Risks of induced farrowing

Risks	Precautions
Injection of wrong sow (produces abortion)	Sows must have reliable identification
Expense: about £2 per sow. Not all sows will respond. Some would farrow at desired time anyway	Selective usage Ensure injection enters muscle and not fat or connective tissue
Neonatal immaturity	Service dates must be reliable Calculate mean gestation length for herd Do not induce >3 days early
Neonatal mortality (piglets are slightly immature)	Ensure high birthweights by individual feeding of sows and good nutrition Good environment and skilful care
Side-effects on sows	Ensure injection is hygienic and not intravenous. Ensure pen cannot be damaged
Human health hazards: droplets may be inhaled or there may be absorption through intact skin	Prostaglandins should not be used by people with asthma, or women of child bearing age. Wear gloves when handling
No financial return! Up to 0.6 extra pigs (£9–12) *may* be weaned per litter	Results vary greatly Piglets must be saved by extra care Prostaglandins cannot substitute for good management and health!

restlessness, increased respiration, frequent urination or defecation, vigorous nesting behaviour, injection site reactions. These effects may appear as early as 10 minutes after injection, or be delayed for a few hours. Sows have been known to damage pen fittings in a distressed reaction.

The use of prostaglandins on pig farms in the UK is governed by a code of practice. Prostaglandins have to be prescribed by a veterinary surgeon, who should issue clear written instructions to the client regarding usage and precautions. The veterinarian should also obtain a signed statement from the client that they will keep the product under lock and key, use it only themselves, account for all doses used and dispose safely of needles and syringes after use.

Induction with prostaglandin and oxytocin

Prostaglandins do not provide sufficient control to avoid some farrowings outside working hours. With prostaglandins alone, 75% of sows farrow over a 12-hour period. However, if an intramuscular injection of oxytocin (10–20 iu) is given 15–24 hours after the prostaglandin, the interval from

---

Example of induced farrowing programme

Thursday (9 a.m.):

Inject sows due to farrow on Friday, Saturday, Sunday

Friday:

Sows farrow as follows:	before 7 a.m.	26%
	7 a.m. to 5 p.m.	71%
	5 p.m. to 7 p.m.	3%
		100%

Farrowing times based on production of first piglet

---

prostaglandin to farrowing is reduced by about 6 hours and the variation in farrowing time is reduced. Typically 60–80% farrow within 10–240 minutes of oxytocin. Some people give a second dose after 4 hours, if there is no response. A variation of this treatment is to give 5 iu of oxytocin plus 1.5 mg of the β-blocker carazolol 20 hours after prostaglandin.

Oxytocin seems to work in these situations by shortening the first stage of labour. However, the first stage is important for dilatation of the cervix and general preparation of the birth canal for delivery. Indeed it is considered very bad obstetrical practice to administer this hormone without first checking that the cervix is open. There have been some reports of an increased prevalence of dystocia and stillbirth when oxytocin is used in conjunction with prostaglandins, but some farms seem to have used it without problem. Some treated sows start farrowing, deliver one or two piglets, then stop. A more selective use of oxytocin has been recommended in which only those sows from whom milk can be expressed are treated. However, should a jet of milk be present, the sow's own oxytocin is very active and supplementation could produce overdosage and spasm of uterine muscle. An adequate duration of first stage of labour is particularly important for gilts, so it would certainly seem unwise to use it in these animals, at least, unless it is known that the cervix is open and that no piglet is stuck there.

Impending farrowing

If the sow is to farrow in a crate, with minimal bedding, then a farrowing room temperature of 18–20°C is important. The creep area for the newborn piglets will need to be much hotter, about 30–35°C. It is common practice to reduce feed intake by about 50% in the last few days before farrowing, and for the first couple of days afterwards. Some people add bran to prevent constipation. The reasons given for these practices are that they reduce duration of farrowing, stillbirths, constipation, over-milking and mastitis.

The sow should be installed in her farrowing quarters about 5 days before she is due. Moving her too late risks a farrowing in an unsuitable 'dry sow' area. Moving her too early could contaminate the farrowing pen unduly with detriment to health of the neonates and predisposing to udder or genital tract infection during farrowing. Before moving, the sow should be treated for internal and external parasites and cleaned if dirty, particularly her udder.

Twice daily checking for signs of imminent farrowing is important. This ensures that creep heating and light for the newborn piglets will be switched on in time and helps to ensure that farrowing will be supervised. Farrowing can be predicted using the following signs:

- 85% farrow on days 114–116 (first day of heat is day 0),
- 60% farrow at night,
- *Drops* of milk can be expressed from teats 24–48 hours before,
- *Jets* of milk can be expressed 12–24 hours before.

Supervision of farrowing

As piglets are born, it is helpful to move them away from the still-farrowing sow to a cardboard box (disposable) in the creep area. When the sow's labour has ended and she is ready to suckle, the litter can then be directed to her teats and assisted in obtaining that vital first suck of colostrum. This suckling will hasten delivery of the afterbirths remaining in the sow. The only exception to this would be when uterine inertia develops and no jet of milk can be obtained from the teats. In this situation, putting piglets already born to suckle can stimulate oxytocin release. If first-born piglets are left with the sow, there is a risk of them being injured by leg movements during straining and also that there will be little colostrum remaining for the last-born piglets.

Modern sows have to deliver litters that are two or three times the size of those of their wild ancestors, so supervision of farrowing and prompt assistance has become important to the welfare and performance of sow and litter. On the other hand, too much disturbance of the sow can interfere with the natural process of parturition. Unless sows are accustomed to close human contact, they will progress better if left quietly alone and just monitored from a distance.

When should assistance be given? First let us consider the gilt at the beginning of farrowing. Her birth canal has never passed a piglet before and she seems to require more time to open up and deliver a piglet than an experienced sow. My practice is to allow an hour from the onset of straining before investigating why no piglet has appeared. In the case of a sow I would expect some result within half an hour of onset of straining. Once the first foetus has been delivered, a delay of more than 20–30 minutes before the next birth indicates an opportunity for skilled assistance to avoid the sow becoming exhausted (especially towards the end of farrowing), to reduce stillbirths and to reduce the chance of piglets being crushed by a weak and unsteady sow.

The dangers of interfering too early during farrowing are that the natural progress of parturition may be disturbed and that manual intervention may damage the delicate tissues of the birth canal and uterus. However, leaving the sow too long can also increase internal damage due to prolonged unproductive straining and a tendency for the birth canal and uterus to close down and become very dry.

To determine if farrowing has finished the following questions should be asked:

- Has sow stopped straining?
- Has sow stood up and urinated?
- Is sow interested in litter and willing to settle to suckling them?
- Has a large mass of afterbirth ('cleansing') been passed?
- Do umbilical cords in afterbirth match number of piglets born?

Retained afterbirth is uncommon in sows. The membranes should be removed as soon as they are passed so that they are not in the way of the piglets and the sows cannot eat them.

Dystocia (difficult or delayed birth)

Strategic approach

The first question to ask when investigating why a sow is not making progress is 'Is she straining?'. If straining has ceased, two initial steps can usefully be taken. The first is to get the sow up and get her to move around. This helps to reposition the uterus and foetuses and gives her a break from a painful and exhausting experience.

The second step is to ascertain if sufficient oxytocin is circulating to stimulate powerful uterine contractions. Can a jet of milk be expressed from the teats? If not, are there some piglets already born that could be put to suckle to stimulate natural oxytocin release? If it is necessary to inject synthetic oxytocin, the birth canal must be checked before administering this powerful uterine stimulant. It should only be given if the cervix is open and there is no piglet in the birth canal. If none of these actions prompts recommencement of straining and there is no obvious indication that farrowing has finished, an internal examination of the birth canal is indicated. Other treatments to aid uterine contractions such as calcium and glucose might also be required.

If a sow has been straining too long without result, or if she cannot be prompted to recommence labour, then an obstetrical examination is indicated. Obstetrical assistance should be as hygienic as possible, with particular emphasis on keeping particles of dung or bedding from entering the genital tract. Washing the sow's vulva and the stockperson's hands with clean antiseptic solution is ideal, but sometimes a clean disposable arm-length glove is more practical. Farm buckets of water, in dusty conditions, may add as much debris as they remove!

Obstetrical assistance

- Check birth canal is open as far as bifurcation of uterus.
- Remove any piglets within reach.
- Ascertain if uterus is contracting normally.
- Check teats for signs of natural oxytocin release.
- Supplement oxytocin if necessary.

Particular problems with prolonged farrowing or repeated manual assistance are swelling and drying of the sensitive birth canal tissues. Both these phenomena make delivery increasingly difficult and increase the chance of postpartum pain and illness. For these reasons, the most important, yet neglected, tip in porcine obstetrics is to use liberal quantities of a good obstetrical lubricant (available from veterinarians, agricultural merchants or pharmacists). Soap is no substitute for this and substances like liquid paraffin must never be used.

Uterine inertia

Uterine inertia is the commonest type of farrowing problem. Uterine contractions either never really get started (primary uterine inertia) or they start normally but then stop (secondary uterine inertia). Secondary inertia can arise from the large number of foetuses to be delivered or because there is some obstruction to delivery of a foetus. It can be viewed as a form of 'exhaustion' of the uterine contraction process. When major uterine contractions cease, reflex abdominal straining ceases also.

Both types of inertia can arise from undue disturbance of the sow during farrowing. Sows need to feel safe while farrowing and should as far as possible be left to quietly get on with the farrowing process. Monitoring and assistance with farrowing should be as unobtrusive as possible. Yorkshire veterinary surgeon Neville Kingston has drawn attention to the importance of good stockmanship skills in achieving good farrowing results. He noticed that in herds with a low level (about 5%) of stillbirths, he could enter the farrowing house with little or no reaction from the sows, whereas in herds with a higher prevalence of stillbirths the sows would jump up and react fearfully whenever someone entered the farrowing room. Nutritional and metabolic factors probably also play a part in uterine inertia. If oxytocin does not stimulate uterine contractions, intravenous calcium salts and glucose may help. The β-blocker carazolol (Suacron) is reported to prevent the inhibitory effect on farrowing of adrenaline released by stress (Bostedt *et al.* 1984).

Relative foetal oversize

Relative foetal oversize is the situation when a foetus is too large for the birth canal. This may be because a foetus is particularly large, e.g. in small litters, or it may be that a gilt was rather small when mated, so her birth canal is too small for what is in fact a reasonably sized piglet. A rather more rare problem is when the foetus is monstrously deformed.

An oversized foetus can usually be delivered if the sow's efforts are aided with manual traction. Only rarely will it be necessary to resort to a caesarean operation. Plenty of lubrication and a steady pull are usually all that is required. The principal problem is to get sufficient traction on the slippery foetus in a very narrow birth canal. If the piglet is coming in posterior presentation (backwards) it is a matter of getting a good grip on the hocks with the fingers. The piglet in anterior presentation is more tricky. Ideally the head is encircled with the hand and traction can be safely and effectively applied via the head and neck. Sometimes, however, it is not possible to get a hand around the head. In this instance traction has to be carefully applied to the lower jaw, but *great care* is necessary to avoid breaking the jaw. At the earliest opportunity transfer grip to the whole head. Other possibilities with an oversize anterior presentation are to use a snare or special forceps to grip the head.

Ventral deviation of the uterus

Ventral deviation of the uterus is a condition that was described by a Cambridgeshire-based veterinary surgeon in the first major study of dystocia in sows (Jackson 1972). It is a situation where a 'log-jam' of foetuses builds up, below the level of the sow's pelvis. The solution consists of reaching deeply downwards into the uterus where a pool of foetuses has accumulated, and 'fishing' them out one by one. Allowing the sow some freedom to move around before and during farrowing may be important in preventing this problem.

Care of newborn piglets

When farrowing has finished, it is time to check how many functional teats a sow has and make arrangements for fostering, artificial rearing or split-suckling of any excess piglets that the dam cannot hope to rear. It is advantageous to supervise the initial suck of colostrum and render assistance or supplementary feeding where necessary. Piglets weighing less than 1 kg at birth have a reduced chance of survival and therefore warrant particular checking and assistance. On average, newborn piglets weigh about 1.7 kg, but they vary enormously. It can be advantageous, if contagious disease is absent, to 'pool' litters born at the same time and divide them into artificial litters of similar sized piglets, relating the number in each litter to the number of functional teats of the sow. It must be borne in mind that some older sows' teats may not be functional in that they are not exposed when she is lying suckling.

Techniques for saving piglets

- Make sure creep heaters are on before farrowing
- Place extra creep heater at rear of sow
- Check farrowing sows frequently, note time of births
  As piglets born:
  - remove any membranes
  - dry with straw or old towel
  - check umbilical cord for bleeding: clamp or tie
  - give 0.5 ml iron dextran if pale
  - 20% glucose solution administered to weak piglets
  - place in box in creep area
- Ensure suck of colostrum at end of farrowing
- Prompt fostering of surplus piglets onto another sow

Ideally, piglets receive colostrum from their dam or the sow that will rear them, but there may not be enough. In this situation, deep-frozen (preferably) or artificial colostrum can be given. Piglets that are too weak to suck will need colostrum by stomach tube.

Lactation

Duration

Wild pigs lactate for approximately 3 months and weaning is a gradual process. The traditional age for weaning domesticated pigs used to be 8 weeks, but this is rarely seen these days. The most common average weaning ages in commercial intensive pig units, both indoor and outdoor, are in the range 3.5–4 weeks. A few units wean at around 2 weeks with the aid of expensive controlled-environment weaner housing and very expensive weaner diets. There are a few units weaning at 5–6 weeks. Attempts have been made to wean as early as 2–4 days but these have not been a commercial success.

Lactation seems to have an important stabilizing action on ovarian function after parturition. In the absence of lactation ('zero weaning'), endocrine disturbances and cystic ovaries are common. Lactations of less than 3 weeks' duration are followed by increased weaning-to-oestrus interval and increased embryo losses (Table 7.9).

Feeding (Table 7.10)

Too high a level of feeding immediately after parturition can result in agalactia, so it is usually advised that feed levels should be gradually increased to *ad libitum* over a period of 3 days. Some restricted feeding may be appropriate for third-litter sows or older but, particularly in young sows, weight loss during lactation must be kept to a minimum in order to ensure a short weaning-to-oestrus interval with good ovulation rate and farrowing rate. Young sows are particularly vulnerable to excessive weight loss because they are still growing and their feed intake capacity is limited by their small body size. In conditions of inadequate energy intake, sows

Table 7.9 Effect of lactation length on subsequent litter size (from Clark and Leman 1984)

	Weaning age	
	3 weeks	4 weeks
No. of sows	1768	5688
Farrowing rate (%)	81	83.5 ($P<0.025$)
No. born alive	9.5	10.1 ($P<0.001$)

Table 7.10 Nutrient requirements in lactation (from Mullan *et al.* 1989)

Requirements	Stage of lactation			
	Week 1	Week 2	Week 3	Week 4
Energy (MJ ME/day)	63	80	93	97
Nitrogen (g digestible N/day)	92	119	133	134

Energy requirements of first-parity animals are higher. The ME range 63–97 is equivalent to DE range 66–102.

continue to lactate but at the expense of their fat reserves. Excessive weight loss can be avoided by using a high-energy lactation diet (e.g. by adding fat, which also increases palatability), feeding to appetite twice daily and encouraging appetite by keeping farrowing house temperature down to 18°C. Feeding pelleted or wet food also increases feed intake. Sows with feed intakes of more than 2 kg (26 MJ DE) daily during pregnancy have reduced appetite during lactation (Cole 1990), so it is important that sows are in good condition at mating to obviate high feed levels in pregnancy. Ideally sows should gain about 12 kg liveweight during each breeding cycle for the first three parities.

Sows fed 3 kg of feed daily during lactation have been found to have lower embryo survival in the next pregnancy than sows fed 7 kg daily, despite similar ovulation rates (see review by Einarsson and Rojkittikhun 1993).

Weaning

Pig farms often wean on one day of the week so their quoted age of weaning (e.g. 3 weeks) represents a range of times (e.g. 18–25 days) for individual litters. Very large units may need to wean on more than one day per week to spread the workload for both boars and humans. Wednesday or Thursday are popular days for weaning because the sows are likely to require serving between Monday and Friday of the following week.

Weaning of some individual litters may need to deviate from usual herd policy. A litter might be weaned early to free the sow for fostering pigs from a sow that has died or had lactation failure. If a litter is sick, or the piglets undersize, it is helpful if weaning can be delayed.

It is not necessary to starve or withhold water from sows at weaning in order to dry them off. On the contrary it is important to maintain or improve body condition in this period, particularly in sows that have just had their first litter.

In some herds, newly weaned sows have no boar contact for the first few days. Research indicates that this can delay the postweaning oestrus. The presence of another sow in oestrus has also been shown to stimulate postweaning oestrus.

In recent years it has become the practice in some herds to 'split-wean' litters. In this system the heaviest pigs are weaned several days earlier than the rest.

Planning a breeding programme

Batch breeding

Much of the success of modern intensive pig production hinges on skilful control of the production process (often referred to as 'pig flow'). The aim is to have a constant and even flow of batches of pigs served, batches of sows farrowing, batches of litters weaned and batches of pigs ready for sale. This achievement allows optimum use of resources at all times and a planned marketing operation. Particularly key resources are housing (especially farrowing housing, which is usually the most expensive housing on a pig unit), boars, labour, cash flow and working capital.

The benefits of breeding sows in batches are:

1. AI: batch insemination cheap and convenient.
2. Oestrus detection: more concentrated and efficient.
3. Mating supervision: more concentrated and efficient.
4. Farrowing:
    (a) supervision more cost-effective,
    (b) cross-fostering of piglets easier,
    (c) batching of management tasks,
    (d) 'all-in, all-out' housing,
    (e) batch weaning helps sow grouping.
5. Weaner health and performance improvement:
    (a) variation in weaner age/size decreased by batch farrowing,
    (b) mixing litters at weaning facilitated,
    (c) 'all-in, all-out' housing.

Control of breeding

In wild pigs, groups of four or five females are often synchronized at the onset of the breeding season. Boars are usually living separately at this time. Environmental triggers, such as day length and food availability, may be significant in this synchronization but it is believed that behavioural or pheromonal interactions between the females are also important. Even with commercial breeds, pigkeepers have been known to add a female in oestrus to a group of anoestrous gilts or sows with some reputed success. Certainly, cycling is known to occur more readily when pigs are grouped rather than isolated.

Introduction of the boar to gilts of pubertal age gives a degree of synchronization. Provided that the gilts are ready for puberty, they will typically show oestrus 10–14 days after first contact with the boar. More reliable and precise control can be obtained with the progestagen altrenogest (Regumate, Roussel-Uclaf, France) added to feed each day for 18 days to suppress natural cycles. On withdrawal of medication, most pigs will be in oestrus 5–7 days later. The gilts or sows must already be undergoing oestrous cycles for this drug to work.

In sows, oestrus can be conveniently synchronized by weaning them on the same day. Under a given set of husbandry conditions, the interval from weaning to oestrus is fairly constant (typically 3–7 days).

Prostaglandins are widely used to synchronize oestrus in cattle, but they cannot be used for pigs in the same manner because porcine corpora lutea are not susceptible to their effects until day 12 of the cycle (only 2 days before they would regress naturally).

Breeding performance

Recording performance

The principles and techniques of recording performance are described in detail elsewhere (Davies *et al.* 1985; Radostits and Blood 1985). As herd sizes grow, there is a trend towards increasing sophistication, computerization and expense of recording systems. The investment of time and money involved in recording is growing and the choice of system and supplier is an increasingly crucial business decision that can be difficult to reverse. Time spent in researching and critical evaluation of the alternatives can be amply repaid.

Monitoring performance

Breeding performance can be monitored in many ways. Economic success can be measured by return on capital invested, or by 'profit margin per sow place'. The latter measures of efficiency of use of capital invested in housing plus efficiency of output in terms of pigs sold per sow. Performance success can be measured in general terms, such as pigs reared (or sold) per sow per year, or in more specific areas such as farrowing index (number of litters per sow per year).

The farrowing index is the mean number of litters produced per sow per year. The interval (in days) from one farrowing to the next is referred to as a 'reproductive cycle' (not to be confused with oestrous cycle) or as the 'farrowing interval'.

High productivity is not always linked with high profitability; a low-performance herd can sometimes achieve good profitability by the strategy of keeping capital investment and costs to a minimum. However, provided that the costs of extra production are controlled, increased output of progeny will usually increase profit and producers should constantly be monitoring the potential for increasing productivity of the breeding herd.

How is it judged what scope there is for improvement? There is no fixed standard by which all pig herds can be judged, because of differences in such things as husbandry system, amount of money (capital) invested and business culture (e.g. high risk or low risk, conservative or progressive). The most relevant and directly useful evaluation is to compare current performance levels with what the herd has achieved in the past. If the difference (regardless of whether better or worse) can be related to changes in the herd management or situation, then this could be the key to improving (or regaining) performance. Other ways of evaluating performance are summarized in Table 7.11. It can be helpful to employ a variety of comparisons; some will be worth doing more frequently than others. Table 7.12 summarizes some breeding performance achievements.

Improving performance

If a herd is already achieving good performance, is there anything that can be done to boost performance further? The answer is invariably yes, but the questions that follow are rather more tricky: How can it be done and will it be cost-effective? Pigs sold per sow per year can be calculated directly from number of pigs sold and average herd size. In order to improve it, we have to consider the two components: pigs sold per litter and farrowing index.

Pigs sold per litter

Rearing and finishing performance are beyond the scope of this chapter, so we will be concerned only with number born alive per litter. There are

Table 7.11 Evaluation of current herd breeding performance (adapted from Meredith 1983)

Reference values for comparison		If current performance
Terminology	Definition	and reference value differ:
Herd reference values	What the herd has previously achieved	What management/health changes account for this?
Population reference values ('standards')	What other herds achieve with: 1. similar resources* 2. different resources*	1. What differences in management/health account for this? 2. Should resources be changed?
Target values ('goals')	What the herd should aim for	Intensify efforts or set more realistic goals
Tolerance values (action limits/interference levels/decision boundaries)	Values beyond which remedial action is required	Institute investigation into reason for unacceptable performance level
Theoretical potential	Biological maximum of pig	Consider new management techniques/new technology

* Resources are relatively fixed aspects of the farm such as capital invested, manpower, herd size, weaning age, housing system, genotype, health status, geographical location.

Table 7.12 Breeding performance achievements (from Pigplan Management Services 1994)

Performance parameters (averages)	Outdoor herds		Indoor Weaning <25 days		Indoor Weaning 26–32 days	
	Average	Best third*	Average	Best third*	Average	Best third*
Total sows and gilts/herd	467	675	328	354	190	197
Unserved gilts (%)	8	9	7	9	8	8
Sows per boar	13	13	16	17	18	17
Sow replacements/year (%)	43	42	44	41	47	49
Sow mortality (%)	3.1	2.8	4.6	4.4	4.6	3.5
Service success rate (%)	89	89	86	88	84	90
Non-productive days	43	36	40	29	36	19
Litters/sow and gilt/year	2.22	2.30	2.27	2.35	2.22	2.34
Cost of sow and boar feed/ sow/year (£)	213	207	199	196	199	199
Total litter size	11.6	11.9	11.7	12.0	11.7	12.2
Born alive/litter	10.8	11.0	10.8	11.1		
Born dead (%)	6.5	7.4	6.7	7.0	6.6	7.0
Weaning age (days)	24	22	22	22	27	27
No. reared/litter	9.6	9.9	9.6	10.1	9.5	9.9

* Best performing herds judged on the basis of pigs reared per sow per year

two main components of this: the total number of foetuses produced and the proportion that die during or shortly after birth.

The number of foetuses delivered per farrowing can usually be increased by increasing the number of matings per oestrus. It is not enough just to formulate a herd policy of aiming for two or three matings per oestrous period; the actual service records must be examined to determine how many gilts or sows are only receiving one service. If sows do not appear to be in oestrus long enough for more than one service, it is advisable to check if some sows have poor follicular development (often of nutritional origin) or are affected by problems in detection of oestrus.

Western breeds of sows can occasionally bear extraordinarily large litters. A British Saddleback sow recently produced 31 live piglets, and the record before that was a Wessex sow producing 30 live young. However, these litters are well above the norm! Western breeds have difficulty producing more than 15 live piglets, particularly when young, and even when they do they often have great difficulty rearing them. Genetic selection is continuing to improve this fecundity, but heritability is low and progress is slow. The use of crossbred sows is of some help in commercial herds because heterosis results in greater litter size than with pure-bred sows.

The drive to increase litter size is resulting in increasing use of the hyperprolific Chinese Meishan breed in breeding programmes. Meishan litter size is three to five piglets greater than the Western breeds. Carcass quality and growth rate of the Meishan is too poor for most pig industries, so usage is generally as crossbreds. Dilution of Meishan prolificacy genes seems to be compensated for by the beneficial effect of heterosis (hybrid vigour) in F_1 crosses with Large Whites. Use of Meishan genes will be facilitated by a new 'genetic fingerprinting' test for breeding nucleus pigs. The test detects a genetic marker for litter size in blood samples or hair follicle cells from piglets of either sex. The marker is on the oestrogen receptor gene and can account for as much as 1.5 piglet difference in litter size.

Why do Meishans have larger litters? Young gilts of the Meishan and Large White breeds have similar ovulation rates, but in older gilts and sows there is an increasingly higher number of ovulations in Meishans. However, the main reason for higher litter size in Meishans is a higher rate of embryo survival. This effect is due to the unusually high uterine capacity of the mother and not the genotype of the embryo (Haley and Lee 1993). F_1 Meishan × Large White crosses have a lower ovulation rate and fewer embryos than pure-bred Meishans, but a lower level of foetal loss allows them to produce litters of similar size.

Embryo losses are a significant loss of potential offspring in all pig herds. This loss occurs mainly between days 10 and 25, particularly between days

12 and 18. At these times, any steps that can be taken to avoid stress of pregnant females could pay dividends.

Mortality of piglets at birth can usually be reduced by increased supervision and care of farrowing sows and newborn piglets. There comes a point, however, where time spent is not repaid with increased survival rates.

Farrowing index

Several approaches are possible for obtaining more farrowings per sow per year. The pregnancy period is often considered unchangeable, but some minor shortening is obtained when farrowing is induced with prostaglandins. Although farrowings are only induced 1 or 2 days before the due date, it must be borne in mind that some sows would naturally have delivered after the due date.

The second largest component of the farrowing interval is the lactation period. Hence the trend over many years now towards earlier weaning. Although earlier weaning can increase the interval from weaning to oestrus and reduce subsequent litter size, these effects are not particularly marked unless weaning at 3 weeks or earlier. This correlates with research indicating that it takes about 3 weeks for the sow's uterus to recover from pregnancy and parturition. However it is likely that this involution time could be beneficially influenced by improved care during farrowing and regular suckling by a vigorous litter.

The vital strategy for lactation length seems to be to monitor the results of current policy for weaning age and, in the light of current performance or change of circumstances, periodically review the possibility that it might beneficially be adjusted. In any herd there is always a spread of weaning ages occurring that can be analysed for comparative performance.

Factors that favour earlier weaning include:

- increased litters per sow per year,
- less housing and labour for suckling sows and litters,
- *small herds*: more pregnancies allows for more efficient boar use,
- direct feeding of litter more efficient than feeding via sow but higher quality feed needed,
- reduced fighting injuries when weaners are mixed.

Factors that favour later weaning include:

- environmental requirements of weaners are less exacting,
- creep and weaner diets can be of lower quality,
- less care and skill required for managing the weaners,

- less care and skill required for rebreeding sows,
- less risk of postweaning growth check, *Escherichia coli*, streptococcal meningitis and respiratory disease,
- less postweaning anoestrus,
- lower throughput means less demand on hygiene,
- decreased litter size.

If weaning age is reduced, the increased production of pigs per year requires one of the following choices to be made.

- Reduce sow numbers, so that housing requirements for growing pigs and annual output of sale pigs remain constant.
- Maintain sow numbers, increase housing for growing pigs and make arrangements to sell more pigs per year.

Unfortunately, producers have a tendency to maintain sow numbers without providing extra housing for growers. The resultant increase in stocking densities can have dire consequences for health and performance.

Another approach to improving farrowing index is what is termed 'split' or 'fractionated' weaning. This involves weaning (at around 3 weeks) the largest pigs in a litter a few days earlier than their littermates. The benefits are a reduction of about 1 day in the weaning-to-mating interval, plus lower postweaning mortality.

For decades people have attempted to breed sows during lactation to improve farrowing index. Usually pigs are anoestrous during lactation, but follicular growth and ovulation can be induced, after the third week, by a variety of techniques (Varley and Foxcroft 1990):

- partial weaning,
- multiple suckling and boar exposure,
- treatment with eCG alone, or in combination with hCG,
- GnRH treatment,
- oestrogen administration,
- opioid modulation.

Multiple suckling involves mixing groups of sows and litters together at about 10 days after farrowing, with boar contact and high feeding levels. Sows come into oestrus at around 34 days after parturition and an average litter size of 11.1 has been achieved. Endocrinologically, the requirements for follicular growth during lactation are a major increase in episodic LH secretion and a sufficient level of plasma FSH.

Culling of sows after service adversely affects calculations of farrowing index (Table 7.13). Most of these cullings are because of repeated returns

Table 7.13 Effect of non-farrowing sows on farrowing index (from *Meat and Livestock Commission Newsletter*, March 1980)

Time components	Mean time per sow (days)	
Sows that farrowed again		
Lactation	25.0	
Weaning to first service	7.8	
First service to successful service	3.8	
Pregnancy	114.9	
Farrowing interval/index	151.5	= 2.4 litters/sow/year
Sows that failed to farrow		
Culled before service	1.7	
Culled after service	7.8	
Deaths	0.7	
Abortions	1.2	
Total non-productive time	11.4	
All sows (farrowing and non-farrowing)	151.5 + 11.4	= 162.9
Overall farrowing interval/index		= 2.24 litters/sow/year

or 'not in pig', i.e. neither returning after service nor farrowing. This emphasizes the importance of efficient detection of non-pregnant pigs and making prompt decisions about culling.

Clinical examination of boars

Before examining a boar, information regarding his breeding and health history should be reviewed. How much has he been used, how has he behaved with sows and what has been the outcome of matings? Next, a general clinical examination is undertaken, with particular attention to legs, feet and external genitalia (prepuce, penis, size and consistency of scrotal contents). Congenital testicular hypoplasia and acquired degenerative testicular atrophy are not uncommon problems. If the boar is to sire breeding females, his number of teats will also be relevant. It must be remembered that the boar has a preputial diverticulum, which sometimes fills with urine. This has been mistaken for an abscess or umbilical hernia!

The third stage of the examination, where possible, is to test him with a female for sex drive and capacity for erection, mounting, intromission and ejaculation. The final step would be to undertake an assessment of semen quality (Tables 7.14 and 7.15). If an unsatisfactory ejaculate is obtained, a second sample should be checked, preferably on another day, before concluding that the boar is unfit for breeding.

Table 7.14 Sperm concentration from semen colour (from *Merck Veterinary Manual* 1991)

Colour	Sperms/ml	Indication
Creamy	$1{\times}10^{9}$	Good
Milky	$3{-}5{\times}10^{8}$	Satisfactory
Watery	$<20{\times}10^{7}$	Unsatisfactory

Table 7.15 Guidelines for satisfactory semen quality (from *Merck Veterinary Manual* 1991)

Abnormalities of sperms	Volume of ejaculate (ml)	Percentage of motile sperms	Total sperms per ejaculate
<10% of heads <5% of acrosomes <5% of midpieces <5% proximal cytoplasmic droplets <25% single-bent	100–300 at 8–12 months old 100–500 if >12 months old	>70	$10{\times}10^{9}$ to $40{\times}10^{9}$

Clinical examination of females

Females for breeding should have a minimum of 12 teats (preferably 14) that are neither damaged nor inverted. They must walk soundly and not have excessively straight legs. Vulval conformation should be checked for normality and freedom from discharge. In gilts it is wise to check that there are no features of intersexuality such as clitoral enlargement, or a preputial vestige just caudal to the umbilicus. All females can be checked with a speculum for absence of vaginal defects or discharge (Meredith 1981). The genital system of sows can be examined by rectal palpation in much the same way as cattle or mares, but greater care is necessary and small hands are an advantage (Meredith 1977).

Breeding problems

General approach

Why do problems occur?

Problems are an unavoidable part of pig breeding, and can be looked on as an opportunity to demonstrate skill, learn and gain experience. However, repeated mistakes threaten financial failure and can be detrimental to human and pig welfare. Good breeding performance requires quality (genetically and health-wise) breeding stock and quality housing, equipment, feed and personnel. These items do not come cheap and the commercial success of a breeder lies in maximizing these contributors to high performance while keeping costs in check. In theory, spending can be sensibly allocated on a basis of anticipated cost-effectiveness. However, in practice, herds are often under-capitalized and risks are constantly taken in selecting areas for under-spending in order to concentrate funds on priorities. There may also be an 'enterprise culture', which focuses on areas for reducing expenditure rather than optimization of investment.

Table 7.16 Sources of breeding problems

Problem source	Prevention
Lack of capital	Financial advice, partners
Innovations in management and technology	Preplanning, advice, common sense, research, monitoring implementation
Ignorance/out of date	Keep informed
Unwise risks with performance/health	Fix underlying pressures (finance?), acquire training/experience/advice
Incompetence	Staff recruitment, aptitude, management and training
Mistakes	Reduce work pressures, manage/train staff, better communication, sort personal problems

What constitutes a problem?

Infertility problems must be considered at two levels. Firstly, at the level of the individual affected animal, how are suboptimally performing individuals detected and treated? Secondly, at the level of the herd, how is it recognized that too many individuals are breeding suboptimally so that control measures need to be applied to the herd in general? At both levels an infertility problem can be defined as a discrepancy between observed and expected performance.

In the initial approach to a problem it is useful to check three points.

1. Are the *observations* of performance reliable (e.g. personal accounts, calculations from records)?
2. Are the *expectations* of performance reliable, bearing in mind factors like genotype, system of husbandry, geographical location and amount of capital invested in the enterprise?
3. Is the observed *discrepancy* in performance statistically significant or just part of normal variation (within the normal range)?

Alternative approaches

One way of approaching a problem is to check all the aetiological (causal) possibilities. Commonly this is done by investigating all the areas of husbandry that might have an influence on the problem, or by going through a 'checklist' (differential diagnosis) of *known causes* of this type of problem. Another type of approach is the 'structured investigation' in which further information about the problem is obtained (e.g. the epidemiological pattern, or the pathological changes in the genital organs) and allows progressive focusing on a particular area of aetiology. A third type of approach is the 'risk factor' analysis in which a number of factors influencing occurrence of the problem are identified, usually by statistical analysis of breeding and health records. In the risk factor approach the emphasis is often on improving an aspect of breeding performance rather than finding or understanding the causes. Any of these three approaches, and often a combination of them, may be appropriate for a particular situation; some examples are given for specific problems considered below.

In an epidemiological investigation the key questions are:

- Can onset or fluctuations of problem be linked with changes in management, feeding, staff, etc.?
- Does it affect particular groups or parities of pigs?

Delayed puberty

When gilts fail to come into heat, the first step is to ascertain their age and decide whether or not they should be allowed more time. Generally speaking gilts are expected to show their first oestrus before 200 days. If this has not occurred enquiries should be made about exposure to the boar since this is a vital factor in stimulating puberty. Exposure should be for at least half an hour per day for at least 3 weeks. The boar must not be one that the gilts have previously become habituated to.

If boar stimulation has been satisfactory, there is no possibility of pregnancy and the gilts are in good condition, it is useful to check whether or not their ovaries are cyclic despite their history of anoestrus. This can be done by determining blood progesterone level with an enzyme immuno-assay kit, taking vaginal biopsies or examining the genital organs of culled gilts. Another technique is to determine the depth to which a speculum or AI catheter can be inserted into the genital tract. When the ovaries are inactive, the genital tract is much shorter than in the luteal phase of a cycle; some shortening also occurs during oestrus. The depth of insertion can be compared with that in gilts which are known to be cyclic or in early pregnancy. As a last resort, ovarian function can be checked by culling some of the affected gilts. Whatever technique is used, it is important to check ovarian function in a number of gilts because it often varies within a group.

There have been reports of gilts with cyclic ovaries failing to show oestrus despite good facilities for detection (so-called 'silent oestrus' or 'behavioural anoestrus'), but my experience is that environmental or social factors interfering with detection can usually be found.

The factors involved in delayed puberty are:

General factors:
- large group size,
- high stocking density,
- dominance–subordination interactions.

Ovaries inactive:
- insufficient male stimulation,
- genotype,
- high ambient temperature,
- obesity,
- poor growth rate,
- short photoperiod (< 6 hours),
  deficiencies of:
  - energy intake,
  - protein intake,
  - vitamin A,
  - vitamin B_{12},
  - manganese.

Ovaries cyclic:
- oestrus detection problems.

Persistent corpora lutea:
- pregnancy,
- mycotoxicosis,
- exogenous hormones.

Cystic ovaries:
- congenital,
- stress,
- exogenous hormones.

A commonly applied remedy for gilts with delayed puberty is to increase male stimulation. This may be done by providing contact with a different boar, more than one boar ('rotating boars') or with a vasectomized boar run with the gilts. Another traditional remedy is to move the gilts to a different environment or mix them into new social groups. The theory of this is that mild stresses stimulate puberty, but a scientific basis is absent.

Prevention and cure of ovarian inactivity lies in identifying and correcting the cause(s) of the problem. However it may take some time to implement the necessary improvements and for currently affected pigs to recover. As an interim measure, hormone treatment may be necessary to bring gilts into heat. A wide variety of hormone preparations are effective in doing this (particularly the combination of eCG plus hCG) provided that the ovaries are definitely inactive. If the ovaries are affected with some other abnormality, or are in fact functioning normally, then at best this treatment will be wasted and at worst the state of anoestrus will be prolonged. Another problem to beware of when inducing ovarian activity artificially is that of encouraging the transfer of genetic factors to the next generation of breeding stock. There is also a risk that pigs that do not conceive at the induced heat may relapse again into anoestrus. With some hormone treatments there may be low fertility or low litter size at the induced heat.

Vitamin treatments (particularly A, B, D or E) are sometimes used for anoestrous pigs, but the indications for using them seem to be quite limited. Biotin, which is important for proper utilization of dietary energy, may be helpful where diets are low in availability of this vitamin.

In all herds occasional gilts are encountered that are anoestrous as a result of congenital intersexuality. External signs are not always present, but an enlarged clitoris or the presence of a rudimentary sheath caudal to the navel may be revealing.

Dyspareunia

Dyspareunia is the term for pain experienced during mating or AI. The pain may impair or prevent successful insemination. There may also be haemorrhage into or from the genital tract. Gilts are most commonly affected, but acquired lesions are occasionally seen in sows.

Dyspareunia in gilts and sows is the result of vulval or vestibule/vaginal lesions (Meredith 1982). Vulval lesions may be caused by bite wounds or traumatic injuries from fittings and fixtures. Vestibule/vagina lesions may be caused by the penis or when the AI catheter fails to penetrate the vaginal ostium and traumatizes the wall of the vestibule and/or enters the urethral orifice. Factors involved are:

- narrow vaginal ostium,
- hymen remnants (common in gilts),
- poor alignment of vaginal ostium with vulva,
- poor alignment of penis (disparity in size of male and female, leg weakness, poor mating position),
- damage (e.g. adhesions) from previous farrowing,
- not introducing catheter along dorsal wall of vestibule.

Service success rate problems

Service success rate problems are often referred to as 'conception rate' problems, but conception is something that cannot be detected directly. The success of services can be judged only by the subsequent returns to service, the pregnancy rate when a pregnancy test is used, the number of sows found to be 'not in pig' as farrowing approaches, and the farrowing rate. The farrowing rate gives the best indication of success in getting pigs pregnant but, because of the 4-month delay for this result, the return rate and pregnancy rate give a quicker indication of any problem in the service programme.

Returns to service

In herds with good performance, about 10% of mated or artificially inseminated sows return to service. Returns to service can be subdivided into those that occur after a 'regular' interval of 18–24 days (equivalent to a 'normal' cycle length) and those that occur after 'irregular' intervals, which are shorter or longer than a normal cycle. Increased returns to service may take the form of:

- increased regular returns (e.g. low boar fertility),
- increased irregular returns (e.g. oestrus detection problems),
- increase in both regular and irregular returns (e.g. embryo death problems).

Regular (18–24 day) returns

A regular return indicates that the genital tract has not recognized a pregnancy. It is considered 'normal' for 5–9% of mated sows to return to oestrus after a regular interval.

There are a number of reasons for regular returns. Firstly, there may be insufficient sperms at site of fertilization due to:

1. Poor semen quality (boar or AI).
2. Sperms not reaching uterus:
   (a) failure of intromission (mating technique, impotence, leg weakness),
   (b) failure of ejaculation,
   (c) failure of AI technique,
   (d) dyspareunia,
   (e) obstruction of lower genital tract (developmental/acquired).
3. Impaired sperm transport to oviduct:
   (a) obstruction of upper genital tract:
      (i) congenital (intersex, aplasia, cysts),
      (ii) acquired (adhesions, abscesses),
   (b) endocrine disturbance (exogenous hormones/ovarian cysts).
4. Death of sperms (endometritis, salpingitis).

Secondly, ova may not be reaching the oviduct due to:

1. Ovulation failure (followed by follicular atresia or follicular cysts):
   (a) exogenous hormones (e.g. to treat infertility),
   (b) stress,
   (c) intersexuality,
   (d) early weaning (prior to 2 weeks),
   (e) genetic?
2. Ova transport impaired:
   (a) tubal obstruction/adhesions (peritonitis, oophoritis, salpingitis),
   (b) developmental defects of oviducts.
3. Death of ova (salpingitis).

Thirdly, failure of fertilization (all ova) may be due to dead or defective spermatozoa or ageing of gametes (poor timing of insemination relative to ovulation).

Finally, death of all embryos before day 12 may be causing returns to service (see 'irregular returns' for causes of embryo death).

Irregular returns

In herds with good performance, irregular returns to service occur in 2–4% of sows served and typically account for 20–35% of all returns to service.

The reasons for irregular returns are complex and depend on the interval before return to service. Where the interval is <18 days (uncommon), this may be due to:

- short luteal phase,
- inseminated when not in oestrus,
- date or sow number recording error,
- total ovulation failure (see under 'regular returns' for causes).

Where the interval is >24 days, this may be due to:

- inactive ovaries,
- undetected return to oestrus (interval often 36–48 or 54–72 days),
- ovulation failure (luteinized cystic follicles),
- embryo death (less than five embryos at 12–15 days or total loss at 16–35 days):
    genetic defects,
    heat stress,
    infectious agents,
    mycotoxins (zearalenone)
    pyrexia,
    other stress (mixing, fighting?).

Failure to farrow ('not in pig', NIP)

'Failures to farrow' are inseminated females that neither farrow nor return to oestrus. In some cases they may have been positive to an early pregnancy test. However, as farrowing time approaches, it becomes clear that they are not showing the usual abdominal enlargement and udder development. A prevalence of up to 1% of inseminated pigs is considered quite usual; a higher prevalence indicates that investigation is required.

Surprisingly, the genital organs of most culled NIP sows are found to be normal, with cyclic ovaries. It is not possible to say if detection of oestrus was the primary problem in all these sows, but it is apparently at least a secondary problem. Important factors may be that the occurrence of oestrus has been unpredictable and that the sows, assumed pregnant, were in housing conditions that were less than ideal for detection of oestrus. This situation emphasizes the need to ensure that sows are securely pregnant before moving them away from the service area. Sows are susceptible to embryo loss and delayed return to oestrus up to day 30 after mating. It is unwise to move them from good facilities for the detection of oestrus earlier than this. This is also a good time to apply a pregnancy test if there is any problem of empty sows not being detected as returns to heat. However, pregnancy tests can give false positives, particularly A-mode ultrasound instruments.

Less common NIP problems arise from sows whose ovaries become inactive after an unsuccessful service, and from sows that develop persistent corpora lutea, which may be due to:

- unexpected pregnancy (recording error, pregnancy diagnosis error),
- exogenous oestrogen (therapeutic/growth promoter/mycotoxin),
- total mummification of litter *in utero* (e.g. due to porcine parvovirus).

'Summer infertility', 'autumn infertility'

Seasonal infertility is a widely used, but vague, term referring to a seasonal decline in reproductive performance, typically occurring in late summer and/or early autumn (Figure 7.5). Seasonal infertility problems reported on different farms and in different countries may be quite different in effects or causation. Indeed, even on the same farm, some groups of pigs may be affected while others remain completely unaffected. Most pig herds seem to suffer slight seasonal declines in breeding performance, but in some herds these become quite serious. In Australia, a 10% reduction of farrowing rate for a period of 4 months is not uncommon. Seasonal infertility may take one or more of the following forms:

- increase in delayed puberty,
- increase in postweaning anoestrus,
- reduced farrowing rate,
- 'autumn infertility' may be an outbreak of maternal-failure type abortions,
- reduced litter size.

Some pigs suffer embryo death at 20–25 days of gestation and exhibit delayed return to oestrus 25–35 days after mating. A particularly common manifestation is an increase in females NIP after service. In some episodes of seasonal infertility, high environmental temperature may be a significant factor. Early embryo death followed by either delayed or undetected return to oestrus is believed to be a major factor in this type of problem. In other seasonal infertility episodes a seasonal fall in temperature (particularly at night) may place strain on the pig's adaptive mechanisms, particularly energy balance.

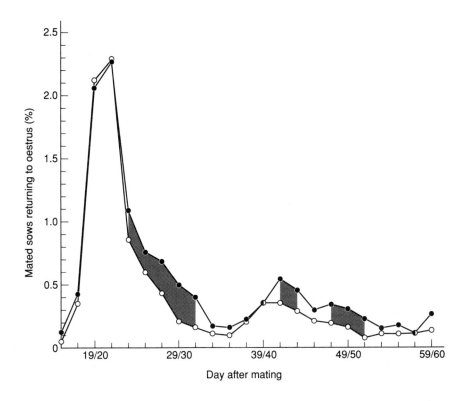

Figure 7.5 Times of return to oestrus after mating for sows mated during the period of seasonal infertility (weeks 1–15) (●) or during the remainder of the year (weeks 16–52) (O). The number of sows returning for each 2-day interval was expressed as a percentage of the total sows mated in each period. The shaded area indicates where the two groups are significantly different ($P<0.05$) (from Love *et al.* 1993).

A partial explanation for seasonal infertility may lie with the European wild pig ancestors of the domestic pig. Wild pigs are seasonal breeders, breeding when day length shortens in the late autumn/early winter and usually farrowing a single annual litter in the spring. In domestic pigs, plasma concentrations of melatonin are high during summer and autumn or when pigs are kept in constant light, and low during winter or when pigs are kept in constant darkness (Love *et al.* 1993). Melatonin implants have been found to reduce farrowing rate in sows. Although produced particularly at night, melatonin secretion in pigs seems to be higher if there is exposure to high light intensity during the day. It is also increased if feed intake is restricted during exposure to long photoperiods. It has been suggested that *ad libitum* feeding during the first few weeks of pregnancy may prevent this increase in melatonin. In fact availability of abundant foodstuffs (beech mast and acorns) seems to stimulate the onset of the breeding season in wild pigs. Indeed, under commercial management conditions, wild pigs can produce more than two litters per year.

Supplementary lighting (increased photoperiod) is sometimes provided in an attempt to prevent seasonal infertility in pig herds. However, pigs, unlike sheep, may be unable to respond to sudden changes in photoperiod; they appear to require incremental changes in day length to affect mela-tonin levels (Paterson *et al.* 1992). There appears to be some association between high melatonin and high LH levels. In some studies, seasonal infertility has occurred in group-housed sows (particularly if group size exceeds six), but not sows in individual stalls on the same farm. Where seasonal infertility appears to be of climatic origin, cooling facilities may be helpful in the form of water-misting devices or wallows. Some farms simply serve more replacement gilts or reduce culling rate during expected periods of seasonal low fertility, in order to maintain a consistent number of farrowings per week.

Farrowing rate

The ultimate measure of service success is the percentage of inseminated sows that subsequently farrow. High performance herds can achieve 85–90% farrowing rate. A rate consistently less than 85% merits investi-gation. Farrowing rate can be influenced by sow mortality and culling of sows after service for reasons other than infertility, but usually farrowing rate data are the most reliable guide to fertility patterns and for analysing the influence of risk factors (see below). Unfortunately they can only relate to services undertaken 4 months or more previously. More recent services have to be analysed by return rate or by pregnancy rate (using a pregnancy test at a specified time after service).

Embryonic mortality

A certain amount of embryonic mortality appears to be inherent in the reproductive process. It has been speculated that this may arise from competition between embryos for available uterine space and nutrients. In recent years attention has also been directed to the factor of embryonic diversity (Pope *et al.* 1990) within litters. Porcine embryos vary in devel-opmental stage as a consequence of natural variation in follicular and oocyte maturation and in ovulation time. The more retarded embryos are less able to survive because the more advanced ones synthesize oestradiol and induce a uterine environment that is asynchronous for their less fortunate littermates!

The second week of pregnancy is a particularly critical time for embryo survival. At this time, spacing of embryos in the uterine horns is finalized, the trophoblast (early placental membrane) elongates enormously, uterine attachment and embryonic oestrogen synthesis begins, maternal recognition of pregnancy occurs, uterine blood flow increases and histotrophe secretion begins. Vitamin A (retinol) is essential, particularly at around day 12, for normal embryo development.

It is known that an ambient temperature exceeding 30°C, between days 8 and 16 after mating, can increase embryo losses, as also can certain infectious agents such as B. suis and porcine parvovirus. Mycotoxins (e.g. the trichothecenes) have also been incriminated.

Very low lactation feed levels can be detrimental to embryo survival (reviewed by Einarsson and Rojkittikhun 1993). It has been suggested that this results from lower LH release at the oestrus after weaning, resulting in inadequate luteinization of corpora lutea (some cystic follicles might also result) and low progesterone levels in early pregnancy. Injection of GnRH at oestrus has been found to increase progesterone and improve embryo survival rates.

Mixing sows and dominance–subordination relationships are suspected of influencing embryo losses. At a high stocking density, mixing older pregnant sows with young, recently mated sows reduced the pregnancy rate of younger sows (Love et al. 1993). Decreasing photoperiod during late summer and autumn may also increase early embryo death.

The consequences of embryonic death are summarized in Table 7.17.

Risk factor analysis

Many factors have been identified that can influence success rate of services (Table 7.18). Genetic differences between individual breeds and lines have been demonstrated, but they are small. Heterosis (crossbred sows) can improve conception rates by 2–3% and a similar improvement is possible if crossbred boars are used.

Investigations into the influence of housing on success rate of services have produced contradictory results. Sometimes group housing has given better results and sometimes individual stall housing has given better

Table 7.17 Consequences of embryonic death (from Love et al. 1993)

Day of gestation	Consequences
13	Return to oestrus in 25–30 days
22	50% sows return to oestrus, 50% pseudopregnant
30	Pseudopregnant

Table 7.18 Service success rate problems: risk factors

Risk factor for sow	Usage examples
Genotype	Is there a genetic basis for the problem?
Ear no./date acquired	Service failures may be related to particular batches of replacement gilts
Parity	Gilts are usually managed separately
	Primiparous sows prone to bullying
Total born (previous litter)	Delayed uterine involution more likely after large litters
No. born dead (previous litter)	Potential indicator of dystocia/uterine problems
No. mummified (previous litter)	May indicate parvovirus immunity
Lactation length	Short lactations can be detrimental
No. weaned (previous litter)	Suckling large litters may link with weight loss
Disease history	For example, occurrence of vulval discharge
Return interval (for repeat services)	Irregular intervals may have a poor prognosis, e.g. in cystic ovarian disease
Weaning-to-service interval	Sows coming into oestrus very soon after weaning may not be mated early enough in their heat period
Farrowing-to-service interval	Short intervals may not be enough for the uterus to regain normal function
Service number (first/second/third)	Service success rate may progressively decrease, e.g. with damaging genital diseases, or be positively correlated with service number, e.g. when there is a problem with postpartum uterine involution
Service location	Service success may be better in one service house than another
Date of service	Periods of poor success can be identified. These may relate to, e.g. periods of stress, feed change or high ambient temperature
Weekday served	For example, services on Mondays may have lower success because some of the sows were on heat at the weekend, but not served until Monday
AI/natural service	If both are in use, is there a difference in success rate?
Inseminator or service supervisor	Can the problem be related to personnel?
Boar usage frequency, age of AI semen	Semen quality problems may be identified
Boar genotype	For example, pure-bred boars, cf. crossbred boars
Boar(s) identity	Identifies boars of low fertility
No. of services per heat	How much of the low fertility is due to sows being served only once?

results. It seems that there are too many unquantified variables involved for findings to be consistent but there is a tendency for reduced service success when sows are housed individually. An Australian study (Hemsworth *et al.* 1989) found that farms where the stockperson's treatment of sows induced a high level of fear tended to have lower service success rate.

Vulval discharges

Diagnosis of genital tract disorders in the live pig is difficult and an obvious symptom such as vulval (vulvar) discharge attracts attention. The discharges that are seen are only a small proportion of those that occur and the proportion detected will be influenced by type of housing and extent of human observation. A good place to look for signs of discharge is the undersurface of the tail, where it makes contact with the vulva. A speculum is helpful for detecting discharge and also for locating the site of origin. Microscopic examination of discharges is vital, particularly for identifying chemical sediments (oxalates or phosphates) from the urinary tract, which are very common and often mistaken for infections of the genital tract (Meredith 1991).

Normal discharges

The genital tract is in a constant state of discharging desquamated cells, mucus and fluid secretions, but there are particular times when these can be grossly obvious. In pro-oestrus and oestrus there is a slight discharge, typically of watery consistency, slightly sticky and of clear or cloudy appearance. In the first few hours after mating, seminal fluids are expelled. Later (8–48 hours), a small amount of thick tenacious material of white, grey or yellow colour may be seen, which may be a reaction to the foreign material (including bacteria) introduced into the uterus during mating or insemination. It is also common for a discharge of similar appearance, probably of cervical origin, to occur during pregnancy. Perhaps this serves a protective role. These discharges are usually flushed away during urination, but can particularly be seen at autopsy or on speculum examination.

After parturition, there is a lochia that can persist for up to 5 days after farrowing. At the same time there are normal histological changes in the endometrium that resemble endometritis. It can be difficult to differentiate between normal lochia and an abnormal degree of endometritis in the first few days after farrowing. I regard foul-smelling discharge exceeding 15 ml (externally visible at one time) as indicative of an abnormal degree of uterine infection.

Abnormal discharges

A specific syndrome of increased discharges in sows after service has been described (Muirhead 1986). This was characterized by occurrence of discharge in at least 1% of sows in the period from 7 days after service, a return rate (to all services) of more than 7% and farrowing rate of less than 87%. Vaginitis and/or endometritis was diagnosed post mortem in many of the affected animals. Some sows had cystitis or both cystitis and endometritis.

Vaginitis can best be diagnosed by vaginal biopsy and there might be fewer field diagnoses of this problem if biopsy was used more frequently. All too often the diagnosis is based only on the presence of slight discharges and some of the affected sows being pregnant. Biopsies must be taken when progesterone levels are high, because false negatives can occur in the follicular phase of a cycle and false positives are likely in metoestrus.

Experimentally mild vaginitis has been produced by inoculating *Staphylococcus aureus* into the upper vagina of gilts. However the infection resolved quickly and spontaneously. Vaginitis can occur in association with endometritis and the question then arises as to which developed first. In experimental inoculations of bacteria into the uterus descending infections of the genital tract are often seen, but ascending infections may be important in the field. The vaginal part of the cervix is frequently affected also in cases of vaginitis.

Bacterial genital tract infections: postulated risk factors

- dystocia
- parturient injury/disease
- retained foetus/afterbirth
- prolonged recumbency
- absence of suckling (delayed uterine involution)
- chilling environment
- service/AI injury
- poor hygiene
- urinary tract infection
- water intake restriction
- foreign material introduced during service
- insemination when not in oestrus
- death of embryos
- specific infections, e.g. *B. suis*

Many veterinarians believe that vaginal discharges can spread venereally, although no particular microorganism has been identified. This has led to attempts to control this type of problem by medicating the sheath or, more particularly, the preputial diverticulum of the boar with antibiotics. The theory seems to be that the boar's sheath becomes over-populated with bacteria and antibiotic treatment will restrict this. In fact it seems that the boar's preputial flora re-establishes within days of antibiotic treatment. However, ulcers are seen quite frequently in the prepuce of boars and it is conceivable that they may be a source of pathogenic bacteria for the sow. It is difficult to say whether or not field problems that 'respond' to this treatment would have resolved spontaneously anyway. Some field problems certainly do not respond to this treatment. Typically, sheath treatment involves squeezing out the contents, then introducing an intramammary antibiotic (e.g. oxytetracycline) and massaging the diverticulum to disperse it. Treatment is repeated at intervals ranging from weekly to every 3 months.

Prevention of bacterial genital tract infections

- **hygiene** (cleaning, drainage, all-in all-out occupation of rooms, use of bedding materials, wash perineum if badly soiled, avoid housing where sows sit or lie in dung/urine, minimize time spent in farrowing pen prior to parturition);
- **minimize recumbency** (attention to locomotor problems, prolonged farrowing and sow illnesses);
- **service hygiene** (supervise and assist matings to reduce contamination of penis, AI hygiene);
- **farrowing hygiene** (when assisting farrowing);
- **urine flushing** (constant access to drinking water, flow rate at least 1 litre/minute);
- **prompt attention to dystocia**;
- **supervision of mating** to avoid genital injury.

Abortion

Abortion has been defined as the expulsion of recognizable foetuses before day 110 of gestation, if none of the foetuses survives more than 24 hours. An occurrence of 1 per 100 sows served is considered quite usual; higher prevalences can signal a problem. Abortions can be categorized clinically and pathologically into two classical types:

1. 'Maternal-failure' type, where luteolysis (failure of ovarian maintenance of pregnancy) is the initiating event. This is the most common type of abortion, yet often the most difficult to explain. At worst these abortions are similar to normal parturition in character and duration, but may be less marked. Expelled foetuses are of 'fresh' appearance and may even be alive. Unless the abortion followed systemic illness, the sow is healthy, recovers quickly and there is a good chance of successful rebreeding. Maternal failure type abortion can be caused by pyrexia (erysipelas infection, heat stress, procaine penicillin); seasonal abortion (late summer/autumn); sunburn; mycotoxins?; systemic illnesses/endotoxaemia initiating prostaglandin release.
2. 'Placentitis' type, where infectious processes in the uterus are the initiating event. Typically these abortions are slow, unpleasant affairs, with expulsion of degenerate foetuses and possibly toxaemia of the sow. Recovery may take a few days and the prognosis for future breeding is poor. Placentitis type abortion can be caused by bacteria (e.g. *B. suis*, *Leptospira*); chlamydia; fungi; viruses (e.g. Aujeszky's disease).

One of the commonest clinical types of abortion is the seasonal ('autumn') epidemic of maternal-failure type abortions. The reason for these abortions is still not entirely clear. They are not related to body condition, but it is believed that increased energy losses in the cooler autumn months may be a factor. At this time of year there can be a sharp temperature fall overnight to which sows are not yet acclimatized. Sows with restricted movement in housing that is poorly ventilated or draughty are particularly vulnerable. Preventive success has been claimed for housing improvements and increased feed levels.

During abortion, foetuses become contaminated with microorganisms from the lower genital tract of the sow. The warm watery tissues of foetuses facilitate rapid multiplication, so microbiological findings in foetuses must be interpreted with great care.

Low total piglets born per litter

Total piglets born per litter includes those born alive, stillborn and mummified. In intensive commercial production using improved white breeds average total litter size should exceed 9.5 for gilts and 10.5 for sows. Litter size is extremely variable so, in monitoring or comparing breeding performance, the number of litters involved must be taken into account before concluding that a difference in litter size is significant (Table 7.19).

Judgements about litter size must always consider the genotype of the

Table 7.19 Differences in litter size required for 95% confidence that the difference is not due to chance (data from Dr M. Bichard)

Number of litters in each of two groups compared	Significant difference in mean litter size
25	1.6
50	1.0*
250	0.5

*, Minimum significant change in litter size from one month to next in a 260-sow herd with 2.3 litters/sow/year.

sow. F_1 hybrid sows with backcrossed litters can be expected to produce about one-half to one pig more per litter than pure-bred sows. Differences in litter size also occur between pure breeds and between lines within breeds. Unfortunately heritability of litter size is low so the response to genetic selection is very slow. Interest has been shown in the crossing potential of some of the prolific Chinese breeds in recent years. These pigs can produce an average of about 14 pigs born alive per litter, have 16–18 teats and are early maturing, reaching puberty at 60–100 days. They are said to have slightly shorter oestrous cycles and longer heats. On the debit side they have slow growth rate, high fat content, small carcass size and low killing-out percentage. The boar can also have a genetic influence on litter size, although the exact mechanism of this is not clear.

Litter size is greatly affected by parity, so it is important to examine the parity profile of a herd before making judgements about litter size performance. Obvious examples are the recently formed or recently expanded herd. Such herds will not have optimum litter size because of the prevalence of low-parity sows. Ideally litter size should be examined for each individual parity group within a herd. Normally litter size increases progressively up to the fourth to sixth litter. Occasionally herds are seen where there is either no increase or actually a decrease in litter size at the second litter. This can arise when sows lose excessive weight in first lactation or there is insufficient compensation in the weaning-to-service period so that ovulation rate is depressed at the postweaning oestrus.

Mummification of foetuses

If embryos die before day 35, they degenerate and are said to undergo 'resorption' although it is possible, when all the litter dies, that remnants pass down the reproductive tract and are flushed out in urine. At about day 35, calcification of the skeleton begins and foetuses that die are either aborted or retained. Dead foetuses that are not aborted undergo 'mummification'. In this process they become shrivelled, dehydrated and

---

Total piglets born per litter: determining factors

The total number of foetuses is determined prior to day 35 of pregnancy, so attention can usefully be focused on circumstances before oestrus or during the first month of pregnancy.

Affecting ovulation rate

Genotype
Hybrid vigour
Insufficient energy intake in previous lactation (second litter sows)
Sow age/parity (rate increases up to fourth litter)
Nutrition before and during oestrus
Zearalenone mycotoxin
Follicular cysts (ovulation failure)
Exogenous hormones

Affecting fertilization rate

Fertility of boar semen
Number of services per heat
Time of insemination

Affecting embryo death

Bovine viral diarrhoea virus
Genetic defects
Porcine parvovirus
SMEDI enteroviruses
Length of lactation (see p. 310)
Heat stress
High energy intake (controversial)

Mode of effect unclear

Biotin deficiency
Individual housing (litter size tends to be lower)

---

become brown or black in colour. The time of death can be estimated by radiographic study of the development of centres of ossification. If the mummified piglets in a litter vary widely in size (age) it is an indication of viral aetiology with intrauterine spread. Mummified piglets of similar size suggest a more ubiquitous factor such as sow illness or exposure to something toxic.

A 0.5% prevalence of mummification in piglets born is considered quite usual; higher levels indicate that a significant problem may be present. The commonest cause of mummified foetuses is porcine parvovirus, although this situation may change now that parvovirus vaccines are becoming widely used. The first viral causes to be found were the 'SMEDI' entero-viruses and this led to misleading use of the term 'SMEDI problem' to refer to any infertility syndrome involving low litter size and mummifica-tion.

The known causes of mummification are:

- bovine viral diarrhoea virus,
- *B. suis*,
- *Chlamydia psittaci*,
- encephalomyocarditis virus,
- erysipelas,
- infectious bovine rhinotracheitis virus,
- Japanese encephalitis,
- leptospirosis,
- mycotoxin (zearalenone),
- porcine cytomegalovirus,
- porcine (SMEDI) enterovirus,
- porcine parvovirus,
- pseudorabies (Aujeszky's disease),
- swine fever,
- swine pox virus.

Stillbirths

In practice 'stillborn' pigs include neonatal deaths that have occurred in the interval from birth to the time when the litter is inspected and recorded. Therefore, three types of stillbirth can be distinguished: prepartum and intrapartum (true stillbirths) and postpartum. In practice these categories and their aetiologies are not rigidly distinct, but they are nonetheless diagnostically useful. Most intrapartum deaths are in the last piglets to be born; it is speculated that the umbilical cord of these piglets is more likely to rupture before they reach the vulva because they originate higher up in the uterus. Placental separation is also more likely to be more advanced in these piglets.

The acceptable level of stillbirths in a herd is open to opinion, ranging from 5 to 7%. Some of the best pig units keep their level of stillbirths down

Stillbirths

Prepartum (rare, died in the few days prior to parturition)
Autolysis and haemolysis may be apparent (skin discoloured, eyes sunken, reddened fluids in body cavities). Ascites and oedema suggest viral infection.
  Causes:
  • *B. suis*
  • chlamydiosis
  • erysipelas
  • F-2 mycotoxin (zearalenone) exposure in late gestation
  • foetotrophic viruses (see causes of mummification)
  • leptospirosis
  • *Leucaena glauca* poisoning
  • manganese deficiency
  • pyrexia
  • riboflavin deficiency
  • toxoplasmosis (infection in last month of pregnancy)
  • vitamin A deficiency

Intrapartum
Meconium expelled as a result of anoxic distress. Lungs may be partly inflated.
  Causes:
  • dystocia, especially uterine inertia
  • 80% are in last third of litter to be born
  • ageing of the dam (parity >4)
  • carbon monoxide poisoning
  • congenital abnormalities
  • eperythrozoonosis
  • large litter size (prolonged parturition)
  • low haemoglobin levels in the sow
  • overweight dam
  • premature farrowing
  • sow illness
  • vitamin E deficiency (in last 4–5 weeks of pregnancy)
  • weakened or dying due to prepartum factors

Stillbirths *continued*

Postpartum (pseudo-stillbirths, neonatal mortality)
Lung tissue floats in water. Soft pads ('thimbles' or 'slippers') over the claws will be worn away if the pig has walked.

Causes:
- born weak due to intrapartum factors
- born weak or low birthweight due to prepartum factors, e.g. severe restriction of energy or protein during mid or late gestation (Einarsson and Rojkittikhun 1993)
- crushed or injured by sow
- haemorrhage from umbilical cord
- hypoglycaemia (starvation)
- hypothermia
- trapped in foetal membranes

---

to 5% or less. Important control measures centre on checking sows frequently during farrowing so that parturition can be aided when necessary and that piglets can be assisted to survive. Induction of farrowings so that they occur during working hours can be very helpful. Autopsy of stillbirths is important in determining the stage of parturition at which death occurred and to identify any congenital abnormality, which may be helpful diagnostically. For example, in vitamin A deficiency there may be ascites, renal abnormalities or microphthalmia.

Should a sow be culled if she has a litter with several 'true' stillbirths? Research by the Pigtales recording service in the USA found that a correlation between current and previous stillbirths occurred only in sows of fourth or greater parity.

Postweaning anoestrus

Over 90% of sows usually show oestrus within 10 days of weaning. Individual sows taking more than 10 days can be regarded as anoestrous. Many of these pigs will have inactive ovaries and can be brought into oestrus with a gonadotrophin injection (e.g. 400 iu eCG/PMSG and 200 iu chorionic gonadotrophin). A high level of feeding is important in these cases, because excessive weight loss in lactation is a common factor. Sows are especially vulnerable to excessive weight loss in their first lactation.

In other sows, *undetected* postweaning oestrus results in apparent anoestrus. These sows may not respond to hormone treatment because they are in the luteal phase of a cycle. Indeed there is a danger of prolonging a luteal phase if hormone treatments are used. It would be preferable to wait for the second postweaning oestrus at about 4 weeks after weaning.

If less than 90% of sows show oestrus within 10 days of weaning, action on a herd level is indicated. A crucial, but often overlooked, step is to ascertain the state of ovarian function in the affected pigs. Rectal palpation is the best method of determining ovarian function in anoestrous sows, but blood progesterone assay can also be used.

The risk factors for inactive ovaries postweaning include:

- biotin deficiency (contradictory reports)
- choline deficiency
- high feed levels in previous pregnancy
- inadequate energy intake in lactation
- inadequate protein intake in lactation
- insufficient male stimulation
- season of year (summer and autumn)

Boar infertility

Detecting infertility in the boar can be problematical. Complete infertility may be apparent on clinical examination, or as returns to service if single-boar matings are practised. However, subfertility is more common and likely to be missed if cross-mating (more than one boar) is practised. Even with single-boar matings, low fertility is difficult to detect because only one to three sows will be mated per week, so it may take 6 months to accumulate data on say 50 matings for an assessment of fertility. There seems to be a case for periodic laboratory checking of semen samples from boars.

Low-fertility boars are commonly culled rather than treated. Newly purchased boars will usually be replaced by the breeder. Rapid genetic progress means that replacing an older boar is not really expensive.

Physical contact with other pigs in the prepubertal period is important for development of sexual behaviour. Boars deprived of this contact have shown later puberty, decreased courtship behaviour and fewer copulations. Even adult boars have shown decreased sexual behaviour and lower ejaculate volume when kept isolated from sows, though total sperm production appears unaffected (Colenbrander and Kemp 1990). Prolonged undernutrition can decrease libido in boars, but nutritional influences have otherwise not been reported.

Spermatogenesis takes approximately 5 weeks. The resulting spermatozoa then need a further 10 days for epididymal transportation before they attain optimum fertilizing capacity. Consequently, when the testes are affected by environmental or pathological factors, it can take up to 6 weeks for a boar to recover fertility. Severe damage may lead to permanent low fertility or, more rarely, complete sterility. Boar fertility seems to be quite resistant to low-temperature environments, but temperatures of 33–38°C for 4–7 days can reduce fertility.

The factors affecting semen quantity and quality include:

- high environmental temperatures
- febrile illnesses
- season of year (sperm production may decrease in spring and rise in midsummer)
- social environment
- nutrition
- breed
- age
- testis size
- specific infections e.g. *B. suis*, Japanese encephalitis or porcine parvovirus

Breed differences in non-return rate, testicular size and semen parameters have been widely reported. Boars over 9 months of age not surprisingly show better semen production than boars less than 9 months. Daily sperm output increases with age. The percentage of abnormal sperms gradually decreases during pubertal development but subsequently increases with age, while pregnancy rate and litter size decrease.

In wild pigs the breeding season is late autumn and winter. This corresponds with the period of higher semen volume, increased testicular size and increased sperm concentration in domesticated boars in temperate latitudes. Artificial changes in photoperiod can mimic these natural seasonal fluctuations but constant supplemental lighting does not appear to benefit semen production or semen quality.

Low ambient temperatures (−10°C) are not detrimental to sperm output but high ambient temperatures (>29°C) for as little as 3 days decrease sperm motility and sperm production. Longer exposure can reduce fertility for a period of about 2 months. Increased numbers of morphologically abnormal sperms occur typically 2–6 weeks after an episode of heat stress.

Zearalenone mycotoxin has a detrimental effect on sperm production and semen quality, as also does an episode of febrile illness, e.g. swine erysipelas or Aujeszky's disease.

Specific diseases

Bovine virus diarrhoea (BVD)

There have been some rare field reports incriminating BVD infection in porcine infertility problems and experimentally it has been shown to be pathogenic for porcine foetuses. It is a possible cause of embryo death and mummification where pregnant pigs are kept in association with cattle.

Brucellosis

Brucella suis is found in pig populations throughout the world, but is becoming increasingly uncommon. Britain, Ireland, Canada, the former Czechoslovakia and Denmark are free from the disease, which incidentally is an important zoonosis. *Brucella abortus* and *B. melitensis* can infect pigs but are only mildly pathogenic. There are five biovars (biotypes) of *B. suis*: biovar 1 is widely distributed, biovar 2 is mainly found in Europe and maintained in the wild hare, biovar 3 is found in the Americas and Southeast Asia, biovars 4 and 5 are not known to be pathogenic for pigs.

Pathogenesis and epidemiology

Oral (most common) or venereal infection is followed by intracellular multiplication in local lymph nodes, bacteraemia lasting several weeks and localization in joints and genital tract. There may be a delay of up to 2 months from infection to the appearance of detectable antibody. Some pigs remain persistently infected.

Infection enters herds most commonly via infected pigs. Hares, meat products, semen and embryos are alternative sources.

The organisms are resistant to drying and freezing and can survive in the environment for months. However they are killed by common disinfectants or by a few hours of sunlight.

Clinical signs

The principal clinical signs are infertility, abortion, orchitis, lameness and posterior paralysis. Pyrexia or death is rare. Abortion can occur at any time, as early as day 17 of gestation (following service by an infected boar) and particularly at 4–12 weeks. Early abortions are likely to go undetected because the conceptuses are small and there is little or no vulval discharge; affected pigs may only be apparent as returns to oestrus at 30–45 days. With late abortions there is considerable blood-stained or purulent discharge and afterbirths may be retained. Some sows produce mummified, stillborn or weak piglets at term. Most affected females shed organisms for less than 1 month and experience temporary infertility but ultimately recover from infection. Some individuals are more persistently infected.

Infected boars are often asymptomatic but they may develop loss of libido, infertility, orchitis and epididymitis within 7 weeks of infection. Ultimately there may be testicular atrophy. Infection of the accessory glands can result in highly contaminated semen.

Genital pathology

Catarrhal endometritis is the most common lesion in sows although there may be miliary abscessation of the endometrium. Cystic endometritis, necrotic endometritis or pyometra are also possible. There are usually few specific changes to observe in aborted material. Placentae may be congested and oedematous with possibly yellow or brown exudate and ecchymotic haemorrhages. Histologically there is diffuse suppurative inflammation. Foetuses may have haemorrhagic subcutaneous and peritoneal fluids or be autolysed. Boars may have abscessation of the testes, epididymes or accessory glands.

Diagnosis and control

The clinical signs are typical and isolation of the organism is conclusive. *Brucella suis* forms 1–2-mm domed colonies after 2–4 days of aerobic incubation on blood agar. Serological diagnosis is widely used, but low titres commonly arise in unexposed pigs and false positives can arise from cross-reactions with *Yersinia enterocolitica*, *E. coli* and *Salmonella* species. A fluorescent antibody technique can be used for diagnosis on aborted material.

Slaughter and restocking are the only sure way to eradicate the disease.

Encephalomyocarditis virus infection

Encephalomyocarditis virus (EMCV) is a picornavirus found in pigs in the USA, Central America, South Africa and Australasia. Antibodies have been reported in Britain, but the disease has not been diagnosed. Rodents are the reservoir host. Affected pigs (mostly young stock) are usually found dead from heart disease but there may be a brief period of illness with depression, inappetence, cyanosis, pyrexia, trembling, staggering, paralysis, vomiting or dyspnoea. The characteristic lesions at autopsy are white areas 2–15 mm diameter in the right ventricular myocardium. Reproductive effects are foetal mummification, stillbirths and neonatal deaths. Affected foetuses may show non-suppurative encephalitis, focal myocarditis, myocardial haemorrhage and excess pericardial fluid. Definitive diagnosis is by virus isolation, demonstration of rising antibody titres in the dam or by detection of antibody in foetal sera or thoracic fluids.

Japanese encephalitis

Japanese encephalitis (JE) is caused by a mosquito-borne flavivirus. It occurs in India and the Far East and has a wide range of avian and mammalian hosts. It causes human disease as well as reproductive problems in pigs. Adult pigs are not clinically affected, but transplacental infection results in mummification, stillbirths (possibly with subcutaneous oedema and hydrocephalus) and weak piglets with nervous signs. In boars the virus can produce infertility and testicular lesions.

Leptospirosis

Aetiology

Many serovars of *Leptospira interrogans* have been associated with reproductive problems. Serovar *pomona* is the most common leptospire of pigs worldwide, although it is absent from Britain, where the *L. australis* serogroup, *L. canicola* and *L. icterohaemorrhagiae* are the most commonly isolated. In Northern Ireland *L. australis* serovars (*bratislava* and *muenchen*) have been found in 71% of aborted piglets and on 68% of farms. In Eastern Europe serovar *tarassovi* is widespread.

Pathogenesis

Leptospiral infection can result from ingestion, inhalation, through skin abrasions, or from conjunctival or venereal exposure. Only a few organisms are required to establish infection and become disseminated throughout visceral organs within 7 days. A serological response is seen from 5 to 10 days, followed by localization in the kidneys. In the kidney tubules the organisms are protected from antibody and there is transient or protracted (up to 2 years) urinary shedding. With *pomona*, abortions occur about 4 weeks after infection in vulnerable (in the last third of pregnancy) sows. After abortion sows are immune.

Epidemiology

Rodents are reservoirs of infection, but inapparent renal carrier pigs are believed to be the main source of infection for pigs. Leptospiruria begins about 2 weeks after infection. Urine may contain over 1 million organisms/ml. Semen can transmit the infection. Leptospires can survive several hours in voided urine and for some weeks in infected soil. They can survive freezing, but are killed by drying or acidic conditions. *Leptospira pomona* has been shown to survive 15 days in surface water. Infection may come from contact with other animals (particularly their urine), e.g. rodents, cattle, sheep, horses, deer, skunks. Leptospires may be spread by feeding farrowing-house material to animals before breeding. Infected pigs are a disease risk to humans.

Clinical signs

Pigs of any age can be infected. Most infections are inapparent. In the leptospiraemic phase (2–10 days after infection) of acute infections there may be depression, pyrexia, inappetence, jaundice, haemoglobinuria, nervous signs or diarrhoea. The signs usually last only a few days and are usually mild. Reproductive effects of leptospirosis are returns to service, abortion, mummification, macerated foetuses, stillbirths and neonatal weakness. Abortions occur particularly in the last third of pregnancy.

Diagnosis

Clinical and pathological findings are often non-specific, but infected sows may show jaundice or renal lesions (grey cortical foci 1–3 mm in diameter, possibly surrounded by congestion, seen after stripping the capsule) would be suspicious. Similar foci may be seen in the liver of foetuses (said to be pathognomonic of *L. pomona*). Leptospires can be grown (very slowly) on special media or identified by dark-ground microscopy or immunofluorescence. Serological diagnosis requires an antibody titre of 1:100 or greater (preferably rising in paired samples). In acute infections with *pomona* the peak titre may reach 1:100 000. Titres decline slowly and may be detectable for some years. The *australis* serogroup does not stimulate high titres (infected animals may be seronegative) indicating that they are well adapted to the pig (maintenance host). Cross-reaction between serovars can occur.

Control

Infected animals (including carriers) can be treated with streptomycin or tetracyclines. Penicillins and tiamulin are also of value. A single dose of 25 mg/kg dihydrostreptomycin intramuscularly has been shown capable of terminating the carrier state for *pomona* in adult pigs. However, a second dose 2 weeks later is advisable and some pigs may still remain infected.

Antibiotics can also be used to protect animals at risk. Vaccination can be used to prevent illness and reproductive effects but it will not be possible to protect against all serovars and regular revaccination is necessary. In the UK there are only vaccines against *L. canicola*, *L. hardjo* and *L. icterohaemorrhagiae*, but in other countries *L. pomona*, *L. tarassovi*, *L. bratislava* and *L. grippotyphosa* vaccines are available.

Control of wildlife sources of disease, isolation of infected animals (preferably followed by slaughter) and good hygiene are important in any control programme; *pomona* infection often enters a herd via infected pigs.

Mycotoxicosis

Zearalenone (F-2 toxin) is an oestrogenic trichothecene mycotoxin produced by *Fusarium roseum* (*Gibberella zea*) growing in pig feedstuffs (particularly maize and barley). It can have wide-ranging effects on the reproductive system at concentrations as low as 3–5 ppm. In prepubertal gilts there is a syndrome (sometimes referred to as vulvovaginitis) of hyperoestrogenism with vulval swelling, mammary development, tenesmus and rectal and vaginal prolapses. Boars may develop preputial swelling and show slight rise in percentage of abnormal spermatozoa. In sows there can be embryo death, early pregnancy abortion, foetal mummification, stillbirth, small litters and weak piglets. Sows may also show excessive vulval swelling. Oestrogens are luteotrophic in the pig and persistent luteal function (extended cycles or pseudopregnancy) is another possible effect.

Exposure to zearalenone in the last 2 weeks of pregnancy can produce stillborn, weak or splay-legged piglets. The toxin also passes into the sow's milk. Newborn piglets naturally have some vulval enlargement, but this is enhanced in zearalenone poisoning.

Deoxynivalenol (vomitoxin) and T-2 are trichothecene toxins that can produce returns to service (embryo death). Aflatoxin is produced when *Aspergillus flavus* contaminates feedstuffs, particularly maize and groundnut meal. It can produce abortion or agalactia. Ergot (*Claviceps purpurea*) can contaminate wheat, oats or rye and cause agalactia and birth of small weak piglets.

Porcine enteroviruses

These are the original 'SMEDI' viruses. They are widespread in pig populations and can occasionally cause identical infertility problems to porcine parvovirus (PPV). They have also been linked with cases of abortion. In contrast to PPV, colostral immunity is short lasting so in herds where these viruses are endemic breeding stock usually become infected and immune before breeding. Problems are more likely to arise from entry of a new serotype into the population. Infected sows are subsequently immune. Diagnosis is by virus isolation from the lungs of affected foetuses, paired serum samples from the dam or serology of foetal fluids (a titre of 1:32 or more indicates infection).

No effective vaccine is available (many serogroups are involved), so control depends on preventing introduction of infection or exposing gilts to infected material prior to breeding. Likely sources of infected material are afterbirths and foetuses from affected litters or faeces from recently weaned pigs.

Porcine parvovirus

Porcine parvovirus is a small DNA virus, stable over the pH range 3–10, resistant to a temperature of 56°C but killed by exposure to 80°C for 5 minutes. It is enzootic in most large pig herds throughout the world. Isolates of the virus are all antigenically similar.

Pathogenesis

The virus is infective via the oral, nasal or venereal routes. The oronasal route is believed to be more common. After infection there is viraemia, but no clinically apparent disease in non-pregnant pigs. The virus replicates in tissues with a high mitotic index, especially lymphoid tissues. Disease occurs when seronegative dams are infected in the first half of gestation and the virus crosses the placenta. Transplacental infection takes about 10–14 days after infection of the dam. Within the uterus the virus may spread from foetus to foetus. Conceptuses die if the virus reaches them before they become immunocompetent at about 70 days of age. If they die before 35 days, the embryos degenerate and disappear without trace (resorbed). Foetuses dying later (death takes a period of time) are mummified or stillborn. Foetuses infected after the development of immunocompetence do not usually die, but may be born weak and stunted with coexistent viral infection and high levels of neutralizing antibody. In rare cases foetuses infected before they have attained immuno competence may become immunotolerant and remain infected for up to at least 8 months after birth.

Epidemiology

In most herds PPV is enzootic and young animals become susceptible to infection once their passive immunity has waned. Most adults are immune in infected herds. Clean herds may acquire infection from recently infected introduced animals, semen, embryos or fomites. Infection is thought to be principally by the oronasal route. Virus is shed for only about 2 weeks after infection, in faeces, urine, semen and nasal secretions. The greatest source of infection are the fluids and foetal membranes of parturient sows. The virus can persist for 4 months or more in the environment.

Newborn piglets acquire high titres of antibody from their dam's colostrum if she is immune. These titres mostly wane by 3–6 months of age, but can persist until shortly before first breeding, leaving gilts vulnerable to infection during pregnancy.

Clinical signs

Infection of postnatal pigs occurs without detectable clinical signs. In pregnant pigs the clinical picture is variable depending on the stage of gestation when infection occurs. There may be increased returns to service, failure to farrow (due to either missed irregular returns or total mummification of the litter *in utero*), small litters, mummified foetuses, stillbirth, neonatal death and weak piglets. Abortion seems to be an uncommon feature. Quite often only part of a litter is mummified and this may sometimes prolong gestation. In boars, PPV can temporarily disturb spermatogenesis.

Diagnosis

Clinically a history of small litters (less than five piglets), returns to service (particularly at irregular intervals), mummifications (>1% of births) and stillbirths, particularly affecting young sows and with no maternal illness is suggestive of PPV infection. The stillbirths may be seen first when sows at a range of stages of gestation are exposed to infection. Abortions are rare with PPV.

Serological diagnosis is usually based on the haemagglutination-inhibition (HI) test; HI titres can develop as early as the fifth day after infection and can last many years. Titres of >1 : 256 indicate that there has been active infection, but because antibody levels are persistent only rising titres can incriminate PPV in a current problem. The antibody can also be detected in the sera of unsuckled newborn piglets and in the fluids of stillborn or late mummified foetuses.

Conclusive diagnosis lies in isolating the virus from mummified foetuses of less than 70 days of age (<16 cm in length) or by the fluorescent antibody test on frozen sections of their lung or liver.

Control

A number of inactivated and live vaccines are available to prevent PPV infection. One of the latest killed vaccines can be used from 5 months of age and two initial doses (3–4 weeks apart) gives protection for 2 years with HI titres of up to 1:2000. It is important to vaccinate boars as well as sows if control is to be effective. Other ways of stimulating immunity in replacement breeding stock, feeding farrowing-house material or providing contact with adult animals are unreliable and may spread other diseases.

Herds free of PPV must take precautions about the sources of introduced stock, semen or embryos. Bought-in animals should be isolated for at least 3 weeks in case their source herd has recently become infected. Purchase of pregnant pigs should be avoided because of the risk of infection by endemic virus. Farm perimeter security and control of possible fomites is important. Some disinfectants are ineffective against PPV, but it can be killed with sodium hydroxide, sodium hypochlorite, 8% formaldehyde or 2% glutaraldehyde.

When an outbreak of disease is in progress, pregnant sows should be isolated until after parturition, then exposed to infection. Sows whose litters have been affected by PPV infection should be retained because they will subsequently be immune, while replacement gilts are likely to be vulnerable. Herds with a high replacement rate are particularly vulnerable to PPV.

Porcine reproductive and respiratory syndrome

Porcine reproductive and respiratory syndrome (PRRS) has previously been called mystery swine disease, swine infertility and respiratory syndrome, syndrome HAAT, Seuchenhafter Spätabort der Schweine, blue ear disease and porcine epidemic abortion and respiratory syndrome. It is characterized by a capacity for epidemic spread and effects on the respiratory and reproductive systems (Meredith 1994). It was first reported in the early 1980s in the USA but has since spread worldwide. A new group of RNA viruses, termed PRRS viruses, has been isolated from affected pigs and shown to reproduce the disease. The first PRRS virus was isolated in The Netherlands in 1991 and called 'Lelystad virus'. It is becoming clear that PRRS is a multifactorial disease; in some circumstances PRRS viruses infect pigs without causing any obvious ill effects. Other agents, particularly some strains of swine influenza virus, can cause a clinically similar disease syndrome. Serological tests are widely used for diagnosis.

The disease can affect pigs of any age. Clinical effects primarily involve the respiratory and reproductive systems, but there is also enhanced susceptibility to other diseases. The most serious effects in acute outbreaks in breeding herds are on pregnant sows (illness, abortion, premature farrowing, stillbirths, mummifications) and on sucking piglets (illness and death). In herds where there are no breeding stock or in breeding herds where the disease has become enzootic the most serious effect is usually respiratory disease in young growing pigs. Most pigs, particularly older ones, usually recover from PRRS, but some die from secondary infections.

Clinically affected farms can lose about 10% of their annual output of pigs in an acute outbreak of the disease, primarily through abortions, stillbirths and neonatal deaths. Deaths in older pigs are less common, but can arise from secondary infections. The effect of these viruses on individual pig herds is extremely variable, ranging from about 50% of animals being affected at one extreme, to no obvious effects at the other extreme. PRRS viruses tend to persist in infected populations and can give rise to continuing problems in both growing pigs and breeding stock. Continuing problems in weaners and growing pigs seem to centre on secondary infections (particularly respiratory disease) rather than the primary disease effects of the PRRS viruses.

PRRS viruses mainly spread from one pig herd to another by transfer of infected animals or by local (within 3 km) airborne spread. Spread via semen and AI also occurs. Semen from boars that have recently been infected may contain virus for up to 6 weeks, but there is no indication as yet that boars may become persistent semen shedders of the virus as occurs with the similar disease, equine viral arteritis.

There are no reports of this disease affecting humans or any other animal species, but PRRS viruses can infect some species of birds. Killed and modified live vaccines are available in some countries. Antigenic variation in the viruses may pose problems for serological tests and vaccines.

Pseudorabies (Aujeszky's disease)

Pseudorabies is caused by a herpes virus that is widespread in the world and enzootic in many countries. It has been eradicated from Switzerland, Britain and Denmark.

Pigs less than 4 weeks of age may show vomiting, diarrhoea, depression, pyrexia and nervous signs. Mortality is very high. Older pigs have longer illness, lower mortality, and constipation and respiratory signs are more of a feature. Skin lesions resembling human 'cold sores' are occasionally present on the face. In adult pigs infection may be subclinical or there may be similar signs to growing pigs.

Pregnant pigs are vulnerable to abortion and there may also be foetal mummification or maceration. Necrotic foci, 2–3 mm in diameter, may be seen in the liver, spleen and lung of aborted foetuses. Sows infected before 30 days are prone to embryo death and return to service. Infected boars may suffer deterioration in semen quality with lesions in the seminiferous tubules, prepuce or penis.

Carrier pigs are the main means of virus spread, but airborne spread is also possible. Boars that travel round a number of herds are a particular risk. The virus may contaminate semen or embryos used to introduce genetic material. The virus can persist for up to 7 weeks in contaminated buildings or slurry and can be spread over 2 km by aerosol. Rats may act as a reservoir.

Once the disease becomes endemic in a herd the reproductive effects become more sporadic. Diagnosis and control measures are considered elsewhere (Taylor 1989). In the acute phase of an outbreak immunoglobulin can be used to protect pregnant sows for 1 or 2 weeks.

SMEDI syndrome

In 1965 the late Howard Dunne introduced the term 'SMEDI' viruses to refer to a group of enteroviruses that produced a syndrome of Stillbirth, Mummification, Embryonic Death and Infertility.

These enteroviruses are not thought to be of much practical importance today, but the disease syndrome is familiar and the term 'SMEDI' has unfortunately lingered on and become a 'dustbin' term applied to all manner of vague infertility problems. It would be preferable to abandon this term in favour of a specific description of the clinical and pathological features of a particular herd problem.

8 SHEEP BREEDING AND INFERTILITY
H Ll Williams BSc (Agric), MSc, PhD, FRAgS

Systems of sheep production

In many areas of the world sheep are agriculturally important because of their capacity to withstand the harsh physical environment and fluctuations in food supply. They can produce a wide range of commodities, the main being meat, wool and milk. The principal commodity produced in any geographical area is usually dictated by the physical environment, which directly influences the availability of food and the choice of breeds. When meat and milk production are the principal objectives, reproductive performance has a marked effect on productivity; in wool-producing flocks reproductive rate is not as critical and it is not unusual for up to one-third of the flock to be wethers (see Table 8.1).

The reproductive performance of sheep can vary from one lamb from a proportion of the breeding ewes at a particular season and for a limited number of years, to a litter of lambs at a low lambing interval, free of seasonal considerations and for a long breeding life. Given this wide range of reproductive potential it is imperative that appropriate targets of performance are set for a particular environment and for the breed chosen for that environment.

In this chapter particular emphasis will be given to the relationship between management and reproductive performance in various systems of production, using the systems found in the British sheep industry as examples. The methods of approach to the improvement of performance are also relevant to systems found in other parts of the world.

In the hill and upland areas dominated by rough grazing, the combination of climate, topography, low soil fertility and inaccessibility places severe limitations on the choice of livestock enterprise. There are vast areas where only sheep can be considered and, in addition, only a limited range of breeds. In the lowland environment a full range of species, and breeds within each species, can be considered for livestock enterprises. On many lowland farms sheep use uncultivatable or surplus land; in the traditional dairying areas they are secondary to the dairy enterprise and often managed by staff whose primary expertise is dairy husbandry.

Sheep are much more dependent on grass and its conserved products, hay and silage, than other farm animals. This high level of dependence usually means that the general system of husbandry is extensive rather than intensive and often with little or no housing. Winter housing or short-term housing over the lambing period is associated with lowland flocks with a high level of performance in terms of animal output and/or land use.

Since 35% of the UK farmed land is uncultivated rough grazing, it is not surprising that the majority of breeding ewes are in hill and upland flocks. The UK breeding flock comprises approximately 20 million ewes and ewe lambs; it has increased by 42.6% since 1980.

A well-established interdependence has developed between hill/upland and lowland flocks. It is a unique feature of the British sheep industry and involves the annual movement of a vast number of breeding stock and store lambs to lowland flocks. This integration allows greater efficiency of land use and provides the lowland flocks with a range of genotypes, mostly halfbreds (F_1), each breeding season. This vast migration of breeding stock includes ewes that have had three lambings on hill farms, and unbred two-tooth ewes and ewe lambs from upland areas. Most of these animals are sold through special regional sales. Although a wide range of advantages arise from this system, problems arise in terms of national disease control. The potential buyer of breeding stock would benefit from knowing their health status. Much interest is currently shown in the national health schemes for sheep, which include monitoring flocks for enzootic abortion of ewes.

In addition to this main movement, replacement ewe lambs from hill flocks are moved to lowland dairy farms for their first winter, returning to the hills in the subsequent spring. Breeding stock also move temporarily between farms in the lowlands.

During the last decade, there has been an increase in the number of large breeding flocks. In the UK almost 50% of breeding ewes are now in flocks of over 500 and approximately 10% in flocks of over 2000. The number of breeding animals in the care of one person is considerably higher than in cattle and pig units. A full-time shepherd is expected to look after a flock of 500–700 ewes. Because the key events of the sheep production cycle are uniquely seasonal, extra help is usually provided during peak lambing, shearing and dipping (Williams 1994a).

Systems of husbandry are markedly different between hill/upland and lowland units. In the former, the pattern of grass growth dominates the timing of the key events of the production cycle: mating, lambing, weaning. Lambing is timed so that lactation coincides with the start of the grazing season and this grass supports lactation and the early growth and development of the lamb. Since there is little scope for the provision of other crops and a reluctance, for economic reasons, to feed concentrates, shortage of grass during the approach to the breeding season not only significantly depresses fecundity but also provides the breeding animal with inadequate body reserves to draw on during the winter. Most losses of breeding ewes in hill flocks occur during late pregnancy/early lactation. Common grazings are a feature of some hill areas. Their use imposes restrictions on husbandry particularly in relation to breeding, for bye-laws state the date on which rams can join flocks grazing such pastures.

In lowland flocks there is more freedom of action. Protection can be provided during adverse weather conditions and the nutritional requirements of all classes of stock can easily be provided at any time of the year. However, in pastoral areas, most lambings occur in late winter/early spring. As a consequence of high stocking rates, alternative methods of wintering breeding stock have resulted in many flocks being housed. The longer the period of housing, the more likely it is for winter shearing to be adopted. This allows higher stocking density, better working conditions for staff and improved surveillance. Although winter shearing increases appetite this does not fully account for the increase of approximately 0.5 kg in the birth weight of lambs from shorn ewes. This may lead to an increase in assisted lambings but not necessarily an increase in neonatal mortality. Ewes housed at high stocking densities demand a high standard of hygiene and a high level of surveillance.

The marked seasonal change in market price for fat lambs, which reflects the supply of lambs to the fatstock market, has generated considerable interest in recent years in early lambing. Dorset Horn and Poll Dorsets have traditionally provided 'Easter lamb' through their natural capacity to lamb in the autumn. Early lambing from crossbred flocks usually means January lambing, and this allows well-managed lambs to be marketed off the first flush of spring grass. Only a proportion of crossbreds have the reproductive capacity to meet this requirement and therefore most flocks undertake some form of treatment. Interest in reducing lambing interval through the production of three crops in two years has waned in recent years and is rarely practised. The high demand on stockmanship and marginal economic benefit make it unattractive compared with once-a-year lambing.

There is an increasing interest in breeding from ewe lambs. In 1980 approximately 30% of ewe lambs retained for breeding were put to the ram; by 1988 this had increased to 47%. The increase is partly due to economic pressure coupled with a better understanding of factors affecting fecundity in these young animals.

The importation and development of prolific breeds has given considerable impetus to the study of neonatal problems of large litters. The development of appropriate methods of intensive care, and the availability of improved ewe milk replacements, have considerably eased the husbandry problems.

Selection of breeding stock

In self-contained flocks breeding stock can be selected at several stages prior to entry to the flock. A high proportion is retained at the early stages and this allows some of those that are eventually surplus to requirement to be sold as sound breeding stock. The traditional terms used to describe sheep in the British system are listed in Table 8.1.

Where lambs maintain a high rate of liveweight gain through to the point of marketing as meat animals, the final selection of breeding stock can be delayed to this stage. In many situations there is no penalty imposed on the carcass value of entire animals when sold prior to 5 months of age.

Performance data are usually derived from flock recording schemes operated by the Meat and Livestock Commission (MLC), sometimes in conjunction with a breed society. The data usually relates to one or more of the following: lamb growth, mature size, litter size and maternal ability. Indices are produced to predict animal breeding values and every animal in the flock is given a scaled index and this provides a sound basis for selection decisions.

Certain criteria will apply only to a particular environment or a particular objective. In a hill/upland situation particular attention has to be given

Table 8.1 Traditional sheep terms

Periods	Uncastrated male	Castrated male	Female
Birth to weaning	Tup lamb, ram lamb, pur lamb, heeder	Hogg lamb, wether lamb	Ewe lamb, gimmer lamb, chilver lamb
Weaning to shearing*	Hogg (also used for the female) Hogget (also used for the female) Haggerel or hoggerel Tup teg, ram hogg, tup hogg	Wether hogg, wedder hogg, he teg	Gimmer hogg, ewe hogg, sheeder ewe, ewe teg
First to second shearing	Shearing or shearling or shear hogg Diamond ram Dinmont ram One-shear tup Two-tooth; four-tooth ram or tup		Shearing ewe, shearling gimmer, theave Two-tooth ewe or Four-tooth gimmer
Second to third shearing	Two-shear ram or tup, six-tooth; full mouth ram or tup		Two-shear ewe, six-tooth; full mouth ewe
Afterwards	Full mouth } ram or Broken mouth } tup		Full mouth ewe, broken mouth† ewe
Ewe not in lamb			Barren, eild, Yeld
Ewe sold for further breeding			Draft

* First shorn in May/June at approximately 15 months of age.
† One or more teeth missing.

to survival and thus the type of birth coat and quality of the fleece is of considerable importance. In flocks producing terminal sires selection can concentrate on growth rate and carcass quality. In a self-contained flock producing fat lambs all the attributes of high performance relating to reproductive efficiency, growth rate and carcass quality have to be taken into account. In these flocks it is highly desirable to adopt a system of identification that prevents inbreeding.

In crossbred flocks there is far more opportunity to gradually change the type of breeding ewe when buying in the annual consignment of replacement ewes. The breed of ram can also be readily changed. The mature size and weight of both the breeding ewes and flock sire is

Criteria for selection of breeding animals

Stage	*Criteria*
Neonatal period	Physical soundness
	Type of birth coat (hill/upland breeds)
	Breed colour markings
	Sex: Surplus rams may be castrated
8/12 weeks of age	Physical soundness
	Breed characteristics
	Number in litter
	Performance since birth and contemporary comparisons
Fatstock weight (approx. 50% of potential adult weight)	As above
Prior to the breeding season	Ram and ewe lambs: final selection prior to first breeding. A more rigorous selection procedure including criteria listed above.
	The annual review of rams and ewes: physical soundness, with particular attention to reproductive capability in rams. Performance and progeny tests; contemporary comparisons

important in relation to potential stocking rate and potential carcass weight of the offspring. These lambs are marketed for meat at approximately 50% of their mature weight, which is usually taken as the mean of the parents. Selling lambs at this stage minimizes downgrading due to over-fatness.

Examination of breeding sheep for clinical soundness (see p. 421) is an important component of selection procedure; in crossbred flocks this is the only criterion of selection once the decision regarding type of crossbred ewe or breed of ram has been made.

Puberty

Puberty is the stage at which reproduction first becomes possible; it requires the display of oestrus in ewe lambs and the attainment of mating competence in ram lambs.

Ewe lambs

Puberty is determined by complex interactions involving growth, develop- ment and the ambient photoperiod. Ewe lambs require a period of long day lengths before ovulatory cycles can be initiated. A sequence of long and short days is provided by the increasing and decreasing pattern of daylight during December–June and June–December. Autumn-born lambs are considerably older than spring-born ewe lambs by the time they are exposed to shorter days from late June onwards, and consequently they are heavier at puberty than spring-born lambs. Growth-related cues also play an essential role in the initiation of puberty (Foster *et al.* 1985). The interrelationship between the photoperiodic and growth-related cues in Suffolk ewe lambs is illustrated in Figure 8.1. It is evident from this illustration that lambs with high growth rates are heavier at puberty largely because of the need for adequate exposure to a stimulatory photoperiod; growth-retarded lambs are either later to show activity or remain in anoestrus until the subsequent year. Flockmasters have considerable scope to manipulate growth rate. The target weight for puberty is approximately 50% of the potential adult weight. After achieving this target weight ewe lambs should be exposed to vasectomized rams; breeding is usually delayed until they reach 65% of adult weight.

Control of puberty in ewe lambs, with the exception of manipulating growth rate, is not advised for commercial flocks. It remains to be seen whether melatonin treatment may be considered as an alternative to photostimulation for autumn/early winter born ewe lambs.

Ram lambs

Recent investigations have established that there is a marked difference between ram and ewe lambs in so far as the photoperiodic control of puberty is concerned. In the ram lamb onset of sexual maturity begins before the longest day. Light treatments, which have a retarding effect on puberty in ewe lambs, do not have such an effect on ram lambs.

Higher rates of liveweight gain (250–300 g/day) than shown above, but which do not result in excessive fatness during the late prepubertal period, coupled with exposure to females, should result in slightly earlier attain-

demonstrated in Table 8.3. Body scoring is easy to learn and to use. It does not require any equipment and may be quickly carried out by moving amongst the ewes in a pen. Scoring is not affected by differences in size or by the stage of pregnancy and in these respects it has clear advantages over lists of liveweights.

Table 8.2 The performance of ewes (lambs born per 100 ewes to ram) according to condition score at mating (from MLC 1981)

	Body condition score at mating						
	1	1.5	2	2.5	3	3.5	4
Hill ewes							
Scottish Blackface		79			162		
Hill Gritstone			75	103	119	109	
Welsh Mountain	60	65	105	116	123		
Swaledale		78	133	140	156		
Lowland							
Gritstone (Lowland)				132	154	173	
Masham				167	181	215	
Mule			149	166	178	194	192
Greyface			147	163	176	189	184
Welsh Halfbred		126	139	150	164	172	
Scottish Halfbred			148	170	183	217	202

Table 8.3 The performance of treated and untreated ewes following body scoring (from Pollott and Kilkenny 1976)

	Treated flocks*			Untreated flocks		
	Poor ewes	Rest of flock	Differ ence	Poor ewes	Rest of flock	Differ ence
Average condition score 6 weeks before mating	1.7	3.0	1.3	1.7	2.9	1.2
Average condition at mating	2.8	3.2	0.4	2.3	3.0	0.7
Lambs born per 100 ewes to ram	147	160	13	135	160	25

* Raised plane of nutrition.

The technique involves palpation of the lumbar vertebrae with particular attention given to the sharpness of the spinous processes, the prominence of the transverse processes and the amount of tissue covering them, the amount of muscular and fatty tissue underneath the transverse process, and the fullness of the muscle and fatty tissue in the angle of the spinous and transverse process.

Body condition scoring

Score *Description*

1 The spinous processes are felt to be prominent and sharp. The transverse processes are also sharp, the fingers pass easily under the ends, and it is possible to feel between each process. The eye muscle areas are shallow with no fat cover.

2 The spinous processes still feel prominent, but smooth, and individual processes can be felt only as fine corrugations. The transverse processes are smooth and rounded, and it is possible to pass the fingers under the ends with a little pressure. The eye muscle areas are of moderate depth, but have little fat cover.

3 The spinous processes are detected only as small elevations; they are smooth and rounded, and individual bones can be felt only with pressure. The transverse processes are smooth and well covered, and firm pressure is required to feel over the ends. The eye muscle areas are full, and have a moderate degree of fat cover.

4 The spinous processes can be detected with pressure as a hard line between the fat-covered eye muscle area. The ends of the transverse processes cannot be felt. The eye muscle areas are full and have a thick covering of fat.

5 The spinous processes cannot be detected even with firm pressure, and there is a depression between the layers of fat in the position where the spinous processes would normally be felt. The transverse processes cannot be detected. The eye muscle areas are very full with very thick fat cover. There may be large deposits of fat over the rump and tail.

Source: MLC (1981).

Since stocking rates on lowland farms have markedly increased in recent years, ewes tend to be in poor condition at weaning. The general condition of the breeding flock 8 weeks prior to mating will depend on the interval from weaning and the quality of the grazings subsequent to weaning. The target mean body score for lowland flocks is 3.0–3.5. This should be achieved with as little variation as possible. Those well below this score 8 weeks before tupping should be segregated and given preferential feeding management. Ewes near this level of condition should be allowed to gradually gain weight during the approach to tupping but not allowed to get excessively fat. No ewes should lose condition at this stage.

Nutrition and feeding

Depending on type of flock and production policy the preparatory phase prior to tupping occurs at different times of the year and at different stages of the grazing season. For the vast majority of flocks lambing in late winter/early spring tupping occurs during the tail end of the grazing season. Usually rested pastures or aftermath grazings provide for the needs of the flock at this stage of the production cycle. Where there is a shortage of grass for some reason or another, forage and root crops or supplementation with concentrates may be used to provide their nutritional needs. Over-dependence on feedstuffs known to depress fertility, such as kale, should be avoided before and after tupping. The general pattern of liveweight change according to stage of the production cycle for the three age groups most commonly found in breeding flocks is presented in Table 8.4. In the case of ewe lambs and two-tooth ewes there is a particular need to achieve the target liveweights at all stages to ensure acceptable levels of fertility and fecundity. In mature ewes there is more flexibility; reserves can be mobilized during mid-pregnancy and thus a lower plane of nutrition can be tolerated during this period.

Table 8.4 Target liveweights (kg) as a percentage of mature weight at conception according to age and reproductive states (from MLC 1981)

	State of pregnancy			Lambing		
	Conception	Day 90	Day 120	Before	After	Lactation (week 8)
Ewe lamb (bearing single)	60	65	70	75	64	62
Two-tooth ewe (bearing twins)	80	85	90	97	80	77
Mature ewe (bearing twins)	100 (score 3)	96	100	112	90	83

Introduction of replacement stock

Replacement stock are normally purchased either at the ewe lamb or two-tooth stage. The latter class has become expensive, so increasingly ewe lambs are purchased and mated in their first autumn. It is advisable to buy two-tooth ewes that have not been bred to reduce the risk of introducing diseases that might depress reproductive performance.

Purchased animals should remain isolated until procedures such as preventive treatments, drenching and foot care are completed. Where there is a flock history of toxoplasmosis ewes should be exposed to a contaminated environment (usually paddocks close to the buildings that cats frequent) 2–3 months before tupping.

It is highly probable that two-tooth ewes will join the main flock prior to tupping and remain with it thereafter. Ewe lambs should be kept separate and tupped later in the autumn, and remain separate throughout pregnancy and during the lambing.

Flock health

Flock health programmes are usually tailored to meet the requirements of the system of production. Particular note is taken of the previous disease history of the flock, the prevalent diseases of the locality and the problems that might arise following the purchase of replacement breeding stock. Preventive treatments are available for the variety of diseases caused by viruses, bacteria and other microorganisms, and external and internal parasites. Since timing of treatment is critical, separate treatment programmes should be drawn up for rams, ewe lambs, purchased stock and the main ewe flock. Dipping for the control of sheep scab should occur during September/October. There is no experimental evidence to show that dipping around oestrus and the early stages of implantation depresses fertility but it would be unwise to disrupt normal flock behavioural patterns during tupping. Dipping should preferably be undertaken before or after this period.

Early detection of ill health during the pre-tupping period is imperative; particular attention should be given to foot care in all classes of sheep.

The breeding season

Breeding seasonality has a marked influence on several aspects of fecundity: the attainment of puberty, postpartum interval to oestrus, prolificacy in females, and semen production and quality in rams. It is one of the basic considerations in production planning.

Breeding seasonality in relation to geographical location

The breeding season of most breeds kept in high latitudes is restricted to a fairly predictable period commencing during the late summer/early autumn and ending during the winter months. The majority of breeds have more oestrous cycles before the winter solstice than after it. There are marked differences between breeds in the duration of the season, with the majority having less than 10 oestrous cycles per season. Consequently, the majority will have lapsed into seasonal anoestrus prior to or soon after lambing and thus there is little opportunity for rebreeding and of achieving a short lambing interval.

The establishment of a clearly defined breeding season is generally attributed to natural selection having taken place in an environment with distinct annual fluctuations. In a harsh climate and short season of growth, the timing of lambing during the approach to the grazing season improves the chances of survival. Natural selection in such an environment was probably based mainly on the onset of breeding activity and on the lack of activity after lambing—the former to organize lambing at the most appropriate time and the latter to eliminate the possibility of conception during lactation.

Investigations have clearly demonstrated that in the higher latitudes the breeding season is entrained to the local light rhythm. These rhythms have amplitudes greater than 4 hours. The pineal gland, through its release of melatonin during the hours of darkness, relays the photoperiodic time-cues to the hypothalamic centres controlling reproduction, and this plays a key role in the regulation of breeding seasonality. In the case of sheep, long nights are regarded as inductive and short nights as suppressive. Sheep are capable of responding to new light rhythms and this adaptive capacity has allowed the successful establishment of European breeds in the Southern Hemisphere. It has also led to the development of methods of photostimulation.

Breeding seasonality is not considered a disadvantage by the majority of UK flockmasters in pastoral areas; it allows lactation and the early growth of the offspring to coincide with the best phase of the grazing season. The postweaning recovery period also coincides in most seasons with the availability of good grazing or forage and root crops. It is only when autumn or early winter lambing is attempted that problems arise and it is usually due to failure to appreciate the interactions that occur between several factors regulating the onset of cyclic activity.

Photoperiodicity is also important in relation to movements between latitudes. It is convenient to divide a hemisphere into three zones, which differ considerably in their seasonal rhythm of daylight change:

1. Zone 1 (equator to 30°) has a low amplitude that is hardly discernible at the equator where it varies little from a 13-hour day.
2. Zone 2 (30–60°) has a regular seasonal rhythm with an amplitude varying from 4 hours at 30° to over 14 hours at 60°. Throughout this zone there is a daily occurrence of alternating daylight and darkness.
3. Zone 3 (60° to Pole) has a unique light environment in that continuous daylight occurs for a period during summer and the sun does not rise above the horizon for a period around the winter solstice.

In so far as sheep exports are concerned, movement to a comparable latitude in the opposite hemisphere, e.g. from Europe to Australasia, the Falkland Islands or the southern countries of South America, subjects sheep to a rephased light rhythm; full entrainment is usually achieved by the second year. In the first year an advancement of 3 months in the onset of activity compared with the UK occurs, and a further 3 months occurs in the subsequent year when they become fully synchronous, in terms of seasonality, with their new contemporaries. There is some evidence that British breeds maintained around 33°S in Australia have a much shorter breeding season than ewes of the same breed kept at 52°N in the UK.

Transfers from the UK to Zone 1 have occurred intermittently over the years. There are vast areas in this zone where altitude offsets the problems associated with high temperature and is a temperate area ideally situated for the systems of sheep meat production practised in Europe. Unfortunately, information on the seasonality of breeds in the UK gives little indication of their suitability to the non-fluctuating light environment of the low latitudes. The poor breeding performance of British breeds in Kenya and Colombia has drawn attention to the importance of genotype–environment interactions in the selection of stock for export (Williams 1977).

The assessment of reproductive efficiency in several British breeds of sheep in Colombia has shown significant breed differences in incidence of oestrus, lambing rate and degree of rephasing in breeding activity. It has also been shown that rams of breeds with depressed fertility readily produce offspring from local ewes and this suggests that barrenness is largely female dysfunction. The experimental investigation of the direct effects of a simulated non-fluctuating equatorial photoperiod has established that breeds differ in many aspects of reproductive function including proportion exhibiting oestrus, quality of oestrus, duration of cyclicity, incidence of ovulation without oestrus and in postpartum interval to ovulation and oestrus (Williams 1984).

Photostimulation

Considerable interest has been shown in the development of photostimulation as a treatment for out-of-season breeding. It has been clearly shown that ewes adapt to imposed 12-month light cycles and also to 6-month light cycles, provided an amplitude greater than 4 hours is maintained. The best and most predictable response is usually achieved when a period of long days (>16 hours) is imposed during February–March followed by a phase of short days maintained until cyclic activity is initiated in June (Williams 1977). Provided due attention is given to the form of treatment and to its timing, the onset of activity should be as predictable as the normal breeding season and the general performance of the flock in terms of fecundity and milk yield. Photostimulation has the particular advantage over all other forms of treatment in that it initiates cyclic activity with all its attendant advantages. It is acknowledged that photostimulation is a costly treatment largely due to the need to provide long nights during late spring and early summer and it also disrupts traditional management at this time of year. Recent investigations have shown that melatonin treatment may replace the costly long night phase. Sheep are often housed for other reasons during the winter and therefore the application of long days can be readily applied in any sheep building. Thus the combination of long days and melatonin treatment is likely to become an attractive alternative to other forms of treatment for out-of-season breeding (Williams and Ward 1988; Williams 1994b). Melatonin treatments without priming with artificial long days and designed for slight advancement of the breeding season have been investigated (Haresign 1991). Williams and Hanif (1990) reported on its use for rephasing peak reproductive activity in rams.

Duration of the breeding season

The majority of British breeds are capable of displaying up to 10 oestrous cycles per breeding season (Figure 8.2). It is well known that the Dorset Horn and Poll Dorset have a long breeding season (>12 oestrous cycles) and are the only breeds capable of lambing out of season without any form of treatment. The majority of the flocks lamb from October onwards. When tupping is delayed until the autumn individual ewes may relapse into a shallow anoestrus for a short period but it is rare for the majority of the flock to do so at the same time.

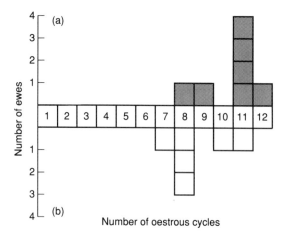

Figure 8.2 The number of oestrous cycles per ewe in a breeding season: (a) 7 Welsh Mountain ewes, mean 10.43 cycles; (b) 6 Border Leicester ewes, mean 8.65 cycles.

The onset of the breeding season

There is, surprisingly, a dearth of information regarding the onset of the breeding season. The distribution of first oestrus and other data presented in Figure 8.3 draws attention to the following features:

- breed differences in mean date of onset,
- considerable within-breed variation,
- low between-year variation in mean onset.

The ewes were exposed to vasectomized rams from the end of June in each year.

There is no doubt that the ambient photoperiod has a dominant influence on the onset and duration of the breeding season. All other factors have only a minor role and cannot be considered as potential treatments where a major shift in the onset of activity is required.

Factors affecting the onset of the breeding season (excluding the physical environment) are considered below.

Nutrition/condition

There is no evidence that the variation in body condition found in flocks during the approach to the breeding season has a significant correlation

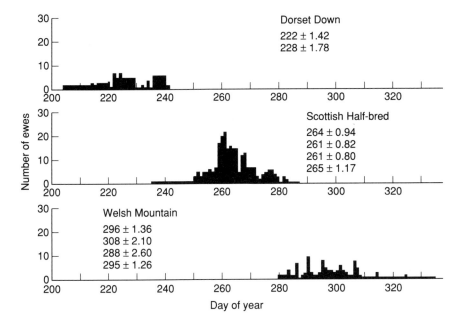

Figure 8.3 The distribution and mean onset (day of year) of first oestrus in three breeds of sheep in successive years.

with the onset of activity. In grossly mismanaged flocks severely emaciated animals may have a higher incidence of ovulation without oestrus. This is unlikely to arise as a flock problem because the attainment of a high mean ovulation rate is a major objective of good management at this time of year and can only be achieved when ewes are in good condition.

Interval from last lambing

Postpartum anoestrus assumes importance only when lambing occurs during the approach to or during the breeding season. The mother/lamb relationship and/or high plasma prolactin levels retard the establishment of normal hormonal interactions. The mean intervals to ovulation and oestrus in two contrasting breeds lambing in October are shown in Table 8.5.

Ram effect

Where rams are isolated from the ewes for a period during the prepubertal phase, late anoestrus or the postpartum period, females will respond to the reintroduction of the rams into the flock. The unaccustomed presence of the ram activates the hypothalamic centres controlling the frequency of

Table 8.5 Postpartum interval to ovulation and oestrus

Ewe breed	Postpartum interval (days)	
	To ovulation	To oestrus
North Country Cheviot	26.4	46.7
Dorset Horn	24.6	39.0

luteinizing hormone (LH) pulses resulting, if the timing is appropriate, in ovulation. This response is known as the 'ram effect' and is primarily a response to pheromones in the wool (Martin *et al.* 1986). Visual and tactile/behavioural stimuli also contribute to the response. The minimum duration of isolation required for a strong response is thought to be 2 weeks. Recent investigations have suggested that pre-isolation of ewes from rams was not required when novel rams were introduced. It is not known whether this applies to all breeds.

In so far as farm practice is concerned it is difficult to predict the nature and uniformity of the response to the unaccustomed presence of the ram at a particular stage of late anoestrus. In all classes of female sheep it is very rare for oestrus to accompany the first ovulation after emerging from anoestrus.

The 'entry of the ram' effect is not as predictable nor as synchronous as that which can be achieved through the use of progestagens; it is best described as non-random distribution of oestrus with a high incidence of oestrus on days 19 and 25 following the entry of the ram. If oestrus has already been initiated in some ewes, due to the lateness of the introduction of the ram, the distribution of oestrus will encompass a much longer period, up to 25 days.

Age

The ewe lamb is the only age group that differs from others in so far as onset is concerned. The mean onset of well-grown ewe lambs is approximately 3 weeks later than adults of the breed.

Planning a breeding programme

The timing of lambing will have a major impact on the seasonal pattern of management, particularly in relation to choice of foodstuffs and to the need for housing during part of pregnancy and lactation. The key events in the UK sheep year are shown below.

	Spring lambing	*Autumn lambing*
Mating	Mid-October	Mid-July
Lambing	Mid-March	Early December
Shearing	Winter or early summer	Early summer
Weaning	Early August	Late January

It can be readily seen that these key events occur at contrasting times of the year particularly in relation to weather and grazing. In the case of late autumn lambing the major part of pregnancy coincides with the grazing season, whereas there is more dependence on hay and/or silage during pregnancy in spring-lambing flocks.

The most appropriate sheep production programme for a particular unit will largely depend on the marketing objectives and the resources available in terms of foodstuffs, buildings and labour supply. Where the marketing objective involves the sale of fat lambs during March–May, the season of high prices, the interval between lambing and sale is dictated by the potential growth rate of the lamb. This is largely governed by the early milk yield of the ewes and the nutritional quality of supplementary feeding. This is the only instance in fat lamb production where the timing of lambing is critical and where a high growth rate is required in order to benefit from the high prices of the early season. The pattern of seasonal price variation has resulted in considerable interest in earlier lambing, partly due to the advent of winter housing resulting from high stocking rates and partly the need to ease grazing pressure later in the grazing season. The attainment of the required effective tupping cycle shown in the production plan presented in Table 8.6 greatly depends on the reproductive capacity of the breed or crossbreed involved, in terms of the onset of the breeding season and its response to manipulation of the non-physical factors affecting onset.

The requirements for compact lambing and high fecundity are:

- All members of the flock cycling
- High ovulation rate
- High level of fertility

Where only a proportion of the flock is expected to lamb early, the rams may be turned in for a restricted period. Where the tupping rate is very high the number of ewes required for early lambing may be met in a few days.

The decision regarding the need for treatment to initiate breeding

Table 8.6 A production plan

Objective	Marketing week	Latest lambing date*	Required tupping cycle
A	5 March	1 December	23 June to 9 July (174–190)[†]
B	30 April	5 January	27 July to 13 August (208–225)
C	4 June	2 February	24 August to 10 September (236–253)
D	25 June	2 March	21 September to 8 October (264–282)

* For twins gaining 250 g/day and yielding a carcass of 17 kg.
† Day of year; refer to Figure 8.3 for data on onset of the breeding season.

activity around the transition from anoestrus depends entirely on whether the production objective involves the whole flock or part of the flock. In the case of the latter, the approach adopted in the previous paragraph is adequate, but when the whole flock is involved the use of an appropriate treatment is advised.

Reference to Figure 8.3 gives a broad indication whether all three breeds listed are likely to meet the tupping requirement, associated with the production objectives listed in Table 8.6, without resorting to some form of pharmacological treatment.

The control of oestrus and ovulation

There are a variety of reasons and benefits for controlling oestrus and ovulation. The physiological reasons include prepubertal, postpartum or seasonal anoestrus, and the unacceptable variation due to transition from anoestrus to breeding season and to distribution of oestrus over 17 days.

The agricultural benefits include the use of artificial insemination (AI), exploitation of superior sires and out-of-season breeding.

Effective treatments must be simple to apply, have a low labour demand, maintain normal patterns of behaviour and produce normal or improved fecundity. The main treatment options currently available, or at the product development phase, are shown in Table 8.7.

Table 8.7 Options for the control of oestrus and ovulation

Treatment	Oestrus response	Synchronization of oestrus	Augmentation of ovulation
Photostimulation	Cyclicity	Random	Ineffective
Melatonin	Cyclicity	Random	Some response
Progestagens/ PMSG	Treatment oestrus	Effective	Some response
PMSG	—	—	Effective but variable response
Progestagens	—	Effective during breeding season	—
GnRH*	Treatment oestrus	—	Ineffective
Unaccustomed presence of ram	Oestrus during approach to normal breeding season	Partial	Ineffective

* Field trials in progress.
GnRH, gonadotrophin releasing hormone; PMSG, pregnant mare's serum gonadotrophin.

Treatments during anoestrus

A combination of progestagen and PMSG treatment is required during anoestrus to initiate oestrus: the progestagen acts as a priming agent and increases the likelihood of oestrus accompanying the ovulation induced by PMSG. Those not responding to treatment and those failing to conceive during the treatment oestrus relapse into anoestrus. The probability of the ewes remaining cyclic after treatment increases when treatment is given near the onset of the breeding season (Gordon 1983).

Treatment during the breeding season

Treatment carried out during the breeding season may utilize the ewe's own feedback system to initiate oestrus and ovulation following progestagen treatment and particularly when synchronization is the only purpose of the treatment. When augmentation of ovulation rate is required, the dosage rate of PMSG should be in the range 750–1000 iu. When PMSG is simply used to achieve better synchrony of ovulation after sponge withdrawal, 500 and 700 iu should be given to small and large ewes respectively. Irrespective of the purpose of the PMSG, it is usually given at the time of sponge withdrawal.

Rams should be released on day 16 at the same time of day as the

---

Treatment schedule

Day 0   Insert sponges.

Day 14   Remove sponges. Inject 500–700 iu PMSG
          intramuscularly.

Day 16   Release rams; 1 ram per 10–15 ewes.

---

sponges were removed. Around this interval from sponge removal (48 hours) the majority of the ewes should be entering oestrus and this reduces the likelihood of rams competing for and exhausting themselves on those first entering oestrus.

Mating behaviour

Ewes in oestrus may seek the ram and a ram may acquire a harem with intense competition between ewes. This is usually very evident when ewes are synchronized. Generally, the ram does most of the seeking and gives an indication of whether or not he is actively involved in detecting oestrous ewes. Shepherds refer to this as evidence of 'working'. During the search, sight, smell and sound play an important part in detection. Rams are capable of displaying a sexual challenge some distance from the ewes, usually by emitting a low-pitched gurgling sound coupled with the extension of the neck and slight rotation of the head. At close quarters the initial approach may involve sniffing the perineal area, and this is often followed by baring of teeth and lip curling (flehmen). Nudging and pawing with the front foot may also occur. Exhausted rams may aggressively butt oestrous ewes if they remain in close proximity.

Rams may mount several times before achieving intromission. A deep pelvic thrust is associated with ejaculation, which lasts only a few seconds. This is followed by dismounting and then the ram stands quietly alongside the ewe with its head lowered. After a brief rest the ram will continue searching.

A comprehensive account of reproductive behaviour may be found in Lynch *et al.* (1992).

Signs of oestrus

Ewes do not normally show signs of oestrus in the absence of a ram and unlike other farm species interactions between females is not used as a means of detecting oestrus. During oestrus ewes stand firmly, will display tail fanning and may look backwards.

Oestrus lasts for 24–44 hours. This duration is imprecise and is affected by the frequency of testing, ram management, breed, age and stage of the breeding season. It is difficult to establish with any precision the onset of oestrus and it is therefore difficult to determine the ideal time for controlled natural service or AI of untreated ewes. The vulva becomes oedematous and there may be some mucous discharge. Histological examination of vaginal mucus can also provide evidence of recent ovarian activity. These changes are of no value in the detection of oestrus.

Detection of oestrus

It is imperative to use a ram to monitor the occurrence of oestrus. Ewes are rarely kept under close observation. Mating occurs on a flock basis and may involve several rams. Presumptive evidence of mating is provided by the use of oil-based colouring paste smeared on the ram's sternum (raddle/keel) or lanolin-based crayons held on the sternum by a harness. The number of ewes colour-marked on the rump should be noted during each inspection. It is a useful method of monitoring the progress of tupping; the more frequently this is done the more accurate the predictions that emanate from these observations. The use of one colour should not exceed the duration of an oestrous cycle, i.e. 17 days.

Ewes are served approximately two to four times during oestrus; the higher the number of services the higher the level of fecundity, an important aspect in deciding on the proportion of rams to be used in the flock.

Management during mating

Subdivision of the flock into tupping groups is usually practised where there is need to identify the sire for pedigree records. Some subdivision may also occur in very large flocks. The average UK flock is kept as one unit throughout the tupping period. The proportion of rams used is rarely less than 1% in large flocks and it is usually in the range 2–3%. Adjustments have to be made in the case of ewe lambs, ram lambs and where the flock or group has been synchronized. In the latter case up to 10% of rams is not uncommon.

Where rams are used in groups, due regard must be given to competition between rams and the establishment of dominance. Daily surveillance will ensure that this kind of problem is detected early, particularly when rams are used in pairs, or when there are age and size differences between rams. One needs to be aware of rape marks particularly when trough feeding is practised. Ewes may be served without being keel marked; this can occur when service takes place during the first and only mount. The factors affecting reliability of keel marking are:

- Frequency of colour change
- Stability of keeling harness
- Length of texture of wool
- Weather conditions
- Texture of crayons
- Number of mounts

Provided the entire flock has initiated oestrous cycles before the ram is turned in there should be random distribution of oestrus over the first 17 days, i.e. approximately 6% of the ewes should be served each day or one-third in 6 days. This pattern of mating is unlikely to arise when the ewes have been partially synchronized before the tupping season by some means or other. The absence of keel marks in a proportion (or all) of a late tupping flock is sometimes perplexing and arises where there has been inadequate control of the rams earlier in the autumn or where uncastrated ram lambs have not been weaned early. Conceptions following an unscheduled overnight stay in the flock can arise in up to 10% of the flock.

Where hand mating is practised, usually in pedigree flocks, ewes should be served following each positive test for oestrus. Reliance on only one service would probably depress fertility and fecundity.

No precise advice can be given regarding paddock size during mating. The majority of lowland farms adopt high stocking rates to ensure good productivity and it follows that the stocking density in a particular area at any time will not involve the rams in excessive walking. In general terms synchronized ewes and ewe lambs should be tupped in smaller fields and this also applies to groups of ewes exposed to ram lambs. In hill and upland areas where tupping cannot be carried out in the enclosed areas around the farmstead a higher ratio of rams is usually used, up to 3%.

Physiology of mating

During ejaculation the swirling action of the urethral process sprays the semen over the os of the cervix; some semen briefly remains as a pool in the anterior vagina prior to entry and passage through the cervix. The cervix forms a barrier to the passage of the semen through to the uterus. Some sperm penetrate quickly and may reach the site of fertilization in the oviduct in 30 minutes. Most sperm are held in the cervical pool, which may take up to 3 days to disperse. Sperm motility is the main mode of transport through the cervix; uterine and tubal peristalsis aid transport after the sperm leave the cervix. Progestagen treatment and oestrogenic pasture may interfere with the time taken to reach the fallopian tube. Sperm are also held back at the utero-tubal junction. Sperm undergo a set of changes (capacitation) during passage through the tract and this enables penetration of the zona pellucida; one sperm enters the nucleus and completes fertilization.

The fertile life of sperm is approximately 30–48 hours and the ovum 16–24 hours. The majority of ova will have reached the uterus by 66 hours. Fertilized ova are at the 2-cell stage by 24 hours and 8-cell stage by 60 hours following ovulation.

Ovulation

Ovulation occurs 24–27 hours after the onset of oestrus. The ovulation rate is influenced by the factors discussed below.

Breed

Most British breeds have a low or moderate ovulation rate in the range one to three. There are several breeds with a higher ovulation rate; the best known are the Finnish Landrace and Romanov in Europe and the Booroola Merino in Australia. In the case of the latter it is thought to be controlled by a single gene and much interest is now being shown in transferring the gene to other breeds through crossbreeding and selection (Land and Robinson 1985).

Age

Peak ovulation rate is achieved at 3–5 years of age and this can be maintained for a further 5 years. Ewe lambs and two-tooth ewes have a lower ovulation rate. The physiological mechanisms associated with the effect of age have not been fully investigated.

Season

In all seasonal breeds the ovulation rate increases over the first three oestrous cycles and is maintained throughout the middle period. It declines towards the end of the season.

Nutrition and body condition

It has long been recognized that ovulation rate and fecundity of ewes can be manipulated by changes in the plane of nutrition. Liveweight and body condition are used as criteria for assessing nutritional adequacy of feeding regimes over a sequence of production cycles or one cycle. In the case of the latter, the period leading up to tupping has attracted most interest. Smith (1985) concluded that both energy and protein content of the diet can influence ovulation rate independently of each other. For maximum response it is suggested that increases in both are advisable. The requirements of breeding stock during the approach to the breeding season, in terms of energy, protein and major minerals, may be found in MAFF (1986). Feeding regimes in relation to the attainment of a high level of fecundity are discussed in another section.

Control of ovulation

Over the last 50 years PMSG has been used to control ovulation (mainly in conjunction with progestagen treatment), to initiate oestrus in anoestrous ewes and to reduce the interval to ovulation following progestagen sponge removal during the breeding season. It is also used to superovulate ewes participating in embryo transplant programmes. Although effective when used alone during the follicular phase of the cycle (day 12–14), for convenience the combination treatment is used more often than not.

The response to PMSG is highly variable particularly at the higher dose levels. Where superovulation is not required the dose rate should be 300–750 iu. This avoids high ovulation rates leading to large litter size with low birth liveweight and poor survival rates (Henderson 1985). Where superovulation is required the dose rate may be increased to 1500 iu.

Artificial insemination

There are clear indications that new developments in sheep breeding techniques are going to play a significant role in the achievement of genetic improvement, particularly in the terminal sire breeds. Improved techniques associated with AI schemes and the use of multiple ovulation/ embryo transfer (MOET) will help to overcome the limitations posed by small size of flocks, long generation interval and low litter size.

The advantages of AI and MOET are:

- higher selection intensity
- shorter generation interval
- improved accuracy of selection in progeny tests
- scope for flock linkage

- fewer rams for synchronized flocks
- reduced risk of infertility
- aid to disease control
- export of semen

Semen collection

Semen may be collected from rams by using an artificial vagina (AV) or by electro-ejaculation. Electro-ejaculation is a convenient method of collecting a single sample of semen as part of a clinical examination and assessment of fertility. In most circumstances it is the only convenient method. It does not require trained rams nor the use of a 'teaser' or a ewe in oestrus. Where repeated collections are carried out the AV method must be adopted. It is more acceptable in terms of welfare and provides good quality semen.

The AV method

The time required to fully train a ram varies according to age, time of year, temperament and libido. Initially, the ram should be conditioned to the semen collecting pen and to an attendant standing alongside during natural service. It is advisable to train rams during the peak breeding season and to use ewes in oestrus. The ewe should be held in a yoked restraining stall with plenty of space on either side. Holding pens for other rams should be within sight of the collecting area and this helps in ram training and during subsequent routine collections. When rams are fully trained any docile sheep can act as teaser during collections. It is quite useful to have ovariectomized ewes as teasers and these can be brought into oestrus by hormone treatment if the need arises.

The electro-ejaculation method

Electro-ejaculation involves the stimulation of the nerve plexus near the pelvic genitalia using a rectal electrode (probe). It is a potentially stressful and painful procedure and the reaction of most rams indicates this. Rams may be stimulated in the standing or lying position. The lying position has the advantage that the rams can be placed on straw bales, and thus raised from the ground, and the legs can be tied together and secured to minimize the physical restraint required during collection.

Guidelines on the use of the technique are available from the British Veterinary Association.

Sheep breeding and infertility

Semen collection by AV is carried out as follows

1. Use purchased ram AV, or bull AV reduced to 17 cm.
2. Add hot water to AV casing to raise temperature to 45°C; do not allow water on to the liner.
3. Use pump to raise pressure; assess subjectively.
4. Lubricate AV (KY jelly).
5. Attach warmed (30°C), insulated collection vessel firmly and protect from damage.
6. Tease ram, by allowing one/two false mounts, to improve semen quality.
7. Hold AV firmly against upper thigh of teaser and manually guide the penis toward it, by grasping sheath, and allow the ram to thrust into it. Do not attempt to place AV over penis during the mount.
8. Take stoppered collection vessel to semen examination area without delay and protect from temperature shock.

Semen collection by electro-ejaculation is carried out as follows

1. Bipolar probes with integral batteries and control switch are available and designed for rams.
2. Check before use, including the voltage output of the batteries. Output in the range 10–15 V is adequate for all breeds and ages. Batteries can be interchanged to vary voltage output. Keep clean between periods of use and service instrument regularly.
3. Lubricate probe and insert into rectum until anterior edge of pelvic rim is felt. Allow the ram to get used to the probe and then bring down on to the floor of the rectum directly over the pelvic genitalia by slightly raising the handle.
4. Stimulate by depressing switch for 4–6 seconds; follow with rest of equal or longer duration and stimulate again. Semen is usually obtained following three or four stimulations. Total stimulations should be restricted to five or six.
5. The person operating the probe should have a good view of the prepuce and semen collection vessel. The semen collector should direct the semen into a prewarmed collecting vessel and also massage the penis in a forward direction from the flexure during the rest period following each stimulation.
6. Avoid temperature shock to semen prior to examination and processing.

384

Semen evaluation

There is wide variation in semen quality between rams of the same breed and between age groups (ram lambs and aged rams are inferior to other age groups) and between seasons of the year. No assessment can predict fertility with a high degree of accuracy. A combined examination of clinical soundness and semen quality improves the probability of achieving good fertility and fecundity in the flock. Poor rams can be culled and the moderately good can be paired with the better rams. Only rams producing best quality semen should be selected for AI programmes, particularly where the semen is deep frozen.

The examination and evaluation of semen involves the assessments described below. It is imperative that samples are carefully handled during these examinations and that particular attention is given to the glassware, which must be sterile, dry and warm. A water bath (32°C), warming cabinet (35°C) and a microscope fitted with a warm stage are essential equipment for a semen collection unit.

Semen volume and physical appearance

The season of the year and frequency of collection can have a marked effect on volume. The average volume of ejaculate from adult Suffolk rams during September–January and March–August is 1.1 and 0.8 ml respectively. In order to allow for this seasonal fluctuation, and other aspects of quality, the frequency of collections should be limited during these two periods to 20 and five collections per week respectively.

Semen collection vessels are graduated and volume can easily be determined. At the same time, an assessment of colour and consistency can be made and given a score (see p. 386); samples used for AI should be in the range 3–5. There is a reasonable correlation between these visible attributes of semen and sperm concentration; this may be usefully used under field conditions as a guide for dilution rates.

Samples produced by electro-ejaculation are usually lower in volume and poorer in other aspects of semen quality than samples collected by AV. Rams producing a poor sample from the first ejaculate should not be rejected without further evidence from one or two subsequent samples.

Motility

A normal undiluted semen sample should clearly show wave-like motion indicative of good motility.

Where there is need to establish the proportion of sperm showing forward motion, the sample should be diluted, one drop of semen with 20

Semen examination: motility

Score	Class	Description
1	Dead	sperm immotile
2	Poor	sperm motile but no waves present
3	Fair	slow wave motion present
4	Good	moderate wave motion
5	Very good	rapid motion characterized by dark waves

Samples in the range 1–3 should not be used for AI.

Source: MLC (1982)

---

drops of warmed diluent, and then examined under the microscope. This procedure is normally done prior to preparations for deep freezing and also to assess quality following thawing.

Sperm concentration

An accurate determination of sperm concentration is required for the calculation of dilution rate and volume of inseminate appropriate to the method of insemination to be used. The haemocytometer method is accurate but slow; most AI centres would be equipped with a colorimeter, which is a quick and convenient method of assessing sperm concentration. There is a need to complete the overall assessment as quickly as possible after collection so that dilution and preparations for storage can proceed.

Semen examination: consistency and number of spermatozoa

Score	Consistency	Number of spermatozoa ($\times 10^9$) per ml	
		Mean	Range
5	Thick creamy	5.0	4.5–6.0
4	Creamy	4.0	3.5–4.5
3	Thin creamy	3.0	2.5–3.5
2	Milky	2.0	1.0–2.5
1	Cloudy	0.7	0.3–1.0
0	Clear (watery)	insignificant	

Source: Evans and Maxwell (1987)

Semen samples to be deep frozen should have a minimum concentration of 3.0×10^9 sperm/ml. The highest concentration of sperm is usually found in samples taken during the late summer/early autumn and the lowest concentration during the winter months.

Abnormal sperms

When collections take place through the year the proportion of abnormal sperm in the sample is normally estimated once a month. If it is a seasonal activity samples should be assessed not more than 1 week before semen collections begin to be stored or used.

A smear is prepared from a sample of one drop of semen with six drops of warmed nigrosin–eosin stain. At least 100 sperm should be examined and note taken of the number and type of abnormality. The most common abnormalities are bent or coiled tails, detached heads and cytoplasmic droplets attached to the mid-piece of the sperm. Semen with more than 20% of abnormals should not be used for AI.

Semen dilution

The main purposes of semen dilution are to allow more extensive use of the rams and to protect sperm against the chemical and physical changes that occur during cooling and freezing. The dilution rate is governed by the motility rating, the concentration of live sperms and the number of inseminations to be carried out. The majority of samples are diluted three-fold (one part of semen with two parts of diluent). Samples that do not stand this degree of dilution are usually discarded. Semen of exceptional quality for conventional AI can be diluted five-fold. Where the laparoscopic method of intrauterine insemination is carried out, good quality semen can be diluted ten-fold.

The number of sperm per inseminate according to type of oestrus and method of AI is shown in Table 8.8. The volume of inseminate required for intravaginal, intracervical and intrauterine insemination is approximately 0.3, 0.1 and 0.08 ml respectively.

Due regard should be given in determining volume and number of sperm per inseminate to the experience and competence of the operator, to the general standard of management of the flock concerned, and the efficiency of the arrangements provided for inseminating the flock or group.

Semen storage

Fresh undiluted semen may be used within 20 minutes of collection at the rate of 0.05 ml per inseminate. This approach may be quite adequate in certain circumstances.

Table 8.8 The number of sperm per inseminate according to type of oestrus, method of AI and season

Type of oestrus	Method of AI	Sperm per inseminate ($\times 10^6$)*
Natural	Intracervical (short-term storage)	125–150
Synchronized	Intracervical (short-term storage)	200–400
Synchronized (no PMSG)	Intrauterine (deep frozen semen)	20–30
Synchronized (> 500 iu PMSG)	Intrauterine (deep-frozen semen)	100–150

* Upper values for ewes bred out of season.

Diluted semen may be stored for 10–12 hours after cooling. Cooling to 15°C should be done over a period of 30 minutes. A variety of diluents have been used for the short-term storage of semen. The most readily available and easiest to use is ultra-heat treated (UHT) milk. It simply requires to be brought up to 30°C prior to use.

The indications for deep freezing semen are:

- longer storage period (may be held at –196°C in liquid nitrogen for 10 years or more),
- collections can be carried out throughout the year,
- easier distribution from AI centres,
- semen export possible.

Where semen is processed regularly and on a reasonable scale it may be frozen in plastic straws (0.5 ml) or in pellet form (0.1 ml). Filling of straws can be mechanized and it is easier to identify individual straws, whereas pellets have to be stored in colour-coded goblets.

Diluents for freezing semen must contain a cryoprotective agent and a constituent to protect the cell membrane during initial cooling. The most commonly used are glycerol and egg yolk. Detailed information on diluents and on all aspects of AI is given in Agricultural Training Board (1989) and Evans and Maxwell (1987). Both straws and pellets may be thawed rapidly by placing them in dry test tubes placed in a water bath at 37°C. The samples should be assessed soon after thawing to determine the volume of semen (number of sperms) required for the method of insemination to be used.

Insemination technique

Synchronization of oestrus is an essential part of AI programmes. Predictable synchrony of oestrus, and ovulation, can be achieved by the use of progestagen intravaginal sponges for 12–14 days and with 375–750 iu PMSG given intramuscularly at sponge withdrawal. The dose of PMSG is determined by ewe size, time of year and the need to achieve a high ovulation rate. For intravaginal and intracervical insemination the hindquarters should be raised in some way so that it is easier for the operator to locate the cervix. Where a large number of ewes have to be inseminated it is useful to have a custom-built pivoting and tipping crate available. This can be linked to the handling race, and sometimes to the sheep dip, so that the inseminator's platform is at the ideal level for viewing the cervix.

The intravaginal method

Sometimes described as 'shot-in-the-dark' (SID), the semen is deposited in the anterior vagina without the use of a speculum to guide the pipette forward. It requires a large volume of semen and a high concentration of sperm and should be considered only when a small group of ewes have to be inseminated and when plenty of undiluted semen is available.

The intracervical method

Unlike other farm species, full penetration of the cervix is not possible and should not be attempted. The cervix should be located using an illuminated speculum and the semen deposited into the first cervical fold.

The intrauterine method

This involves the use of a fibre-optic instrument to observe and examine the internal reproductive tract. Semen is injected into each horn via a second cannula. This laparoscopic technique was developed in Australia about 5 years ago to improve fertility rates when using deep-frozen semen and to achieve more progeny per ram per season.

The ewe must be fully restrained (head down) on a custom-built examination cradle at 75–80°. The area around the penetration points cranial to the udder and close to the midline must be thoroughly cleaned and prepared as for surgery. The immediate area is then infused with local anaesthetic. With 5-mm canulae no postoperative stitching is required.

A major advantage of the technique is the significant improvement in fertility with deep-frozen semen (70–80% conception rate compared with 30–50% when using intravaginal cervical insemination). It also requires only 10% of the sperm required for intracervical insemination. The technique has now been adapted for the recovery and transfer of embryos and will be used in ovine MOET schemes as well as breed improvement programmes (MLC, 1991).

Time of insemination

Since synchronization of oestrus and the use of PMSG has become an integral part of AI programmes, the timing of insemination is invariably given as the interval from sponge removal. It is a convenient reference point and much research has been conducted into the interval from sponge removal to onset of oestrus, to the LH surge associated with ovulation, and to ovulation. The majority of ewes are in oestrus within 36–48 hours and ovulate about 60 hours after sponge withdrawal. Ewes that have been given high doses of PMSG for superovulation usually ovulate earlier than ewes with a normal ovulation rate. The optimum interval from sponge withdrawal to insemination according to the method of insemination is given in Table 8.9. Travel time and on-farm work routines have to be taken into consideration in making the final arrangements for inseminating the group or flock.

Fertility and fecundity

There is no commercial service, comparable to the cattle and pig industries, available to the UK sheep producer and therefore data on fertility and fecundity is restricted to that provided by those involved in research and development work. The data presented in Tables 8.10–8.12 give some indication of the results that can be achieved using various procedures currently adopted in AI programmes.

The factors affecting fertility and fecundity following AI are:

- diluent and dilution rate,
- number of sperms per inseminate,
- number of inseminations per oestrus,
- type of storage and duration (if short term),
- season of the year,
- type of oestrus (natural or synchronized),
- method of insemination.

Table 8.9 Recommended intervals from sponge withdrawal to AI

Method of insemination	Optimum interval (hours)
Intracervical	One insemination, 56 Two inseminations, 48/60
Intrauterine	
No superovulation	56–64
Superovulation	
Fresh semen	36–48
Frozen semen	44–48

Table 8.10 The effect of semen storage time on fertility and fecundity (from MLC 1982)

Semen age	No. farms	No. ewes inseminated*	No. ewes lambed	Conception rate (%)	Lambs per ewe lambed
<5 hours	4	378	233	62	1.83
24 hours	4	375	212	57	1.76

* Ewes inseminated 57 hours after sponge/PMSG treatment; $150–200 \times 10^6$ sperms per inseminate; a skim milk diluent was used.

Table 8.11 The effects of number of inseminations and volume of inseminate on fertility and litter size (from MLC 1982)

No. inseminations per ewe	Inseminate volume (ml)	No. ewes inseminated	No. ewes lambed	Percentage lambing	Lambs per ewe lambed
2	0.1	31	18	58	1.89
1	0.2	30	10	33	1.90
2	0.2	32	18	56	1.56
1	0.4	32	11	34	1.73

Single insemination at 57 hours, double insemination at 50 and 60 hours after sponge/PMSG treatment.

Table 8.12 The effect of time of intrauterine insemination on conception rate and litter size (from Haresign 1990)

	Interval from sponge withdrawal (hours)		
	48	54	60
Conception rate (%)	58	66	67
Mean litter size (live)	2.13	2.04	2.04

Pregnancy

Duration of gestation

There are significant differences in the duration of gestation between breeds of sheep, for example:

Finnish Landrace	142	±	0.23 days	($n = 249$)
Border Leicester	145	±	0.39 days	($n = 31$)
Oxford Down	146.8	±	0.75 days	($n = 18$)
Welsh Mountain	149.2	±	0.26 days	($n = 79$)

Bradford *et al.* (1972) have provided clear evidence from egg transfer and from reciprocal crossing among these breeds that the genotype of the foetus is the major determinant of the duration of gestation over a wide range of litter sizes (1–5) and sizes of donor and recipient breeds. Forbes (1967) found a significant negative effect of litter size on gestation length with singles, twins and triplets being carried for 147.3, 146.7 and 145.6 days respectively. Sex of lamb had no significant effect on duration of gestation. Spring-born lambs are inclined to be carried longer than autumn-born lambs.

Management during pregnancy

Feeding management

Feeding management during early pregnancy includes the tupping period and that stage of gestation around implantation when the foetuses are at their most vulnerable. The feeding regimen during this critical phase should remain unchanged and if at all possible the flock should be left undisturbed. A marked change of diet to either a lower or higher plane of nutrition is contraindicated; recent evidence indicates that high-plane feeding has a detrimental effect on embryo survival largely due to a reduction in progesterone, the hormone that plays a key role in the maintenance of pregnancy. Over-dependence on foodstuffs known to depress fertility, such as the kale family, should be avoided.

Ewe lambs and two-tooth ewes should remain on the same plane of feeding through the middle period of pregnancy to allow further growth and development (see Table 8.4). Adult ewes may be treated quite differently. During mid-pregnancy there is no harm in allowing a 5% loss of liveweight and a fall in body condition score to 2.5–3.0. This is normally brought about by using the flock to clear up pastures prior to the introduction of the basal diet for winter, either hay or silage. Overfat ewes will benefit from this mild degree of undernourishment in that it reduces susceptibility to metabolic disorders, particularly pregnancy toxaemia. During the early and middle phases of pregnancy all flocks of adult ewes are managed as a unit; thereafter, and particularly during the last 6 weeks, flocks should be subdivided on the basis of:

- time of lambing,
- potential litter size,
- body condition score (ewes below 2.0 should be separated).

Subdivision allows economies to be made without compromising the well-being of the ewes and lambs. It should also improve the efficiency of surveillance. Particular attention should be given to feeding behaviour and provision made for shy feeders. There should be no further major changes of management during the last 6 weeks of pregnancy.

Importance of nutrition during the last 6 weeks of gestation

Ewe	Lamb
Prevention of metabolic diseases	Foetal growth rate and maturity
Fitness and maternal drive	Birth weight
Supply of colostrum	Vigour
Milk yield during early lactation	Neonatal survival

The intake of energy, protein, minerals and vitamins is gradually increased to meet the demands of foetal growth and development. About 70% of lamb birthweight is put on during the last 6 weeks. The increasing nutrient requirement can only be met by limiting roughage intake and increasing the amount of concentrates fed (Table 8.13). This also allows for a decrease in appetite resulting from physiological changes and the physical effects of the foetal burden. Changes in body condition score can give a reasonable indication of the adequacy of the feeding regimen. Where there is some doubt about the quality of the food, even after the conventional routine analyses have been done, the blood levels of glucose, free fatty acid and ketones provide a meaningful assessment of contemporary nutrition (Russel 1985).

Table 8.13 Feeding regimen (kg/day) for ewes in late pregnancy (from MLC 1981)

| | Ewe weight and number of foetuses | | | | | |
| | 50 kg | | | 70 kg | | |
	Single	Twin	Triplets	Single	Twin	Triplets
Six weeks before lambing						
Hay*	0.83	0.83	0.83	1.00	1.00	1.00
or silage	2.60	2.60	2.60	3.50	3.50	3.50
plus concentrates	0.18	0.30	0.34	0.24	0.37	0.44
Four weeks before lambing						
Hay*	0.83	0.83	0.83	1.00	1.00	1.00
or silage	2.60	2.60	2.60	3.50	3.50	3.50
plus concentrates	0.28	0.45	0.51	0.36	0.56	0.66
Two weeks before lambing						
Hay*	0.83	0.83	0.83	1.00	1.00	1.00
or silage	2.60	2.60	2.60	3.50	3.50	3.50
plus concentrates	0.37	0.59	0.68	0.48	0.75	0.86

* Assuming ME concentration in the dry matter of 10.0 MJ for hay and 11.0 MJ for silage and dry matter content for silage of 25%. Roots could be used to replace 75 and 50% of the concentrates on a dry matter basis at 6 and 2 weeks before lambing, respectively.

Winter housing and shearing

Long-term winter housing, often in purpose-built housing, has become commonplace in the UK, largely due to higher pasture stocking rates and the need to rest and protect swards over winter.

The features of good management during housing are:

- good ventilation,
- group size should not exceed 40,
- long shallow pens to allow efficient surveillance,
- provision of pens for individual mothering,
- isolation pens for aborting and sick ewes.

Winter shearing is now widely adopted in the south of England as a consequence of long-term winter housing. It was first introduced to benefit from savings in pen space and trough space per ewe. The potential advantages of winter shearing are:

- more efficient surveillance at lambing,
- easier teat seeking,

- lower incidence of crushing in mothering pen,
- higher birthweight,
- higher early growth rate.

More ewes may need assistance at lambing but this does not lead to more injuries and deaths. It has been established that gestation is 1 day longer in shorn ewes than in unshorn ewes.

Health care

In many flocks dipping against sheep scab coincides with early pregnancy; in autumn-lambing flocks it coincides with late pregnancy or lactation. In tick areas sheep are dipped in late pregnancy. Dipping is stressful and should be carried out with quiet efficiency. Sheep should not be dipped when they are hot, tired, thirsty or full-fed.

General foot care needs more attention during the high rainfall seasons. Every effort should be made to correct all foot problems before the second half of pregnancy and, if housed, before housing.

The timing of vaccinations will be dictated by the expected lambing dates of the flocks or subflocks. To provide a high level of antibodies in the colostrum, vaccination should be done 2–4 weeks before lambing. There may be reasons for drenching the flock during late pregnancy. Both vaccination and drenching should be done with minimal restraint of the ewe and preferably in a small pen. Prolific ewes in late pregnancy find it difficult to negotiate a race.

Embryonic and foetal development

The 8-cell fertilized egg enters the uterus at 3 days after ovulation. In sheep with one ovulation the blastocyst rarely migrates to the other horn. If two ova are released from one ovary, one blastocyst migrates to the contralateral horn.

The early phases of gestation can be summarized as:

- maternal recognition on day 12/13,
- attachment begins on day 14–16,
- attachment completed on day 28–35,
- type of placenta: cotyledonary.

Table 8.14 lists the distinguishable features of embryo and foetal development that may be used to indicate age and normality.

Table 8.14 The development of the ovine embryo and foetus (adapted from Jainudeen and Hafez 1987)

Distinguishable features	Age (days)
Morula	3–4
Blastula	4–10
Differentiation of germ layers	10–14
Elongation of chorionic vesicle	13–14
Primitive streak formation	14
Open neural tube	15–21
Somite differentiation (first)	17
Fusion of chorioamniotic folds	17
Chorion elongates in non-pregnant horn	14
Heart beat apparent	20
Closed neural tube	21–28
Allantois prominent (anchor-shaped)	21–28
Forelimb bud visible	28–35
Hindlimb bud visible	28–35
Differentiation of digits	35–42
Nostril and eyes differentiated	42–49
Allantois replaces exocoelom of pregnant horn	21–28
First attachment (implantation)	21–30(?)
Eyelids close	49–56
Hair follicles first appear	42–49
Horn pits apparent	77–84
Tooth eruption	98–105
Hair around eyes and muzzle	98–105
Hair covering body	119–126

Pregnancy diagnosis

The benefits of pregnancy diagnosis are early detection of barrenness and subdivision of the flock according to expected litter size.

Barren ewes and lambs may be segregated and placed on a low plane of feeding, probably left on pasture during winter, or sold as cull or draft animals. Pregnancy diagnosis is particularly beneficial in ewe lambs because barrenness is more common than in the adult flock.

In the case of the adult flock, subdivision is the main benefit of pregnancy diagnosis.

1. Preferential treatment in terms of feeding and housing can be given to those carrying twins and triplets:
   (a) it reduces ewe losses due to metabolic disorders such as pregnancy toxaemia;
   (b) it leads to better colostral and milk supply, which benefits the lambs in terms of health and growth rate;

    (c) it improves the birthweight and survival rate of lambs from large litters.

2. Ewes carrying singles can be maintained on a lower plane of nutrition for longer; hill ewes known to be carrying singles can be left on the hill until late pregnancy. Dystocia problems from over-weight single lambs can be reduced.

3. Arrangements can be made for cross-fostering.

These benefits can only be realized when positive action follows the diagnosis. A clear and durable method of marking the various categories of ewes should be undertaken at the time of diagnosis and ewes should then be released to their appropriate group. Stress to operators (invariably contractors) and ewes should be avoided through the provision of good handling facilities and labour organization. A high level of accuracy cannot be expected from operators working under adverse conditions. The cost of scanning (50–75p per ewe in the UK) is partly dependent on the type of diagnosis required. The economic benefit of pregnancy diagnosis should be in the range £2–6/ewe. The technique has been rapidly accepted by the sheep industry and it has been estimated that over 25% of the UK national ewe flock is now scanned.

Methods of pregnancy diagnosis

To be of value in current systems of production the method of diagnosis must be accurate, rapid, safe and a practicable means of diagnosing pregnancy and determining foetal number in ewes. It is generally acknow-ledged that only the real-time ultrasonic scanning method meets these requirements. Other methods of diagnosis such as vaginal biopsy, radio-logy, ballottement, laparotomy, laparoscopy, blood progesterone assay, the detection of pregnancy-specific antigens and non-return to oestrus may have a particular role in certain situations. Where flock owners are reluctant to undertake any form of diagnosis involving the use of instru-ments and/or bench technique, the use of non-return to oestrus can be of some value particularly if it is coupled to the use of harnessed vasectomized rams approximately 1 month after the removal of entire rams. Ewes remaining in or having resumed cyclic activity can be detected in this way. Those that have entered seasonal anoestrus or are in anoestrus due to other reasons, such as death of the foetus after implantation, will remain undetected.

Real-time ultrasonic scanning

There is no doubt that the use of this technique has made a significant impact on the management of breeding flocks throughout the UK.

There are two types of instrument: linear array scanner and sector scanner. When used by competent operators both types are capable of a high level of accuracy. The main difference between the two instruments is in the arrangement of the crystals emitting the ultrasound. In the case of linear array, as the description implies, the crystals are arranged in a long row, necessitating a large contact area and scope for moving the probe around over a wide area on either side and in front of the udder in order to visualize the uterine contents. This can only be achieved if the ewe is in a semi-sitting position and with all wool removed from the area to be scanned to allow good contact between probe and skin.

The probe of the sector scanner is different in design and the active elements are located in a small cylinder rotating about a central axis with the probe automatically bathed in oil supplied from a reservoir. The beam of sound is shaped like a fan and provides a wide-angle view of the uterus and its contents from a small contact area, usually the bare area immediately in front of the udder on either side of the midline. This scanner has the added advantage that the ewe can be scanned standing and no preparation of the abdominal skin is required (Figure 8.4).

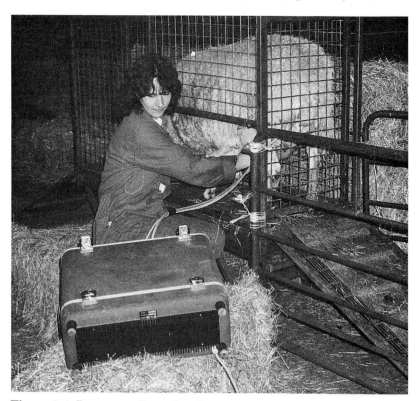

Figure 8.4 Pregnancy diagnosis using a sector scanner.

The highest accuracy is achieved between 50 and 100 days of gestation. It is customary for the whole flock to be done during one visit. To allow for spread of matings, flocks should be scanned 11–15 weeks from the date matings commenced.

The type of diagnosis required will depend on the breed of the ewe and the expected level of performance. In flocks with a low lambing percentage (120–140%) about 60% of the ewes will be carrying singles and the incidence of triplets will be exceedingly low. It would not be economically justifiable to pay the higher charges for distinguishing those carrying triplets from those carrying twins. In flocks with a lambing percentage of 180–200% the incidence of triplets would be over 20% and there would be considerable advantage in identifying the dams.

The following levels of accuracy can be expected:

- diagnosis of pregnancy (99%),
- differentiation of barren, single and multiple (98%),
- determination of exact number of foetuses (96%).

The termination of pregnancy

The need to terminate pregnancy in ewes usually arises early in pregnancy and mainly due to unplanned matings occurring in pedigree flocks. During the first 8 weeks of gestation the maintenance of pregnancy is dependent on an ovarian source of progesterone, and prostaglandin or its analogues may be used for termination. Thereafter corticosteroids may be used but their effectiveness and the interval to abortion is variable. Daily injection of 2.5 mg of flumethasone for three consecutive days resulted in abortion in three ewes, 67, 74 and 51 hours following the first injection, whereas one injection to two ewes on day 125/126 proved ineffective. It has also been reported that only 5 of 12 ewes treated with 12 mg dexamethasone aborted (mean interval from injection, 66.05 ± 4.18 hours).

Prenatal loss

Prenatal loss is the difference between ovulation rate and the number of lambs born (see Table 8.26). It has been estimated that 20–40% of ovulations are not represented by live births. Fertilization failure and embryonic and foetal mortality contribute to this loss. Numerous factors have been shown to influence embryonic death (Figure 8.5). The manipulation of one or more of these factors may slightly reduce the loss but not eliminate it (McKelvey and Robinson 1986; Wilmut et al. 1986). Most of the losses occur during the first month of gestation. Losses from day 30–40 of gestation through to lambing are negligible except in cases of abortion or feeding mismanagement in late pregnancy.

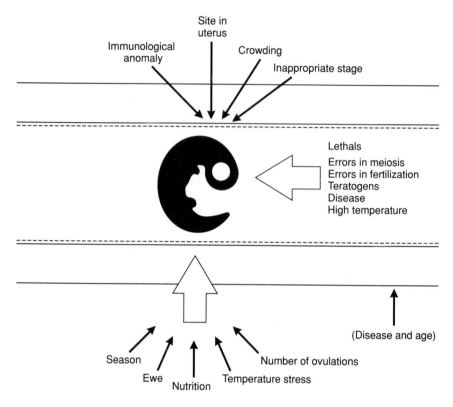

Figure 8.5 Factors associated with prenatal loss in sheep, shown according to the route by which they act. Those at the top of the diagram disrupt the relationship between embryo and mother, those on the right cause abnormal embryos and those at the bottom of the diagram act through the maternal environment (from Wilmut *et al.* 1986).

Failure of fertilization

Few investigations have established the contribution of this form of loss to prenatal loss in served ewes; it is usually quoted at 5–10% of eggs shed. More data are becoming available from units involved in embryo transplants. Results from studies at the Rowett Research Institute show that when ewes are inseminated artificially with 480×10^6 viable sperms at 48 and 60 hours after progestagen withdrawal and PMSG administration, approximately 9% of ova are not fertilized and this value is unaffected by the nutritional status of the ewe (McKelvey and Robinson 1986).

Embryo mortality

There is general agreement that losses occurring between fertilization and day 30–40 of gestation represent significant loss of potential production. Where total loss occurs early, before day 13, the oestrous cycle may be unaffected and the ewe will return to service. At a later stage it may result in delayed return to oestrus and, because of a short tupping period, the ewe will not have the opportunity of being served and will remain barren. Where there is only a partial loss of embryos (as in Figure 8.6) the ewe will go through to term.

The manifestations of embryo mortality are:

- an increase in barrenness rate,
- a reduction in number of lambs born,
- the birth of small lambs, with low survival rate, due to inability of surviving embryo(s) to utilize the placental attachment point vacated by those that die.

Returns to service will extend the lambing period and may result in delayed marketing and lowered productivity.

The incidence of embryo mortality is higher in ewe lambs and old ewes than in other age groups. The survival rate of embryos is linearly and negatively related to the number of fertilized eggs per ewe. The present

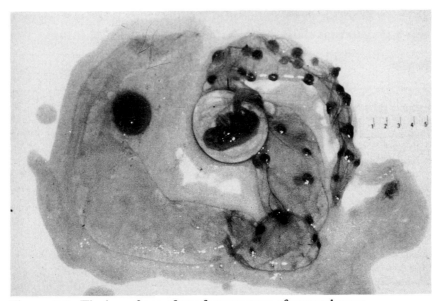

Figure 8.6 The loss of one of two foetuses soon after attachment.

evidence indicates that differences in embryo survival among ewes is small and is unlikely to feature in breed improvement programmes.

Abortion

Survey data show that there are up to 20% of unproductive ewes in recorded lowland flocks; this includes barren ewes, ewes that have aborted and ewe deaths. This is a major loss of production potential in any flock; it is also known that this level is exceeded in some flocks during an abortion storm when 50% or more of the flock become unproductive. It is estimated that infectious abortions cause an annual loss of £20 million to the British sheep industry. Incidence of abortion has increased during the 1980s. The incidence and causes of reported infectious abortions in the UK national flock are presented in Table 8.15. The features of and control measures for the main infectious causes are summarized in Table 8.16. Aitken *et al.* (1990) have presented up-to-date practical advice on the control of enzootic abortion.

All these diseases present a general health risk to personnel associated with the care of flocks and particularly to pregnant women, who should not in any way assist with the lambing of flocks where there is a risk of infectious abortion occurring.

Table 8.15 Infectious causes of abortion in ewes (UK) (from MLC 1989)

Infection	Prevalence (%)	Causal agent
Enzootic abortion of ewes (EAE) ('Kebbing')	22	*Chlamydia psittaci*
Toxoplasmosis	19	*Toxoplasma gondii*
Bacterial		
Campylobacter	8	*Campylobacter foetus*
		Campylobacter jejuni
Salmonella	4	*Salmonella abortus ovis*
		S. montevideo
		S. typhimurium
		S. dublin
Listeria	3	*Listeria monocytogenes*
Corynebacterium	2	*Corynebacterium pyogenes*
Streptococci	1	*Streptococcus pyogenes*
Pasteurella	1	*Pasteurella haemolytica*
Diagnosis not verified	40	

Table 8.16 The main features of infectious abortion

Disease	Source of infection	Manifestation	Control
EAE	Aborting and newly lambed infected ewes	Abortion Stillbirths Neonatal lamb deaths	Vaccination Purchase replacements from *clean* flocks Strict hygiene during lambing: —collect and destroy afterbirths Isolate aborted and suspect ewes
Toxoplasmosis	Oocysts voided by cats, contaminated pasture, hay, straw and stored grain Rodents contribute to cycle	Barrenness Mummified foetuses	Purchase replacement ewes from flocks with known health history. Introduce well before tupping Strict hygiene during lambing and abortions Vaccination
Campylobacteriosis	Contaminated pasture infected by sheep, birds and wild animals	Severe abortion storm	Introduce replacements well before tupping Strict hygiene during lambing and abortions
Salmonellosis	Contaminated pasture and food troughs	Ewe deaths Foul-smelling aborted foetuses Neonatal lamb deaths	Strict hygiene
Listeriosis	Contaminated silage	Abortion preceded by thick brown discharge from vulva	Strict hygiene

Parturition

Understanding the ewe's behaviour around lambing is crucial to competent stockmanship. The behavioural signs include:

- separation from flock,
- restlessness,
- scraping and turning,
- nose pointing to sky during contractions.

The physical signs include:

- distension of udder,
- enlarged vulva,
- appearance of amnion ('water bag').

There is more opportunity for ewes lambing outside to display innate patterns of parturient behaviour than for ewes housed during late pregnancy. In a field situation behavioural signs give the first indication that the ewe is preparing for lambing. Physical signs are difficult to see when the ewe is in full fleece and often some distance away. A housed flock may be winter shorn and then physical signs are more obvious; behavioural patterns are inclined to be disturbed by other sheep in the pen and by routine activities within and around the building.

Ewes usually isolate themselves from the rest of the flock and establish a birth site. It becomes a focal point for the ewe and she may occupy that site for several hours after lambing and it will have a recognizable smell. Early recognition of the offspring and maternal bonding occur at the birth site. Provided weather conditions permit this sequence should not be disturbed. In the case of housed ewes they should be allowed to lamb in their original pen and then taken out and the family placed in an individual pen for 24–48 hours. This allows grooming, recognition and bonding to proceed undisturbed and also allows a high level of surveillance during the neonatal period. Aborting ewes should be taken out of the main pen and isolated as soon as detected. If there is a particular reason (e.g. other ewes displaying premature maternal instincts) for moving ewes during the second stage of labour, contractions normally resume after a short interval. Abnormal behaviour should be noted early. This may include one or more of the following: desertion, delayed grooming, and rejection of one or more members of the litter. These abnormalities may lead to lack of imprinting, colostral deprivation through delayed sucking, hypothermia, or physical injury as a result of butting.

Ewes may lamb at any time of day or night; a higher proportion lamb between 05.00 and 09.00 and 19.00 and 23.00 than at other times.

Assistance during lambing

The stages of labour and timing of related events are shown in Table 8.17. If the ewe has been straining hard with nose pointing to the sky during contractions for 15 minutes and there is no physical sign of progress, she should be restrained and examined internally to establish the cause of delay—inadequate dilatation of the cervix, abnormal presentation or dystocia due to disproportionate size of a foetus. Inadequate dilatation may require more time and/or finger manipulation. Total absence of dilatation ('ring-womb') requires prompt action because caesarean section is usually necessary.

The vast majority of births are anterior presentation with less than 5% posterior presentations. It is difficult to establish the incidence of dystocia; competent shepherds are capable of dealing with the majority of cases and thus only the extremely difficult cases are presented for veterinary attention. Feto-pelvic disproportion, particularly in single male lambs, is generally regarded as the most common cause. Maldisposition increases as litter size increases.

In 15 584 lambings in three Scottish hill flocks over 7 years, Gunn (1968) reported that 3.1% were difficult births; 44% of these difficult births were normal presentations and 59% were given assistance. In contrast, about 90% of abnormal presentations required assistance. The four main types of abnormal presentation were head alone (42%), head and one leg only (29%), breech (17%) and forelegs only (6%).

Blackmore (1960) described the types of dystocia in 100 veterinary cases in lowland crossbred flocks. These are presented in Table 8.18.

The induction of parturition

There are a variety of reasons for attempting to synchronize lambing. It is unusual for it to be attempted on a large group of ewes. There are two important requirements that must be met before contemplating any of the treatments listed in Table 8.19. The first is the need for accurate information on tupping dates and the second is the need for a lambing pen for each treatment ewe. Treatment should be given on day 142 or 143 of pregnancy. Treatment given earlier than 10 days from term leads to an unacceptable level of lamb mortality due to prematurity. An indication of the degree of synchrony following treatment may be gained from the data presented in Table 8.19. The spread of lambing following a synchronized tupping is given in Figure 8.7.

Table 8.17 Stages of parturition in sheep (adapted from Jainudeen and Hafez 1987)

Stage of labour	Mechanical forces	Period	Related events	Average duration (hours)
I Dilatation of cervix	Regular peristaltic uterine contractions	Beginning of uterine contractions until cervix is fully dilated and continuous with vagina	Maternal restlessness Changes in foetal position and posture	2–6
II Expulsion of foetus	Strong uterine and abdominal contractions	From complete cervical dilatation to end of delivery of foetus	Maternal recumbency and straining Appearance of amnion (water bag) at vulva Rupture of amnion and delivery of foetus	0.5–2.0
III Expulsion of afterbirth	Uterine contractions	Following delivery of foetus to expulsion of afterbirth	Loosening of chorionic villi from maternal crypts Inversion of chorio-allantois Straining and expulsion of foetal membranes	0.5–8.0

Table 8.18 Types of dystocia (from Blackmore 1960)

Type of maternal dystocia	Number of cases	Type of foetal dystocia	Number of cases
Failure of the cervix to dilate	32	Lateral head posture	27
Uterine inertia	7	Carpal flexion	15
Other maternal abnormalities	4	Shoulder flexion	11
Abortion	3	Simultaneous presentation	10
Abdominal rupture	2	Hip flexion	7
Prolapse of the uterus	2	Oversize	6
Prolapse of the vagina	2	Dorso-transverse presentation	5
		Monsters	5
		Hock flexion	3
		Shoulder–elbow flexion	3
		Head–breast posture	2
		Rotation of the neck	1
		Lateral position	1
		Hip–stifle flexion	1

Puerperium

The puerperium extends from the time of expulsion of the afterbirth to the time the tract returns to its normal non-pregnant state. It involves the regeneration of the endometrium, uterine involution and the resumption of oestrous cycles.

Degeneration of the surfaces of caruncles, necrosis and sloughing occurs during the first few days following parturition and results in dark reddish-brown discoloration of the lochial discharge. This process continues during the first 2 weeks; the process of regeneration, which involves the re-epithelialization of the caruncles, is usually completed by the end of the fourth week.

The shrinkage of the tract associated with involution is particularly rapid during the third to the tenth day post partum. It then continues at a slower rate and is complete by the end of the third week.

In the majority of British breeds of sheep, parturition occurs in the spring coincident with or after the establishment of seasonal anoestrus. It is rare for spring-lambing ewes to ovulate and display oestrous cycles before the subsequent autumn. Postpartum oestrus occurs in some ewes a few hours after lambing but is invariably anovulatory.

In autumn-lambed ewes low basal LH levels and low LH pulse fre-

Table 8.19 Induction of parturition; treatments and responses

Treatment and dose	No. of ewes	Stage of gestation (days)	Interval from treatment to lambing (hours)	Comments	Reference
Oestradiol benzoate (20 mg)	39	143/144	38.6 ± 20.8	Lambing over 4 days	Boland et al. (1982)
Dexamethasone (16 mg)	41	143/144	44.2 ± 18.1	Lambing over 4.5 days	Boland et al. (1982)
PGF$_{2\alpha}$ (10–25 mg)	40	143/144	83.5 ± 39.8	Ineffective	Boland et al. (1982)
Untreated control	39	143/144	82.9 ± 43.1	Lambing over 8.5 days Lambing over 8.0 days	Boland et al. (1982)
Dexamethasone (12 mg)	20	142	46.42 ± 2.29	Lambing over 3 days	Webster and Haresign (1981)
Untreated control (saline)	11	142	72.00 ± 11.02	Lambing over 5 days	Webster and Haresign (1981)
Epostane (prevents progesterone synthesis) 50 mg in 2 ml ethanol, i.v.	8	138/141	32 ± 1.0	All lambs live and healthy; no postnatal problems; normal birthweights; no lactational problems	Silver (1987)
50 mg in 0.5 ml DMSO, i.m.	8	138/141	35 ± 1.4		
50 mg in 2.0 ml saline, i.m.	4	138/141	About 36 hours		
Betamethasone (10–12 mg)	898	141/142	45.1	95% within 70 hours	Trower (1991)

DMSO, dimethyl sulphoxide; PGF$_{2\alpha}$, prostaglandin F$_{2\alpha}$.

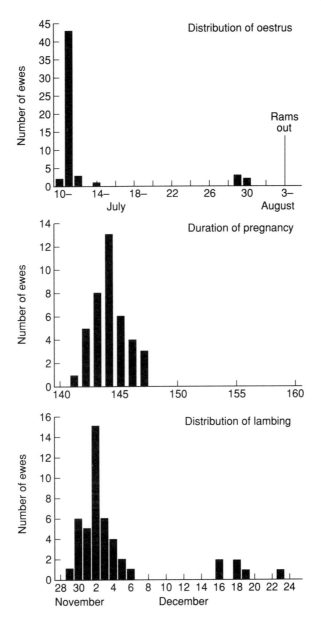

Figure 8.7 The distribution of oestrus in ewes following progestagen/PMSG treatment, subsequent duration of pregnancy and distribution of lambing.

quency fail to stimulate ovulation during the first 3 weeks post partum. The first ovulation occurs soon after the completion of involution but is not accompanied by oestrus. Oestrous cycles are initiated 6–8 weeks post partum. The duration of lactational anoestrus may be influenced by body condition score, level of feeding and number of lambs suckled.

Health problems

Health problems during the puerperium are not a significant problem in the majority of flocks despite the fact that the standard of hygiene at lambing time leaves a lot to be desired in many instances. The incidence of retained afterbirth is very low and the routine use of pessaries or antibiotic treatment after assisted lambing probably accounts for the low incidence of serious metritis.

Neonates

About 20% of lambs born alive in the UK national flock die shortly after birth. A significant reduction in this loss can be achieved by more efficient management and improved stockmanship over the lambing period.

The relative importance of the causes of lamb deaths is shown in Table 8.20; 75% of the losses may be described as avoidable losses in that quick action by skilled personnel during and just after lambing can improve survival rate.

Management

Efficient management during lambing cannot be separated from that discussed earlier for late pregnancy. One is a continuation of the other and they are interdependent.

Table 8.20 The relative importance of the causes of lamb death (modified from Eales and Small 1995)

	Percentage of deaths
Foetal stillbirth	10–20
Parturient stillbirth	10–20
Hypothermia due to exposure	15–25
Hypothermia due to starvation	20–30
Infectious disease	10–15
Congenital abnormalities	5
Other causes	5

The requirements for good lambing management are:

1. Adequate time for surveillance (day and night in prolific flocks with compact lambing).
2. If housed, good access to pens and easy movement of ewes from pens to mothering pens or isolation pens.
3. A well-equipped box of lambing aids (Table 8.21).
4. Good facilities for intensive care, fostering and artificial rearing.
5. A well-stocked and controlled source of drugs and medicines.
6. A clear and simple method of marking pens for animals requiring attention or treatment.
7. A comprehensive recording system.
8. A simple method of identifying families when released to pasture.

In many flocks semi-skilled help is drafted in to help with the lambing. It is imperative that all personnel are well aware of the following points concerning the lambing and the care of the newborn lamb.

The points concerning lambing that should be stressed to assistants are:

- consequences of a protracted birth,
- undesirability of premature assistance,

Table 8.21 Items to be readily available during lambing

Hot and cold water	Lambing ropes
Buckets	Prolapse retainer
Soap	Prolapse harness
Hand towels	Colour marker
Lantern (spare batteries)	Antiseptic pessaries
Disposable surgical gloves	Antibiotics (prescribed)
Lubricating fluid (obstetrical)	Needles and syringes
Frozen colostrum	Disinfectant for lambing pens
Stomach tubes	Lambing record book
100-ml plastic jugs	Heater-box for hypothermic lambs
Bottles and teats	20% glucose solution
'Milton' disinfectant	50 ml syringe/19G, 1 1/2 inch needles
Ewe milk replacement powder	Solution for enema
Disinfectant dip or spray	Oral rehydration solution
for navels	Lamb adoption pen
Lamb-drying towels	Rubber rings and applicator
Digital thermometer	
Calcium borogluconate solution	
Magnesium sulphate solution	
Calcium, magnesium, dextrose (CMPD)	
solution	
Iodine solution	
Foot-paring knife or secateur	
Foot-rot spray	

- techniques for dealing with dystocia,
- methods of resuscitation,
- antiseptic treatment of the navel cord.

The points concerning the newborn lamb that should be stressed include:

- can quickly succumb to hypothermia particularly when exposed to wind and/or rain,
- has only limited reserves of energy so undue delay in sucking or supply of colostrum must be avoided,
- is totally dependent on colostrum for the supply of antibodies. The average lamb requires 250 ml/kg liveweight during the first 12 hours. Vaccinating ewes near lambing ensures wide range of antibodies in the colostrum.

A very comprehensive guide to veterinary care at lambing has been compiled by Eales and Small (1995).

Common problems

The type of problems found in newborn lambs are shown in Table 8.22. In addition to these problems, some lambs are also at a disadvantage due to low birthweight and poor condition. These are usually from ewes in

Table 8.22 Problems in newborn lambs according to age at which they may first be seen (from Eales and Small 1995)

Birth
Atresia ani, Border disease, cleft palate, entropion, fractured ribs, jaw defects, joint defects, prematurity, umbilical hernia

0–5 hours
Congenital swayback, daft lamb disease, fractures, hypothermia (exposure)

5–36 hours
Castration (incorrect), enteritis, hypothermia (starvation), inhalation pneumonia, stiff lamb disease, watery mouth

36 hours
Eye infections, joint ill, lamb dysentery, liver necrosis, navel ill, scad, spinal abscess, tetanus

The number of conditions to be considered increases as the lamb gets older, i.e. for a 4-hour-old lamb only conditions in the first two categories need be considered, but for a 2-day-old lamb all the conditions are possible poor condition, very old ewes or ewe lambs, or are members of large litters. In some cases, low birthweight in singles and twins may be due to the loss of other litter members after implantation when the viable foetus(es) are unable to benefit from the attachment points vacated by the dead foetus(es).

Breeding records

Recording schemes can be quite demanding in terms of time and managerial skill. The level of input required depends entirely on the types of analyses necessary for the assessment of flock productivity and individual performance. The ease with which problem areas can be identified will greatly depend on the quality of the information available. Decisions regarding the type of data to be recorded and the method of recording must be made well beforehand.

Methods of identification include:

- tattooing,
- horn branding,
- ear tagging (metal and plastic),
- ear notching,
- aerosol paint spraying,
- colour branding.

Only tattooing and horn branding are regarded as permanent identification and some breed societies require them. Spraying and colour branding of the fleece are lost during shearing; ear tags are liable to be ripped out and have to be quickly replaced.

The tupping period

Unlike other farm animals breeding ewes are usually tupped during a short period of weeks. Supervised tupping is rarely undertaken and would be confined to pedigree flocks wishing to make the best use of a high price ram or to eliminate any possible doubt about the parentage of offspring. In the vast majority of flocks reliance is placed on presumptive evidence of tupping derived from keel/raddle marks left on the rumps during mounting. Some flocks would have no record of the proportion of ewes tupped over any given period and would only note the date the rams were turned in and the date of removal. There is always the minority who would attempt to recall the date of ram entry from memory, the rams remaining with the flock until near lambing.

The reasons for recording tupping data are listed below:

1. To determine number of ewes keel marked in any given period. The benefits include:
   (a) visual evidence of ram activity and incidence of oestrus,
   (b) refined prediction of lambing.
2. To determine the proportion of ewes returning and remaining unmarked. This gives a first indication of:
   (a) abnormal level of infertility,
   (b) persistent anoestrus.
3. To predict approximate onset and duration of lambing. Benefits include:
   (a) feeding management during pregnancy,
   (b) timing of vaccinations,
   (c) preparations for lambing.

Tupping period: data to record

- Number of ewes in flock/subflock
- Number of rams; also identity of rams if allocated to subflocks
- Date rams turned in
- Date and colour of crayon/raddle
- Number of ewes keel marked during each colour
- Number of ewes not keel marked by end of tupping
- Date rams removed
- Ewe to ram ratio
- Prediction of onset and end of lambing
- Non-return rate (to first keel mark)

The completed record sheet shown in Figure 8.8 is from a subflock in which all ewes had displayed oestrous cycles and the sequence of colour change provides information that is useful at later stages. Where there is doubt about the proportion of cyclic ewes at the start of tupping, and a high incidence of keel-marking around days 19 and 25 is anticipated, the following sequence of colour change is recommended:

The tupping period 1988

No. of ewes: 70
Subflock: A (Suffolk Crosses)
No/identity of ram(s): 2; K54; K58
Date rams in: 1 October 1988

Period	Colour	Total marked 1st 2nd		Lambing period*
1–9 October (8 days)	Yellow 1st mark – 1st October	29		21 February to 6 March
9–18 October (9 days)	Blue	41		1 March to 15 March
18 October to 4 November (17 days)	Red Last mark- 26 October	–	9	10 March to 23 March

Ram out: 4 November

Total with one colour: 61
Total with two colours: 9
Total unmarked: 0

Summary
Ewe to ram ratio: 35
Non-return rate: 87%
(to 1st keel mark)

*Based on pregnancy of 143-148 days

Figure 8.8 Data sheet for tupping period.

Days 1–14	First colour
Days 14–21	Second colour
Days 21–28	Third colour
Days 28–42	Fourth colour

Where tupping occurs unusually early, persistent anoestrus may be a reason for unmarked ewes. It should also be borne in mind that ewes can be served without being marked and that weather conditions can affect the efficiency of the keel-marker.

Many large lowland crossbred flocks, and also upland and hill flocks, record only the dates on which the rams were turned in and removed from the flock. This places great reliance on the selection of sound rams, rams remaining sound throughout the tupping period, and barrenness rate remaining as low as previous years.

Vasectomized rams turned in 3–4 weeks after the completion of tupping will identify cyclic ewes. These can then be removed from the flock and disposed of or held until the next breeding season. This practice is unnecessary where the flock is scanned in early pregnancy.

The lambing period

This is unquestionably the stage of the production cycle when managerial skill and stockmanship are severely tested. It is also the time when there are a variety of reasons for identifying individual ewes and/or their progeny. These reasons may include husbandry and hygiene, breeding records, behaviour, health care and ease of surveillance.

Individual identification allows lists of breeding animals to be drawn up according to breed, year of birth and source. Additional information such as parentage and miscellaneous items can be recorded. These data form the flock register, which would be the main source of animal and lifetime records of fertility, fecundity and lamb survival. These records form the basis of summaries of flock performance. Most of the data stem from the variety of items that are recorded around lambing time.

Important data to record at lambing time include:

- identification number and breed of ewe,
- lamb sire code,
- lambing date,
- lamb identification,
- sex,
- birthweight.

A typical lambing record sheet is shown in Figure 8.9. The wide remarks column may be used to note some or all of the following:

Lambs:	Stillbirths
	Deaths during parturition
	Deaths during first 48 hours
	Notes regarding fostering and artificial rearing
	Physical abnormalities
Ewes:	Parturition
	Abnormalities of teats/udder and colostrum supply
	Behaviour
	Deaths during parturition and early lactation

Lambing record sheet 19					Sheet	

Notes on group/subflock

Ewe		Lamb sire code	Lambing date	Lamb		Birth weight	Remarks
No.	Breed			No.	Sex		

Figure 8.9 Data sheet for the lambing period.

The most appropriate series of items for a particular flock will depend on the type of flock (crossbred or purchased), labour resources and the objectives of the enterprise. Participation in a recording scheme should not be undertaken without careful thought given to the work involved, particularly during lambing. Individual recording is much more demanding than flock recording in terms of time, detail and accuracy. Data processing has been made easier in recent years with the development of computer programs for data storage and retrieval, and for the calculation of indices and summaries. These aids do not remove the need for the discipline required to record the basic information during the frenetic activity associated with the lambing period.

Breeding performance

Breeding performance contributes significantly to the economic performance of any flock; 'lamb sales' accounts for 80% of 'output per ewe', and 'flock replacement costs' account for 35.7% of 'variable costs'. High breeding performance is also beneficial to genetic improvement pro-

Table 8.23 The relationship between lambs sold per ewe and weight of carcass marketed per ewe

Lambs sold per ewe	Total weight of carcass marketed at	
	17 kg	19 kg
1.0	17.0	19.0
1.2	20.4	22.8
1.4	23.8	26.6
1.6	27.2	30.4
1.8	30.6	34.2
2.0	34.0	38.0

grammes. Smith (1991) has recently undertaken a survey of reproductive wastage in 5488 commercial lowland ewes in west Somerset. It is in the interest of all producers, irrespective of the type of flock or location, to achieve a high level of flock fertility and high survival rate of lambs. The most appropriate level of fecundity (lambs per 100 ewes mated) will vary according to environmental and other constraints. On lowland farms the improvement of fecundity is invariably given high priority for it has a direct and major effect on the total weight of carcass produced per ewe (Table 8.23).

The assessment of economic achievement (productivity) requires a system of flock recording, whereas breed improvement programmes and maintenance of pedigree records require the identification of all individuals in the flock and a variety of data about each individual in the flock. Both systems of recording may be used in the assessment of breed performance.

Flock performance

The objectives of flock recording are:

- to identify below average performance,
- to establish the main types of losses and the stages at which they occur,
- to develop effective methods of raising output and of minimizing losses.

The items listed in Table 8.24 provide a comprehensive summary of flock breeding performance. It is an example of the data provided to flock owners under the MLC Flockplan Scheme. The data provided in Table

Table 8.24 Performance data from flocks in MLC Flockplan Scheme (from MLC 1992)

	Lowland spring lambing	Lowland early lambing	Upland spring lambing
No. of flocks	227	48	127
Average flock size (ewes to ram)	569	265	709
Ewe to ram ratio	39	34	41
Ewe lambs in breeding flock (%)	17	11	16
Ewes (per 100 ewes to ram)			
Empty	5	4	5
Dead	4	4	4
Lambed	93	93	93
Lambs (per 100 ewes to ram)			
Born dead	8	10	7
Born alive	158	156	142
Dead after birth	6	7	5
Reared	152	149	137
Retained for breeding	8	6	19
Sold finished	92	133	72
Sold or retained for feeding	48	9	43

8.24 represent average performance in three types of flocks and in contrasting environments. Participation in this and similar schemes allows comparisons to be made with other sheep enterprises in the area, other enterprises on the farm, and other years. It also allows an element of competition to develop between the membership, and participation in discussions regarding the performance and productivity of sheep enterprises in the area. Summaries of performance and productivity according to category of flock are published annually (MLC *Sheep Yearbook*). The summaries also tabulate the attainment of the top one-third of flocks in the scheme; these are usually ranked according to gross margin per hectare.

Detailed information on the breeding performance of a single flock over a series of production years is rarely published. McCrea (1976) summarized the breeding performance of a lowland Clun Forest flock over 13 years. The data are presented in Table 8.25. The inclusion of information on the proportion of ewes lambing to first, second and third service is particularly useful and illustrates the high level of fertility that may be achieved in well-managed flocks.

Ovulation rate and litter size

It is well established that ovulation rate is influenced by breed, nutrition and stage of the breeding season. The data presented in Table 8.26 give

Table 8.25 Flock breeding performance over 13 years (from McCrea 1976)

| | No. | Died before lambing (%) | Infertile, barren, aborted (%) | Percentage of those that lambed pregnant to service | | |
				First	Second	Third
Gimmers lambing						
at 2 years old	346	0.87	11.6	87.4	10.9	1.6
Older ewes	1120	0.62	4.5	89.5	8.9	1.5
All females	1466	0.68	6.2	89.1	9.4	1.5

Table 8.26 Ovulation rate and litter size in adult ewes (from Hanrahan and Quirke 1985)

Breed	No. of records	Ovulation rate	Litter size
Finn	595	3.46	2.65
Galway	147	1.67	1.44
Finngalway	463	2.43	2.02

Table 8.27 The incidence of single and multiple births according to age (from McCrea 1976)

Age of ewe at weaning (years)	Singles (%)	Twins (%)	Triplets (%)	Quadruplets (%)
2	38.2	58.4	3.1	0.3
3	30.4	62.3	6.6	0.3
4	23.8	66.0	9.4	0.8
5	24.1	68.0	6.9	
6	26.2	63.1	9.9	0.7
7	24.7	61.8	13.4	
8	30.0	62.9	7.1	
9	38.8	59.2	2.0	
10	23.1	69.2	7.8	
11	30.8	69.2		
12	33.3	66.6		

a clear indication of breed differences in ovulation rate and the improvement that can be achieved through crossbreeding. It also demonstrates that differences in ovulation rate are far greater than differences in litter size. Embryo survival declines as the ovulation rate increases and this masks genetic differences among animals for ovulation rate. Consequently it is now thought that ovulation rate should be used in preference to litter size for selection purposes. The identification of a gene with a very large effect on ovulation rate in Booroola Merino and Cambridge sheep has recently markedly improved the possibility of increasing performance through breeding.

Culling and replacement rate

In a lowland flock of recorded Clun Forest ewes the average culling rate over 13 years was 17.9% (McCrea 1976); deaths before and after lambing accounted for a further 3.5%, thus giving a replacement rate of 21.4%. The reasons for culling ewes fluctuate from year to year depending on market price of cull ewes and of replacement ewes, and by changes in selection policy. Where it is a firm policy to draft ewes after a given number of lambings, for example after three crops in hill flocks, the replacement rate can be over 40% and necessitates the retention of almost all ewe lambs born.

There is some benefit in keeping breeding ewes under 8 years of age. It can be seen from the relationship between age at lambing and multiple births presented in Table 8.27 that the proportion of single births decreases during the first three lambings, remains stable until 7 years of age and then increases in older ewes. Extending the useful breeding life of ewes without depressing performance will reduce the average cost of replacement.

Clinical examination of breeding sheep

All breeding animals, irrespective of their age, should be carefully assessed for their soundness 2–3 months before the tupping period. Soundness involves the examination of the mouth, feet, udder and external genitalia. In the case of the ewe flock it is usually carried out by the shepherd/ flock owner at or soon after weaning. It is an ideal time for veterinarians involved in flock health schemes to carry out a full clinical examination of a proportion of the flock and, together with the flock record of deaths and treatments, to review the general policy regarding health and preventive treatments.

Examination of breeding sheep may be required for a variety of other reasons, such as private sale of breeding animals, sale by public auction, entry for shows/competitions and export. These will require different kinds of examination and different forms of certification: from qualification on basis of age and freedom from clinical disease to a comprehensive certificate of breeding potential and state of health. The work is inclined to be very seasonal.

Mouth

Examination of the mouth is carried out to establish age, assess occlusion ('bite') of incisor teeth, and to check for dental abnormalities and diseases.

Estimation of age in sheep

Dental formula: $2 (^{I} 0/4, ^{PM} 3/3, ^{M} 2/3)$
I = incisor, PM = premolar, M = molar

Type of incisors	Average eruption age (years, months)	Age range	Recommended description*
Temporary	Near birth or up to 2–3 weeks		Lamb
Permanent First pair			
(central)	1.3	0.10–1.7	Two-tooth
Second pair	1.9	1.6 –2.2	Four-tooth
Third pair	2.3	1.11–3.0	Six-tooth
Fourth pair**	2.9	2.6 –4.0	Full mouth

* to avoid the use of local nomenclature
** sometimes displaced or absent
Bear in mind the most likely month of birth when estimating age.

The vast majority of breeding sheep are sold either at the lamb or the two-tooth stage usually at special regional sales and breed society sales.

The assessment of occlusion or bite is an important component of an examination involving grazing animals that, in many cases, have little or no access to other foodstuffs. Particular attention must be given to the detection of animals with congenital defects before they are bred. All animals that have severely overshot (sow-mouthed) or undershot (parrot-mouthed) jaws should not be approved for breeding. Such abnormalities result in inefficient grazing and affected animals are predisposed to dental problems resulting in low body condition, poor performance and early culling.

Ideally, incisors should meet the pad within 5 mm of the front edge. As animals get older there is a tendency for the cutting edge to drift forward due to change in the slope of the teeth. Mild forms of overshot and undershot jaws may be tolerated in some situations, e.g. in rams to be used as terminal sires in lowland crossbred flocks.

Loss of incisor teeth (broken mouth) is well recognized as the most significant dental problem contributing to the culling of breeding ewes in the UK; it can occur over a wide age range (3–8 years) and may be due to a variety of causes. Spence and Aitchison (1986) have developed a scoring system for incisors that may give an early indication of this abnormality. Misalignment and gaps in the cheek teeth can be detected by palpation through the cheek. A gag is required for a more critical examination of these teeth.

Locomotor system

Lameness is endemic in most flocks in the UK. It is a condition that all breeding animals should be free from particularly during the approach to, and during, the tupping period. Lameness may be due to one or more afflictions of the feet including minor injuries, foreign bodies and ab-scesses, bacterial infection, interdigital fibromas or congenital abnorm-alities.

Particular attention should be given to spinal weakness, poor alignment of legs and gait. Note excessive slope to pasterns. Where there is doubt about gait, manipulate joints particularly of the hind legs and watch for evidence of pain.

Foot-rot is by far the most prevalent disease and is a major cause of lameness. Ineffective or delayed treatment can result in irreparable damage to the claws, sometimes requiring amputation. The health care of any breeding flock must give great emphasis to the control of foot-rot.

Interdigital fibromas should be surgically removed well before the tupping period, in rams preferably 6 months prior to use.

Particular note should be made of corkscrew claws. This is a congenital condition that distorts the outer claws of the hind feet and requires frequent paring to avoid lameness. Breeding animals showing this condi-tion should be culled. Splayed claws should also be regarded as an undesirable weakness. Acute laminitis and post-dipping lameness can arise just prior to, or during, tupping and sometimes involve a high proportion of the flock. Laminitis is usually the result of grazing on very lush pasture or over-generous feeding of cereal grains. Post-dipping lameness can arise when sheep are dipped in stale dip in which *Erysipelothrix rhusiopathiae* has proliferated.

Examination of the female

Udder

First an assessment of size, symmetry and suspension should be carried out. Information recorded during early lactation may also be available. At that time poor udder conformation, excessive size and poor adjustment of teats are more obvious than at any time after weaning.

With the ewe cast and in a sitting position, gentle and thorough palpation of both halves should be undertaken, giving particular attention to:

- surface injuries to teats and each gland,
- nodules and abscesses,
- general suppleness of the gland,
- heat, pain, swelling and surface reddening or blackening associated with mastitis.

Physical defects of the reproductive tract

Abnormalities of the tract (e.g. occlusion of the oviducts) are only occasional causes of infertility and cannot be observed during a clinical examination. Although twinning rate is very high in many breeds the incidence of freemartins is thought to be very low. However, an animal with a small vagina and enlarged clitoris should be given a vaginal examination to establish whether it also has a blind-ending vagina.

Examination of the male

In recent years there has been more awareness of the benefits of examining rams 2–3 months before the tupping period. This should be supported by another more general clinical examination 6 months later, i.e. the stud is checked at 6-monthly intervals. It is imperative that any physical abnormality or disease that prevents or reduces the capacity of rams to search for oestrous ewes, to serve and to yield good quality semen is detected early. This provides opportunity to undertake effective treatment or to replace the rams well before the tupping period. The preparation of the ram or stud for tupping should be given high priority in any flock. Its contribution to the attainment of high performance is undeniably highly significant. A comprehensive guide to the care and examination of rams has been compiled by Boundy (1985, 1992).

The examination should be preceded by note-taking on recent management, stud history and general health care. Some thought should be given to the effects of season on feeding management, prevalence of parasites, nature of the fleece, behaviour and reproductive function. Ambient temperature exceeding 33°C may lead to lethargy and lowering of semen quality.

The majority of clinical examinations will include only general appraisal and examination of the external genitalia. Hindson (1989) states, 'Where a physical examination of the reproductive system has failed to give any evidence of abnormality, then little more need be done.' Where there is any doubt or when the nature of the certificate requires it a semen evaluation should be included.

The clinical examination of the ram should start with a general appraisal, noting identification, breed, estimated age, health, behaviour, posture, condition of fleece, body condition score (ideally better than 3), conformation, gait and soundness of limbs.

Prepuce and penis

With the ram cast and in an upright sitting position the examination of the prepuce and penis should proceed as follows:

1. Examine prepuce for infections, injury or adhesion.
2. Palpate the penis through the skin from prepuce to sigmoid flexure.
3. Extrude penis: grasp near flexure, move forward and out of prepuce. Look for early signs of pain or physical restriction preventing extrusion. Grasp penis near the glans using a loop of gauze, and fully extrude by gentle pulling.
4. Examine penis for lesions and evidence of injury.
5. Examine glans and urethral process for injury (at shearing time) and infection.
6. In prepubertal ram lambs the urethral process may be attached to the glans and only partial extrusion of the penis is possible.
7. Calculi may be found in young ram lambs raised on high rates of concentrates.

Scrotum

The scrotum should be examined for:

- injury and abscesses (ascertain whether affecting only scrotal skin),
- parasites on woolly scrotum,
- scrotal bifurcation,
- evidence of hernia.

The testes

When examining ram lambs and two-tooth rams it is particularly important to note that seasonal and nutritional factors affect testis size. In ram lambs there is a strong correlation between liveweight and testis size. There is a gradual increase in testis size over the first 3 years and a concomitant annual fluctuation during each late winter/spring period. There is also a significant reduction in testis size during the course of the tupping period.

Testis size is an indication of potential sperm output, which has been estimated as 26×10^6 sperm/g per day during the peak season.

1. Establish that both testes are present and can be freely moved within the scrotum. Unilateral and bilateral cryptorchidism, a hereditary condition, must be detected at the ram lamb stage.
2. The testes should be large, ovoid and equal in size. Where scrotal circumference or testis diameter is measured, interpret the data carefully. Note abnormal enlargement, orchitis, misshapen testes and unilateral hypoplasia.
3. Palpate both testes firmly and determine degree of firmness and resilience. Note excessive hardness and sponginess.
4. The scrotum and testes should hang perpendicularly.

The epididymes

Palpate firmly along the length of the testes giving particular attention to the tail, which is near the base of the scrotum and thus vulnerable to injury. Both tails should be large (indicating a good reserve of sperm), firm and resilient. Excessive hardness may be due to epididymitis, a common cause of culling. If detected during stud examination, establish the cause.

Semen collection

It is now generally accepted that clinical examinations of rams should rely primarily on palpation and visual inspection of genitalia. The examination of semen should only be undertaken for specific reasons such as infertility investigations, the assessment of aged rams, rams recovering from illness or recently injured, and for certification purposes.

Rams may be trained to use an AV and this should always be done where repeated collections are carried out for AI and research programmes. Training rams is time-consuming and not all rams respond to training. Examinations are usually carried out before the onset of oestrous activity in the flock. If the rams to be examined are docile and used to being handled the problem of providing oestrous ewes for AV collections would arise. Under field conditions electro-ejaculation is the only method widely available.

It should be noted that, in the UK, the Veterinary Surgeons' Act 1966, Schedule 3, Amendment Order 1982, permits electro-ejaculation to be performed only by a veterinary surgeon in the course of veterinary practice (see p. 383 for techniques of semen collection and evaluation).

The rams should be conditioned to the area where the collection is to take place, preferably under cover to avoid inclement weather, and the handling facilities should be strong and allow easy movement of animals. The rams should be handled quietly before and during collection. Stress can be minimized by carrying out the procedures expeditiously. A minimum of three persons is required during collection: an experienced stockperson, the veterinary surgeon and a trained assistant. With good management and technique, the stress involved can be minimized so that analgesia or anaesthesia is required only in a minimum number of cases; where drugs are used, provision must be made to isolated treated rams for 24 hours and to keep them under observation.

Serving capacity test

A serving capacity test is a means of identifying rams of high mating potential. It involves exposing the ram to a small group of restrained ewes, in which oestrus has been synchronized, in a test pen for a fixed period, usually 20 minutes. The number of mounts and services is recorded and this information, sometimes coupled with testis measurement, is then used to rank the team of rams (Blockley and Wilkins 1984). It is widely used in very large flocks in Australia and New Zealand. Some concern has been expressed about the welfare aspect of this test.

Infertility problems

In flocks given minimal care, with no records relating to tupping, and where pregnancy diagnosis is not undertaken, there may be little evidence of an infertility problem until lambing time. When a new cause of infertility arises in such flocks a very high proportion of the flock may be affected and little can be done to minimize infertility in that production year. This kind of situation should not arise in herds of dairy cattle or pigs, where non-pregnant animals can be readily identified as a result of behavioural interactions between the female members of the herd at any time of the year, and where there is also far greater opportunity to see and assess individual animals daily.

There is ample evidence that infertility and low fecundity make a significant contribution to poor flock performance. Table 8.28 indicates the proportion of flocks, in an MLC survey of lowland flocks, with an unacceptably low level of performance in respect of four criteria of performance. Several flocks were poor in more than one respect; this is a reflection of mismanagement at several stages of the production cycle. This kind of situation is not uncommon and can arise in all the production systems. More often than not these flock owners rarely seek advice unless it is blatantly obvious that a disease is involved. It is generally accepted that, in some extensive systems involving the harshest environments in the UK, poor levels of fertility, high neonatal mortality and high death rate in breeding ewes is inevitable. In these situations little consideration is given to the welfare aspects of the system.

In most flocks there is ample scope to improve the level of reproductive efficiency. This can be achieved without resorting to over-demanding recording techniques. Initially, comparisons can be made with similar

Table 8.28 Variation in level of reproductive performance between lowland flocks

	Average flocks	Top flocks	Poor flocks	Percentage* of all flocks
Barren ewes				
(per 100 ewes to ram)	6	4	>10	22
Ewe deaths				
(per 100 ewes to ram)	4	3	>10	6
Lamb deaths				
(percentage of live lambs born)	13	12	>20	11
Lambs weaned				
(per 100 ewes to ram)	139	154	<120	20

*Applies to poor flocks

flocks by consulting data similar to those presented in Table 8.24. Flock targets can then be set and these improved on year after year following critical analysis of flock performance and adjustments to husbandry procedures and preventive treatments (Hindson and Winter 1990).

A broad analysis of the most critical periods of the production cycle will help to identify the primary areas requiring action. The items listed in the vertical lines of Figure 8.10 will be adequate for this purpose.

The analysis of ewe performance requires a knowledge of:

- number in breeding flock at tupping,
- number at lambing,

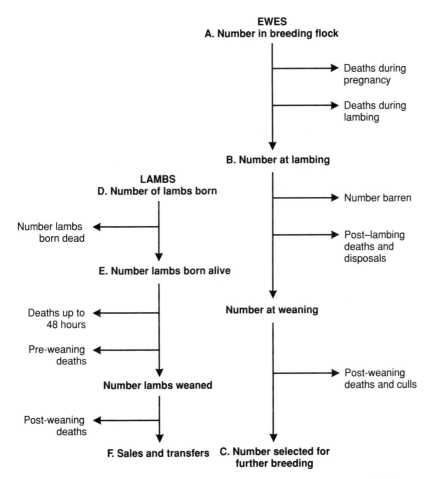

Figure 8.10 The analysis of flock performance and the stages at which losses occur. Replacement rate (%) = (A – C)/A × 100 (to maintain constant no. in breeding flock). % Lambing = B/A × 100. Average litter size = D/B. Potential lambing % = E/A × 100. Lambing % = F/A ×100.

- number of ewes at weaning,
- number selected for further breeding.

As performance improves, more sophistication, more detail and more consultation is required for further improvement. Only where there is good communication and full cooperation between client and veterinarian or specialist adviser will both parties fulfil their role to the benefit of the productivity of the sheep unit.

There is no doubt that the ease with which problems can be resolved will greatly depend on:

- the early notification of a problem,
- the quality of the biological material contributing to the diagnosis,
- the reliability and relevance of the information available.

It is unusual to investigate flock infertility during the early stages of pregnancy. The exception would be obvious disease or malfunction in the rams. The majority of flocks do not undertake a system of management and recording that allows critical assessment and detection at this stage of the production cycle.

Problems during the tupping period

A: Rams 'not working'

Evidence of a ram 'not working' includes the unharnessed ram not seen to tease and mount ewes, harnessed rams not leaving keel marks, and the harem of ewes around the ram not seen since ram turned in.

Consider or obtain information on the following:

1. The age range of the group and previous breeding history.
2. The onset of the breeding season of the breed/crossbreed.
3. The date the ram was turned in. Calculate the interval from (2) to (3).

Compare data with previous years and other similar flocks in the area. Note that ewes in late seasonal anoestrus show peak activity around days 9 and 24/25 following entry of the ram. Ewe lambs that are not as forward as previous years may be anoestrous. Establish ram:ewe ratio and number and age of rams in use.

The examination of rams should check the following:

1. If harnessed, check whether harnesses fitted properly with crayons in place and secured. Check texture of crayons. Poor marking arises when hard crayons are used during wet weather or sudden cold weather.

2. Carry out full physical examination.
3. Consider usefulness of test mating with a receptive ewe; this is difficult to arrange. Observe the rams when they rejoin the ewes.

The examination of a proportion of the ewe flock should check the following.

1. Examine fleece for obnoxious smelling chemicals.
2. Examine external genitalia and vagina for infection (and presence of sponges).
3. Consider possibility of group being already pregnant:
   (a) uncastrated ram lamb(s) running with ewes weaned late,
   (b) ewes purchased at market with no history,
   (c) assurance given in market place that ewes have not run with rams can be quite unreliable.
4. Pregnancy scan if 4 weeks have elapsed since ram turned in.

B: High proportion of ewes returning to the ram

Establish what proportion returned to first or subsequent services and how this was determined.

Check whether rams were raddled or were fitted with harnesses when first turned in. Some do not use raddle during the first 17 days. High incidence of keel marks during the second 17 days would occur when anoestrous ewes respond to the unaccustomed presence of the ram(s), particularly around days 19 and 24/25.

Where majority of ewes are keel-marked during the first 17 days interpret proportion of returns to first service as follows:

>5 to <10%   Very satisfactory; acceptable
>10 to <15%   Moderately satisfactory; acceptable
>20%   Unsatisfactory; unacceptable; investigate problem

The information required for investigating returns includes:

- ram:ewe ratio; number and *age of rams* in use,
- age structure of the group/flock,
- whether synchronized with progestagens/PMSG,
- management history of ewes and rams including foodstuffs used,
- if ram(s) purchased, interval since arrival. Ailments and treatments since arrival. Source of ram. Exposure to endemic diseases since arrival.

Examine those ewes returning to service and a representative sample of flock/group. A general physical examination should pay particular attention to vagina/vulva, condition score and appearance of fleece.

A general physical examination of the ram(s) should pay particular attention to the reproductive tract. A behavioural test should be done using draft ewe(s) on heat from main flock. Check whether intromission is achieved coupled with thrusting. Collect semen and evaluate.

A blood sample should be taken to establish whether the ram has reacted to exposure to a systemic disease. Poor semen quality resulting from pyrexia would most probably be temporary. This should be checked at a later date.

Problems during pregnancy

If many ewes are marked by a vasectomized ram 4–6 weeks after the end of tupping, these ewes should be drafted to a side pen and a representative sample or the whole flock should be available for inspection.

The information required to investigate post-tupping infertility includes:

- general flock history and performance in previous years,
- ram:ewe ratio; number and age of rams used,
- age structure of the flock,
- age range of ewes under investigation,
- the timing and overall duration of the tupping period,
- calculate the number of 17-day periods.

If keel-marking is adopted:

- number of ewes marked for first time during each 17-day period,
- total number of ewes not marked,
- number of ewes returning to first and subsequent services.

Compare the number of ewes marked during the last 17 days of the tupping period and the number of ewes under investigation. Good correspondence indicates that the ewes failed to conceive and continued cycling (prognosis A). Poor correspondence indicates resumption of oestrous cycles following embryo/early foetal death (prognosis B).

Prognosis A   Pursue investigation as for problem B during tupping period with emphasis on examination of ram(s)

Prognosis B   Confine examination of rams to general examination of physical features (see p. 424).

Examination of the ewes should note the following.

1. General physical examination of soundness with emphasis on body condition, vulva and vagina.
2. Prevalence of excessively fat ewes in the group indicates that mismanagement might be a contributing factor.
3. Take blood sample for serological study, particularly if the majority under investigation were new and young introductions to a flock known to have a toxoplasmosis problem.

Where there is evidence that infertility arises during the first 6 weeks of pregnancy and the cause has not been established, consider further investigation during the subsequent season. Progesterone profiles during the first 6 weeks of pregnancy will indicate the nature of the problem. The usefulness of this approach in the investigation of infertility has been reported by Scott *et al.* (1983).

Problems in late pregnancy

In the majority of flocks it is much easier to detect the occurrence of diseases and disorders affecting fertility during later pregnancy than it is in early pregnancy. Abortions, metabolic disorders or severe loss of body condition can be readily detected during the normal surveillance of the flock approaching lambing. Action and further investigation should be carried out without delay following the first occurrence of a problem.

The primary objectives at this stage are to prevent the problem occurring in the remaining pregnant ewes and to minimize the spread of infection to other members of the flock. Where there is early notification of a problem effective preventive measures can be quickly implemented. In some cases this may be only tentative until a positive diagnosis is available following conventional investigative procedures.

Problems during lambing and the neonatal period

There is no doubt that a high level of surveillance and skilled assistance during and after the lambing can minimize loss and injury during these stages.

Reducing lamb losses

Birth injury sustained during a difficult or prolonged birth is an important cause of stillbirth, death during the neonatal period, and morbidity (Wilsmore 1986, 1989). These losses should be carefully recorded so that one or more of the following options can be implemented in an endeavour to reduce perinatal mortality.

1. Provide better facilities and aids for the lambing.
2. Provide further training for those assisting at lambing.
3. Segregate and feed ewes according to expected litter size.
4. Select more appropriate sires in subsequent years.

Surveys of the causes of lamb deaths during the first hours have highlighted the importance of good shepherding and management at this critical time.

In the event of a high incidence of lamb mortality during this time, particular attention should be given to the following:

- resuscitation,
- prevention of hypothermia,
- early detection of abnormal maternal behaviour,
- intake of colostrum during the first 12 hours,
- type and timing of vaccination during pregnancy,
- methods of adoption,
- facilities for artificial rearing.

9

BIOTECHNOLOGY IN ANIMAL BREEDING
D POWELL PhD and I WILMUT PhD

Introduction

Intensive animal husbandry has been practised for several centuries. Over the past century, breeding societies have promoted the careful selection of stock animals. The last 40 years have seen an increasingly scientific contribution to this selection and assessment of breeding lines, using analysis of lineages and artificial insemination (AI) to expand productive populations. Especially during this last phase, there have been dramatic changes in milk yields and growth rates, as well as carcass composition of most domestic species. The recent changes in milk yield, for example, have seen an increase of about 45 litres per cow per annum. Conventional breeding strategies are limited by the long periods required for establishment of breeding lines, the complexity of introducing desirable traits into otherwise productive genetic backgrounds and the limited number of offspring produced from the female germ line. In this chapter we assess the likely impact of novel biotechnological processes on these areas. As these are young sciences, much of the discussion is inevitably prospective, but the importance of these developments for agricultural practice requires that those in the area are aware of the methods and their likely applications.

Developments in the areas of cellular manipulation and molecular biology have provided the impetus for these developments (Church 1987). First, new techniques have been developed in the laboratory that provide large numbers of functional oocytes, enabling the female germ line to be almost as productive as the male. Combined with methods that are already established for semen storage, *in vitro* fertilization (IVF) and embryo storage, the full reproductive capacity of valuable individuals should be realized. Second, techniques for manipulating nuclei open the possibility of generating many progeny using early embryonic nuclei. Third, techniques are being developed to allow the indefinite propagation of embryonic cells for use in expanding breeding lines. Last, molecular biological techniques will allow us to analyse the genetic composition of animals more closely and provide a means for introducing new genes into valuable lines.

Breeding strategies

The major factors contributing to breed improvement in cattle since the Second World War have been the efficient application of progeny or performance tests to identify superior animals and the dissemination of superior genotypes by use of semen dilution, storage and AI. Considerable benefits can also be expected from the application of embryo transfer. Exploitation of embryo transfer depends upon the ability to recover, store and transfer embryos and these procedures are established for the livestock species. In addition to these procedures, several others are being developed to enhance the value of embryo transfer. These include the use of culture to produce embryos suitable for transfer, determination of the sex of the embryo and even the choice of the sex of the embryo (Figure 9.1). Similarly, exploitation of all of the approaches discussed so far in this chapter depends upon the ability to recover, store and transfer embryos.

Embryo collection

Embryos are usually collected from females that have been induced to superovulate by injection of gonadotrophic hormone for several days. Different types of hormone preparation have been used over the years, in different species and in different laboratories. The preparation used in early studies was pregnant mare's serum gonadotrophin (PMSG, now known as equine chorionic gonadotrophin (eCG)) (Newcomb *et al.* 1976). Treatment was certainly effective in promoting follicle growth, but there was a tendency for unovulated follicles to develop and a suggestion that the hormones produced by these follicles disturbed embryo development. More recently, preparations of pituitary follicle stimulating hormone (FSH) have been employed with greater success (Hasler *et al.* 1983; Monniaux *et al.* 1983). The major difference between the FSH and PMSG preparations concerns the number of injections that are required. The

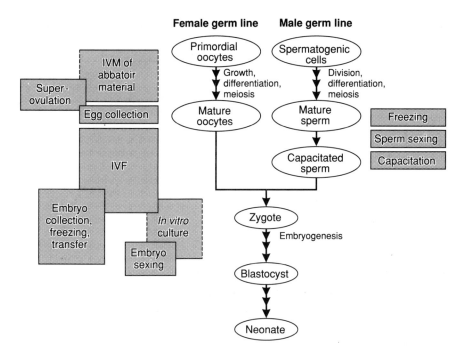

Figure 9.1 Manipulation of breeding strategies. Developmental stages are enclosed within oval boxes and their fates indicated by arrows. For each appropriate stage, the *in vitro* manipulation is indicated by a boxed, capital legend. Not all procedures are available for all species and the more imperfectly developed are delineated by dashed boxes.

PMSG molecule has considerable numbers of sialic acid residues and it is believed that these confer the extremely long half-life. As a result only one injection of PMSG is required. By contrast, pituitary FSH is given daily or even twice daily, depending upon the species of origin. Treatment lasts for 3 (sheep) or 4 (cattle) days and ends shortly before the expected time of ovulation.

The time of oestrus and ovulation are controlled in order to prepare groups of animals for embryo transfer at the same time. In sheep and goats this is achieved by treatment with progestagen administered on intravaginal sponges (e.g. Simons *et al.* 1988). The last injection of FSH is given at the time of, or 12 hours after, sponge withdrawal. In cattle, treatment to induce superovulation is begun in the mid-luteal phase of a cycle and luteal regression is induced by injection of prostaglandin $F_{2\alpha}$ or an analogue (Newcomb *et al.* 1976). In some circumstances, there is a need for even greater control of the time of ovulation and this is achieved by injection of gonadotrophin releasing hormone (GnRH) or an analogue at, or shortly

---

Terms used in breeding strategies

AI: artificial insemination

Blastocyst: stage of embryonic development after rapid cell division characterized by a cellular, fluid-filled cavity partly lined with cells of the inner cell mass, which are destined to form the embryo

Genotype: genetic constitution that defines the inherited characteristics of an organism

IVF: *in vitro* fertilization. After pretreatment (capacitation) of spermatozoa and appropriate maturation of oocytes, carefully regulated mixing, incubation and media formulation can produce efficient fertilization rates in many species

IVM: *in vitro* maturation (of oocytes). The immature oocyte undergoes a complex developmental programme, some components of which can be simulated *in vitro* allowing the use of large numbers of oocytes from inexpensive abattoir material for IVF

Oocyte: the female germ cell that undergoes meiosis and maturation before becoming competent to participate in fertilization

---

before, the expected time of onset of oestrus (Simons *et al.* 1988). Even then there is a spread of several hours in the time of ovulation. This is made up of variation within a female and of differences between females in the time of ovulation.

Normally eggs are collected from donor females after fertilization. There is a need for precise control of the time of insemination and of the quality of the semen if complete fertilization is to be achieved. In cattle this depends upon conventional AI, whereas in sheep and goats insemination into the uterine lumen is routinely carried out by laparoscopy (Evans and Maxwell 1987).

The method for embryo collection varies with species and with the stage of embryo being collected. Collection from the oviduct always involves surgery, usually by mid-ventral laparotomy. In cattle and horses, non-surgical collection of uterine stages is carried out using manual manipulation per rectum to position the catheter correctly and control the flow of fluid (Figure 9.2) (Newcomb *et al.* 1976). Collection from sheep is usually carried out by mid-ventral laparotomy, but laparoscopy is being used by experienced practitioners (Wilmut 1987). By contrast, pig embryos are collected surgically because the great length of the uterine horns makes it impracticable to pass catheters or fluid effectively.

Procedures for egg or embryo collection

Sheep (Simons et al. 1988)

Oestrus synchronization:	Progestagen sponge for 12–16 days	−12 to −16 days
Superovulation:	2 mg FSH s.c., 30 hours before and at sponge removal	−30 hours, 0 hours
Insemination/ oestrus test:	8, 12, 16 and 20 hours after last FSH	+8 to +20 hours
Egg/embryo collection:	Flush during mid-ventral laparotomy	

Pig (Wall et al. 1985)

Oestrus synchronization:	Altrenogest, 15 mg/1.8 kg of feed for 5–9 days, beginning day 12–16 of oestrus	approx −14 to −16 days (−138 hours)
Superovulation:	1000 iu PMSG s.c., 24 hours after last altrenogest feed	−114 hours
	500 iu hCG i.m., 72 hours after PMSG	−40 to −44 hours
Ovulation:	40–44 hours after hCG	0 hours
Egg/embryo collection:	Flush during mid-ventral laparotomy	+18 to +27 hours

Cow (Prather et al. 1987)

Superovulation:	6.5 mg reduced to 4.5 mg FSH over 4 days last day + 2 ml Estrumate (cloprostenol)	−6 to −1.5 days
Oestrus:	36–48 hours after cloprostenol	0 hours
Insemination:	12–24 hours after oestrus	+12 to +24 hours
Egg/embryo collection:	From excised oviducts 40 hours (eggs) to 100 hours (embryos) after oestrus	+ 36 to +120 hours

The main characteristic of the response to superovulation regimens is the variability between females and between treatments in the same animal. This variation may reflect differences in the population of follicles capable of responding to treatment (Monniaux *et al.* 1983). Administration of the same dose of the same batch of hormone to sheep or cattle of the same breed, on the same farm and according to the same protocol may

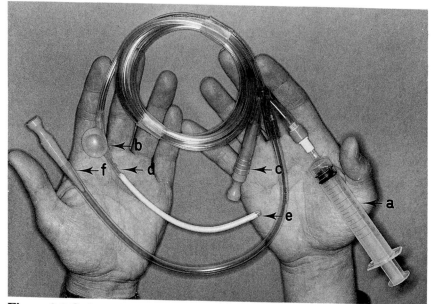

Figure 9.2 Catheter for use in non-surgical embryo recovery in cattle showing (a) the syringe used for inflation of the cuff (b), the inlet point (c) for medium that is introduced into the uterine lumen through the opening at the tip of the catheter (e). The medium and embryos are recovered through outlets immediately anterior to the cuff (d) and collected from the end of the catheter (f). As the catheter is filled with medium before introduction into the uterine lumen the inlet (c) and collection (f) points are closed with spigots to prevent loss of the fluid.

result in anything from zero to 50 ovulations. This variation has major implications for the planning of embryo transfer because embryos must be transferred to females that were in oestrus at the same time as the donor if their survival is to be maximal. Fortunately, the advent of methods of embryo freezing provides an alternative means of achieving the desired degree of synchronization, although at the cost of the 20–30% of embryos that do not survive storage.

In vitro embryo production

An alternative source of cattle embryos has been created by the development of techniques for the *in vitro* maturation (IVM) of oocytes, their IVF and culture to the stage at which they can be transferred to the uterus (Gordon and Lu 1990). While these procedures yield embryos suitable for transfer, only a minority of the oocytes that are cultured become blasto-cysts and, after transfer, the proportion of pregnancies is lower than normal.

Oocytes are collected from the ovaries of slaughtered females by aspir-ation from the follicle before culturing in medium enriched with serum, usually from oestrous cattle. Before spermatozoa are able to achieve fertilization they must undergo specific changes that result in the exposure of the enzymes that are required for penetration into the oocytes. These changes are induced by incubation in the presence of heparin while the spermatozoa are being cultured with the oocytes. Embryo development to the blastocyst stage may be achieved during culture *in vitro* or in a sheep oviduct. Early in the establishment of these procedures the yield following culture in the sheep was substantially higher than after *in vitro* culture, but the use of co-culture with cells recovered from the oviduct has resulted in similar yields in the two methods.

Embryos produced in this way are cheaper than those collected from superovulated donors and may be used for the production of beef calves. Several companies in the UK, Europe and North America now offer commercially prepared IVF embryos. The genetic merit of the donor female is almost certain to be only average as she had been sent for slaughter, but the bull can be selected for high performance. Probably the greatest cost is in travel to the farm to carry out the embryo transfer, rather than in the production of the embryo. This may be reduced by synchroni-zation of oestrus in a group of females, but this in turn carries a cost. Finally, there is, at present, the lower conception rate following transfer, which increases the cost to the farmer. These procedures are very new and their efficiency is certain to increase. In addition, oocytes matured *in vitro* are likely to be used during nuclear transfer (see below).

Embryo transfer

The method required for embryo transfer varies with the stage of devel-opment and the species. All transfers to the oviduct require surgery. Similarly, a surgical method is usually used for all transfers of pig embryos, although some pregnancies have been obtained following non-surgical transfer to the uterus. Sheep embryos are usually transferred by mid-ven-tral laparotomy although there is increased use of laparoscopy (Wilmut 1987). Goat embryos are transferred by laparoscopy, but the cervical canal is large enough to permit non-surgical transfer. In cattle and horses, the routine method for non-surgical transfer is similar to that used for AI.

The proportion of recipients that become pregnant is similar to or slightly higher than that routinely obtained after AI. There are many factors that can affect the establishment of pregnancy, the most important of which is the requirement for synchrony between donor and recipient animals. This probably reflects an interaction or series of interactions between the embryo and uterus that can occur normally only if the embryo and uterus are at particular stages of their development. Measurement of the interval since the onset of oestrus provides a convenient means of estimating these two parameters (Wilmut *et al.* 1985). Other factors that may prejudice the outcome include rough handling of the reproductive tract, the introduction of microorganisms into the uterus and poor health or nutrition of the recipient.

Embryo storage

Embryos may be stored at room temperature, in the refrigerator or in liquid nitrogen. In general, the lower the temperature the longer the period of survival, provided that the embryos can tolerate the lower temperature. During routine transfer, embryos are left on the bench for several hours and provided that the temperature is around 20–25 °C and the medium is protected from contamination or drying out, there is no apparent loss of viability. The response to cooling below room temperature varies with stage of embryo development and species. Pig embryos at all stages studied are killed by cooling in ice, regardless of the medium or the rate of cooling used. Cattle embryos become resistant to cooling during the morula stage of development, whereas sheep embryos appear to be resistant to cooling at all stages. This phenomenon is different from cold-shock death of sperm in that it is independent of the rate of cooling. It has been suggested, but not proved, that at a particular temperature, which is between 10 and 15°C for pig embryos, there is a phase change in the lipids of the cell membrane and that in the susceptible cells the change is irreversible. Whatever the mechanism, fundamental new approaches will be required to develop methods to protect these cells.

Embryo freezing involves cooling and warming the cells at precise rates in the presence of a cryoprotective agent (see Wilmut 1986). Medium containing the agent, usually glycerol at a concentration around 10% (v/v), is added to the embryos at room temperature. After allowing time for the glycerol to enter the cells, the embryos are placed in storage containers, usually straws, and cooled. The rate of cooling above the freezing point of the medium is less important than after ice formation and would typically be around 1°C/minute. Before further cooling, it is essential that ice formation is induced in order to avoid supercooling. This can be achieved by placing forceps cooled in liquid nitrogen against the outside of the straw and watching the ice appear. Controlled cooling devices are then used to cool the sample at a precise rate, usually around 0.3 °C/minute. The straw is transferred to liquid nitrogen for long-term storage once the sample temperature is $-60\,°C$ or below. Storage life is indefinite at the temperature of liquid nitrogen ($-196\,°C$).

Embryo survival depends upon warming the sample and removal of the protective agent. Typically, the straw is warmed by shaking in a water bath. Embryo survival is poor if the embryo is transferred to a recipient in the presence of 10% glycerol, probably because of osmotic shock as water enters the cells. Two approaches have been used to minimize this stress. In the first, cryoprotective agent was removed by passing the embryo through a series of dishes containing progressively lower concentrations of glycerol. While this is effective, it is laborious and cannot be used in the field. More recently, sucrose has been included in the medium to reduce the quantity of agent in the cells. As a result the amount of swelling is reduced and the embryos survive. Dilution in the presence of sucrose has been carried out in the straw before direct transfer of the embryo on-farm. This is very convenient, but undoubtedly results in the transfer of some dead embryos that would have been eliminated during manipulation under the microscope.

The tendency during the development of these procedures has been to strive for speed and simplification. This pattern is likely to continue and in time, by modification of the medium used during cooling, it may be possible to enhance survival, particularly after dilution in the straw. Similarly, methods of cooling as well as warming will be easier to apply in the field. This would be of great value in developing countries where the electricity needed to control cooling machines may not be available.

With present procedures in the best-regulated situations, only 70% of cattle embryos survive freezing and storage and, when considering use of storage procedures, it is important to contrast the efficiency of storage with that of any other solution to the problem. Embryo storage is essential for import/export if tests are to be applied to donor females in quarantine. It also provides an economical means of shipping large numbers of (potential) animals, for hundreds of embryos can be stored in a small canister. There are also many research reasons for embryo storage. Probably the most frequent application is to store the embryo until a suitable recipient female becomes available. In this way it is no longer necessary to synchronize oestrus in a very large group of females in case the yield of embryos is particularly great. Experience shows that better quality embryos are very likely to survive freezing and thawing while those embryos of ragged or slightly degenerate appearance are less likely to survive. Maximum yield of calves may be obtained by transferring such poorer embryos immediately and storing the better embryos.

Sperm sexing

One approach to modifying the ratio of male to female progeny is to isolate X- or Y-bearing sperm. Because the X chromosome is much larger than the Y, methods have been applied based on differences in mass, density or DNA content. Studies have also been carried out to identify differences in antigenic properties (for a review, see Amann 1989). Probably the most promising method is based on cell sorting using vital dyes, which seems to have few deleterious effects on sperm viability or subsequent development (Morrell and Dresser 1989: for a review, see Cran 1992). Johnson and colleagues (1989) used a modified, fluorescence-activated cell sorter to enrich for population of rabbit spermatozoa bearing either X or Y chromosomes. The enriched X-bearing population resulted in birth of 94% females and the enriched Y-bearing population resulted in birth of 81% males in a total sample of 38 offspring. More recently, Johnson (1992) has described similar experiments on the sorting of pig spermatozoa: in this study, spermatozoa enriched for X-bearing cells gave rise to 74% female offspring, and the Y population gave 68% male offspring. The relatively low numbers of spermatozoa that can be sorted efficiently (about 400 000/hour) means that surgical fertilization methods had to be used in both these studies. This low rate of separation is a major stumbling block to the application of this technology.

Cran *et al.* (1993) have used sorting to produce bovine calves of the appropriate sex. In these experiments, they used recently optimized methods of IVM of oocytes and IVF. This work showed that this combination of *in vitro* methods could still lead to successful pregnancies in the recipients. Moreover, IVF allows the use of far smaller numbers of sperm than does surgical insemination, and IVM allows the production and selection of many, synchronized oocytes.

Advances in the use of these methods will depend on increasing the rate of sorting, finding alternative methods of sperm separation, or increased use of *in vitro* methods. First, the numbers of sperm that can be sorted are relatively small and to produce a typical 'straw' used in bovine AI would take about 20 hours of sorting, obviously requiring complex technology. This, allied to the losses that occur when freezing is used, is likely to limit application to more sophisticated centres. Second, production of embryos will probably be more efficient using IVF, where fewer sperm are used. Under such constraints it is likely that current technology will be limited to the most valuable and productive animals.

Embryo sexing

There have been several different approaches to discovering the sex of an embryo (reviewed by Wilmut and Smith 1988), but the most promising involves detection of DNA that is specific to the Y chromosome (Leonard *et al.* 1987; Peura *et al.* 1991; Agrawala *et al.* 1992; see Figure 9.3). A small number of cells are removed from the embryo by biopsy before the DNA is isolated. The polymerase chain reaction (PCR) is then used to amplify the specific DNA sequences, before a labelled probe is used to screen the

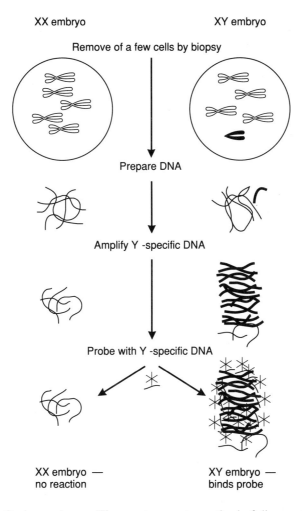

Figure 9.3 Sexing embryos. The most accurate method of discovering the sex of an embryo employs the polymerase chain reaction to make thousands of copies of specific sequences. A small number of cells are removed from the embryo by biopsy and the DNA is extracted. Many copies of the specific sequences are made by application of the polymerase chain reaction. The presence of the Y-specific sequences is then assayed by probing with labelled copies of the Y-specific sequences. The labelled DNA only binds to DNA samples that contain the sequences of interest, as like binds to like.

sample for the presence of the sequences of interest. This test can be carried out within a day, allowing transfer of biopsied embryos without the requirement for freezing and thawing. One factor of considerable practical importance concerns the risk of contamination of the samples leading to false conclusions as the amplification obtained can permit detection of DNA from a single cell. One means of limiting the risk is to carry out the analysis at a central testing station, but this inevitably causes delays and may depend upon an ability to freeze the embryo.

The ability to discover the sex of an embryo will be particularly useful when groups of embryos are being produced by nuclear transfer because the costs involved are spread over a large number of calves. By contrast, when individual embryos are being transferred the costs are considerable. In addition to the actual costs of the tests, if calves of only one sex are desired, the charge for embryo collection has to be doubled because half of the embryos must be discarded.

Manipulating genomes—nuclear transfer

Over 20 years ago, John Gurdon showed that nuclei from the intestine of the toad *Xenopus* would direct development of eggs from which the nuclei were removed, i.e. these intestinal nuclei were totipotent (see Gurdon 1974). In a small percentage of cases, Gurdon obtained apparently normal tadpoles from such experiments, although development to adults was rare. The intense interest that these experiments generated led to many attempts to reproduce such experiments in mammalian systems. The consequences of the principle of cloning are quite spectacular; in theory the most productive farm animals could be replicated indefinitely by nuclear transfer to produce identical brothers (or sisters) each of which carries all the genetic heritage of its valuable 'parent'. As we shall see, such manipulations in mammals have encountered unexpected obstacles.

Nuclear transfer in mammals

A great deal of effort has been devoted to attempts to use embryonic nuclei to direct the development of enucleated eggs in laboratory and farm species (McGrath and Solter 1983; Surani *et al.* 1984; Prather and First 1989; Smith and Wilmut 1990). The principal conclusion from these studies is that there are major differences between the species and that, unusually, the procedures are more successful in farm animals than in mice. Three generalizations are informative. First, as embryonic cells differentiate there is a decline in the proportion of nuclei that are capable of supporting normal development following transfer. However, the rate of this change depends upon the species and the choice of recipient cell. Second, the

Terms used in nuclear manipulation

Blastocyst: stage of embryonic development after rapid cell division characterized by a cellular fluid-filled cavity partly lined with cells of the inner cell mass, which are destined to form the embryo.

Blastomere: cell of blastocyst.

Cytoplast: the residual cytoplasmic and membranous components of a cell after removal of a nucleus or karyoplast. May be used as recipient for donor nucleus.

Chimera: organism composed of cells of two or more genetically different types; typically produced by aggregating cells from more than one embryo into a single embryo.

Karyoplast: the nuclear component (with a small amount of attached cytoplasm and membrane) extracted from a cell by micromanipulation. Used as donor in nuclear transfer experiments.

Oocyte: the female germ cell that undergoes meiosis and maturation before becoming competent to participate in fertilization.

Pronucleus: after fertilization, the male and female genomes are packaged in separate membrane components, the pronuclei, that usually fuse during the first cell cycle.

Totipotency: the ability of a cell, typically an embryonic cell, to differentiate into *all* the tissues of an organism. More restricted developmental capacity is termed pluripotency.

Zygote: the fertilized egg, before the first cleavage division.

pattern of gene expression in the transferred nuclei may be changed by exposure to the cytoplasm of a different cell and this may be essential for normal development. Last, these studies are very new and it is likely that significant changes in techniques will lead to normal development occurring more frequently.

Whereas normal development may occur following transfer of nuclei from intestinal cells of an adult toad to enucleated oocytes (Gurdon 1974), many experiments have shown that nuclei from 4-cell mouse embryos are unable to support development if transferred to zygotes from which the pronuclei have been removed (McGrath and Solter 1983). However, Cheong *et al.* (1993) have shown recently that 2-, 4- or 8-cell nuclei will direct development of enucleated oocytes if the donor nuclei are isolated from the 'early' stages of the cell cycle. It was proposed that proper pronuclear formation and chromatin structure could be formed using such early stages only. Although an accurate assessment of the loss of potency of nuclei in livestock species has not been made, such cells appear to lie between the two extremes of frog and mouse.

Willadsen (1986) first reported successful experiments to transfer advanced nuclei from domestic animals to recipient eggs and obtain viable progeny. He collected eggs from superovulated ewes and 8–16-cell embryos from naturally mated ewes. He then bisected the eggs to produce two halves, one of which contained a nucleus (karyoplast) while the other was enucleate (cytoplast). He then introduced a single blastomere (from embryos at the 8–16-cell stage) under the zona pellucida. He achieved fusion of the blastomere with the cytoplast using either inactivated Sendai virus, which causes fusion of plasma membranes, or electrofusion, in which a short, high voltage pulse causes temporary disruption of the membranes, allowing fusion to occur. In several series of experiments, about half of the manipulated enucleate egg–blastomere fusion products gave rise to blastocysts and three out of four transferred blastocysts gave rise to apparently normal, viable lambs. Willadsen then went on to produce three identical calves using similar techniques in the bovine.

In both Cambridge and Edinburgh, recent experiments have indicated that nuclei from even more advanced embryos can serve as donors for successful development (Figure 9.4). Sun and Moor have used electrofusion to transfer nuclei from 64–128-cell embryos to oocytes and have been able to produce a viable lamb. Similarly Smith and Wilmut (1989) used the methods of Willadsen (1986) to produce a lamb from inner cell mass nuclei of day 6 blastocyst. In general, similar techniques have been used by other workers, although it is now more common to produce enucleated eggs by aspirating the pronuclei from the zygotes or oocytes.

Prather et al. (1987) studied the ability of oocytes of various ages and stages of maturation to support embryonic development. They electrofused blastomere nuclei of various stages to enucleated eggs. The most successful combination they reported was to use oocytes matured in vivo for 36 hours as recipients and nuclei from 9–15-cell stage embryos as donors; under these circumstances they established two pregnancies that carried to term, yielding normal offspring.

Evidence of changes to gene expression following nuclear transfer is of two types: direct and indirect. Indirect evidence arises in two ways. Following transfer of nuclei from sheep 8–16-cell embryos to enucleated oocytes, the reconstituted embryos form blastocysts after the interval required by a recently fertilized egg rather than the period required by the donor embryo (Willadsen 1986). Similarly, following transfer to an

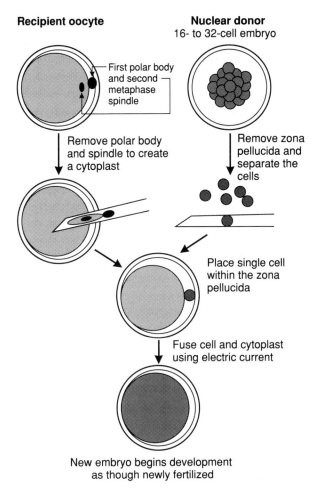

Recipient oocyte

First polar body
and second
metaphase
spindle

Remove polar body
and spindle to create
a cytoplast

Nuclear donor
16- to 32-cell embryo

Remove zona
pellucida and
separate the
cells

Place single cell
within the zona
pellucida

Fuse cell and cytoplast
using electric current

New embryo begins development
as though newly fertilized

Figure 9.4 Nuclear transfer in cattle and sheep. Nuclear transfer involves the removal of the chromosomes from the recipient oocyte by aspiration into a pipette. The chromosomes are revealed by staining with a DNA-specific fluorochrome. The cells of the donor embryo are removed from the zona pellucida and separated. A single cell is placed within the zona pellucida and fused to the recipient cytoplast by passage of a pulse of direct current. The reconstituted embryo begins development as though a recently fertilized egg; chromatin structure and gene expression are modified by the cytoplasm of the recipient oocyte.

enucleated oocyte before activation, there is a characteristic swelling of the transferred nucleus to a volume that approaches that of the early cleavage stage embryo (Tarkowski and Balakier 1980). By contrast, there is little or no swelling following transfer to 2-cell embryos or to enucleated zygotes (Barnes *et al.* 1987).

The only direct measure is of the change in production of the heat shock proteins in mouse embryos following transfer of nuclei from 8-cell embryos to enucleated zygotes (Howlett *et al.* 1987). Heat shock proteins are among the first proteins to be produced following initiation of expression from the embryonic genome during the 2-cell stage in mice. When 8-cell nuclei were transferred to enucleated zygotes expression of the gene was first turned off and then re-initiated at the appropriate stage. This observation provides unequivocal evidence of effects of the oocyte cytoplasm on gene expression; however, it seems unlikely, at least with the present procedures, that such efficient control exists for all the necessary changes.

Manipulating cell lineages

The present procedures for gene transfer have significant limitations (see above). An alternative approach, which has so far been established only in mice, depends upon the manipulation of cells from the early embryo, i.e. embryo stem (ES) cells (Robertson 1987). These cells are isolated from early embryos and maintained in culture in such a way that they divide, but do not differentiate. While in culture, it is possible to apply to such cells all of the procedures of gene manipulation that have been developed for use with tissue culture cells (Figure 9.5). Although these procedures have an even lower efficiency than gene transfer (only around 1 in 10 000 manipulations is successful) and so cannot be applied directly to embryos, it is possible to confirm *in vitro* that the desired change has been made before the ES cell is used for the production of offspring.

When injected into the blastocoel cavity of another mouse embryo, stem cells are sometimes able to colonize that embryo and contribute to all of the tissues of the offspring including the germ line. In this way, it is possible to make changes to existing genes and, in principle, it should also be possible to develop methods for the insertion of genes into specific sites in order to avoid causing damage to endogenous genes and to increase the probability of full expression of the transgene. Furthermore, replacement, repair or modification of the type described above offers new opportunities for subtly altering physiology. There is also the possibility of being able to obtain offspring after the transfer of nuclei from ES cells. The two techniques of nuclear transfer and ES cell manipulation would then be mutually supportive. Embryo stem cells might provide an ideal source of nuclei for transfer when seeking to create large numbers of offspring from élite donor animals, while nuclear transfer from genetically modified ES cells may be a very effective means of introducing such changes into livestock.

Mouse ES cells are isolated by culturing blastocysts upon a layer of feeder cells (Robertson 1987). At this stage the embryo has only two cell types. The outer trophoblast layer will provide the first contact with the mother, while the embryo will form from the inner cell mass. After a period of 5 days in culture, the trophoblast cells have spread along the surface of the feeder cell layer, revealing a clump of cells derived from the inner cell mass. This clump of cells is taken from the first culture well, disaggregated and transferred to a fresh culture well. In some cases the potential stem cells form small colonies that can be recognized by their distinct morphology and grown up to form stable lines. When grown under these

---

Figure 9.5 Five techniques have been developed for generating transgenic mice; of these, microinjection, retrovirus infection and sperm-mediated transfer have been used in livestock species. DNA is most commonly introduced into embryos by microinjection (a). Shortly after fertilization a glass needle is inserted into the larger male pronucleus and 10^{-12} ml injected. The injected embryos are transferred to foster mothers and allowed to develop to term. Approximately one in eight manipulated embryos survives the treatment; of these about one in five contains integrated transgene copies. In a more recent technique, early embryonic cells derived from the inner mass cells of the blastocyst are established in culture dishes (b). DNA can be introduced simply into these embryonic stem (ES) cells *in vitro* and appropriately transformed cells containing the transgene selected, isolated and grown up. A small number of selected cells are injected into a recipient blastocyst where they will divide and may contribute to all the tissues of the resulting animal. If the animals from which donor and recipient blastocysts are derived have different coat colours, then mosaic individuals containing transgenic cells can be identified by patches of donor cell coat colour. The success rates of such manipulations are high—routinely one in two mice contains some transgenic cells. Another method is to use disabled viral vectors (c); by genetic engineering, vectors have been generated that contain only the sequences required for integration of viral DNA into the host chromosome. These deleted viral vectors can carry about 7000 bp of foreign DNA. Using cultured cells, the foreign DNA/viral vector can be packaged into virus particles and these defective virus particles injected into early embryos where they enter the cell and allow the transgene to be integrated into the host chromosome with high efficiency. In sperm-mediated transfer (d), DNA is mixed with sperm in a specially formulated medium. The DNA becomes attached to the sperm (and some may enter). The treated sperm may be used for *in vitro* fertilization or for surgical insemination by intrauterine implantation. For stem-cell replacement (e), a non-germline transgenesis technique, stem cells are isolated from, say, bone marrow, manipulated *in vitro*, and introduced into the recipient. Here cells of only one specific tissue are transgenic.

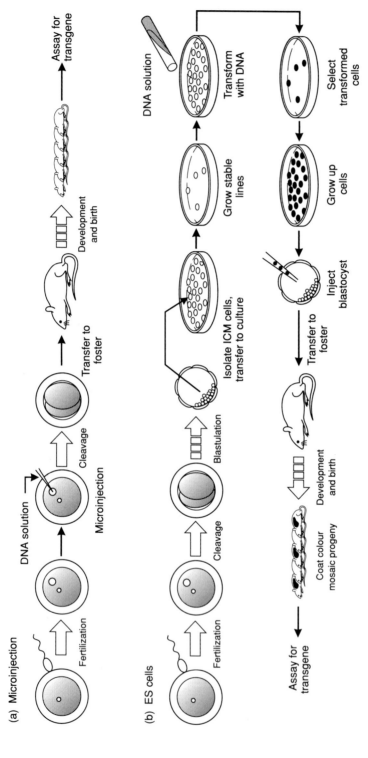

(a) Microinjection

Fertilization

DNA solution

Microinjection

Cleavage

Transfer to foster

Development and birth

Assay for transgene

(b) ES cells

Fertilization

Cleavage

Blastulation

Isolate ICM cells, transfer to culture

DNA solution

Transform with DNA

Grow stable lines

Select transformed cells

Grow up cells

Inject blastocyst

Transfer to foster

Development and birth

Coat colour mosaic progeny

Assay for transgene

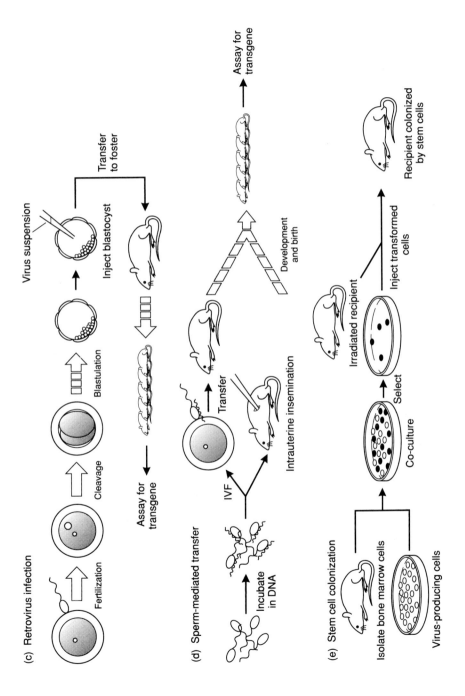

(c) Retrovirus infection

Fertilization → Cleavage → Blastulation

Virus suspension

Inject blastocyst

Assay for transgene

Transfer to foster

Assay for transgene

(d) Sperm-mediated transfer

Incubate in DNA

IVF

Transfer

Intrauterine insemination

Development and birth

Assay for transgene

(e) Stem cell colonization

Isolate bone marrow cells

Virus-producing cells

Co-culture

Select

Irradiated recipient

Inject transformed cells

Recipient colonized by stem cells

Terms used in cell lineage engineering

Blastocoel: the fluid-filled cavity of the blastocyst, into which cells may be injected.

Blastocyst: stage of embryonic development after rapid cell division characterized by a cellular fluid-filled cavity partly lined with cells of the inner cell mass, which are destined to form the embryo.

Blastomere: cell of blastocyst.

Chimera: organism composed of cells of two or more genetically different types; typically produced by aggregating cells from more than one embryo into a single embryo.

Feeder layer: cells attached to a culture dish and then growth arrested using drugs or irradiation. They secrete growth factors and other factors into the medium 'conditioning' it for growth of fastidious embryonic cells.

Germ line: those cell lineages that produce germ cells—sperm and eggs.

Haematopoietic cells: stem cell lineages that produce blood cells.

Inner cell mass: cells, attached to the inner wall of the blastocyst, that are destined to form the embryo proper.

Trophoblast: outer cells of the blastocyst that interact with maternal tissues forming embryonic chorion and placental components

---

conditions such cells divide, but do not differentiate. However, when cultured in the absence of feeder cells a characteristic pattern of differentiation is observed. Furthermore, if they are injected into the blastocoel cavity of another embryo they are sometimes able to colonize the recipient embryo and contribute to all of the tissues of the offspring, including the germ line. One major disadvantage of this approach is that because the young are derived from two embryos they are chimeras. If the ES cell offspring contribute to the germ line, there will be two different types of offspring from such chimeras, one derived from the recipient embryo the other from the ES cell lineage.

Considerable effort has been directed to the isolation of ES cells from embryos of farm animals, but so far there are no reports of the birth of chimeric offspring following the injection of putative ES cells into recipient embryos. It is only by this means that it will be possible to be certain that the cell line is totipotent. When embryos from farm animals are cultured in the conditions in which mouse ES cells are isolated, cells with similar morphology are sometimes seen, but they have proved more difficult than mouse cells to maintain in culture. Cells derived from pig and cattle embryos that resemble mouse ES cells have been maintained in culture for several months but it remains to be confirmed whether or not they are totipotent (Evans *et al.* 1990). The frequency with which cells with stem cell-like morphology are seen is lower with sheep embryos and lines have not been maintained in culture (Handyside *et al.* 1987).

The apparent difficulty in isolating ES cells from farm animals may be a consequence of several effects. The pattern of embryo development in these species is different from that in the mouse. In particular, there is very little cell division in the inner cell mass of such embryos and initiation of division in culture may be less efficient than in mouse cells. There may be species differences in the nature of the growth factors that regulate early development. A factor has been identified that inhibits differentiation of mouse ES cells in culture (Smith, A.G. *et al.* 1988) and it may be necessary to identify a source of an analogous factor for embryos of other species. Certainly this factor alone is unable to maintain ungulate ES cells. Finally, it is possible that embryo development is so different that ES cells cannot be maintained.

The value of ES cells in farm animals would be particularly great if it were possible to transfer nuclei from such cells. In view of the development of normal young following the transfer of nuclei from cells of the inner cell mass of sheep and cattle embryos (as discussed above), it may well be possible to transfer nuclei from ES cells if they could be isolated in these species. This would have enormous implications both for the production of large numbers of young from valuable donors and for the introduction of genetic change in livestock. The opportunity to exploit ES cells by nuclear transfer would avoid the chimeric generation. While the time saved in laboratory animals would not be great, in cattle it would be several years. In addition, it would be possible to obtain several identical offspring from the same line of cells. Production of large numbers of identical transgenic offspring at present would be wasteful because present predictions of the effect of transgenes are inaccurate. However, in the future, as the predictions become more accurate it may be useful to save time by establishing groups of animals. In addition, ES cells may offer the means to the largest pool of offspring that can be produced by nuclear transfer, if serial transfer of nuclei from early embryos proves to be unreliable.

In time, there may also be the opportunity to manipulate other stem cell populations. During development a series of stem cell populations becomes established, each of which has a particular restricted potential for differentiation. In some cases, including the haematopoietic cells, stem cells persist into adult life. Some human conditions have been treated experimentally by removing stem cells, introducing specific genetic changes in them, and returning the modified cells to the donor (French Anderson 1992). In the same way, stem cells that released a hormone could be transferred to an animal. While the biological problems involved in this work seem soluble, the costs of treating each animal would be considerable. There is one potential advantage to the practitioner in that each animal of every generation would require treatment. By contrast, as transgenic animals are expected to transmit the transgene to their offspring the producer need only purchase one such animal.

Manipulation of genes

The mammalian genome encodes some 50 000 genes, each of which can produce an mRNA molecule of, on average, 1200 nucleotides. This accounts for only about 6.0×10^7 base-pairs (bp) of the genome of 3×10^9 bp. A large proportion of the remaining DNA is repeated sequences, many of which, as we shall see, are unique to the individual. A 'typical' gene comprises a protein-coding region that specifies (encodes) the protein product, and a regulatory region that dictates the timing and site of protein synthesis (Gluzman and Shenk 1983; Grosveld *et al.* 1987). In many genes, the protein-coding region is divided into discrete blocks, each separated by non-coding DNA (the function of which is unknown) that is removed during mRNA maturation.

Mammalian genes are thus often organized as two separate functional components and this component structure means that recombinant DNA techniques can be used to alter the patterns of synthesis of individual genes. For example, the metallothionein gene is expressed principally in the liver, whereas the growth hormone (GH) gene, which regulates overall growth rates, is expressed in the pituitary whence the encoded protein passes into the bloodstream to increase growth rate. By fusing the metallothionein regulatory sequences to the protein-coding sequences of the GH gene, several groups have altered growth rates in mice and carcass composition in pigs (Palmiter *et al.* 1982; Hammer *et al.* 1985; Palmiter and Brinster 1986; Vize *et al.* 1988). This principle of combining regulatory elements of one gene with the structural regions of another has now been applied to many mouse model systems.

Terms used in genetic manipulation

bp: Base-pair(s) of DNA, used as a measure of length.

Chromosome map: map of the genome, classically based on location of overt traits identified by their behaviour and association with each other (linkage) in breeding experiments. Recently, RFLPs and VNTRs (q.v.) have provided far more readily mapped markers.

DNA construct: genetically engineered DNA molecules in which, usually, two or more modified DNA sequences are recombined *in vitro*, the intention being to confer modified biological specificity through new combinations of regulatory and protein-coding sequences.

DNA map: restriction enzymes, of which there are over 600, cut DNA at different specific sequences and these cut sites provide reference points along the DNA molecule over lengths of tens of base-pairs to thousands of kilobases. Such reference points can then be used to position functional sequences such as start and stop sites of mRNA synthesis, locations of regulatory regions, etc.

DNA (RNA) probe: DNA (RNA) labelled *in vitro* using ^{32}P-nucleotides is used to detect complementary DNA or RNA sequences in hybridization experiments. The probe, hybridized to its complement, is detected by autoradiography.

Encode: the amino acid sequence of a protein is encoded in the DNA sequence of the genome. Thus a gene encodes (in nucleotide sequence) the corresponding protein amino acid sequence.

Genome: the entire genetic complement of an organism; the genome of most mammals consists of between 15 and 35 chromosome pairs.

Homologous recombination: most often, DNA integrates randomly into the genome. More rarely the construct recombines into the corresponding, homologous sequences in the host genome and may replace or duplicate them. Such homologous events render gene therapy possible, though technically demanding.

kb: 10^3 bases or base-pairs.

Oligonucleotide: a short stretch of DNA sequence usually synthesized chemically.

Terms used in genetic manipulation *continued*

PCR: polymerase chain reaction. Technique for amplifying short stretches of small DNA samples. A series of 30–60 synthetic reactions is performed between two oligonucleotides within the sequence of interest resulting in its amplification of up to 10^{10}-fold. Used for analysing small numbers of, or even individual, cells in, for example, embryo sexing.

RFLP: restriction fragment length polymorphism. Due to DNA sequence variation between individuals, restriction enzyme sites may be present in the genome of one individual but absent from that of another, producing fragments of different lengths in the two individuals. Analysis of inheritance of such differences can be used to construct chromosome maps (q.v.).

Transgene: usually used to refer to a DNA construct (q.v.) after it has integrated into the host genome.

Transgenic cell: a cell or animal in which a DNA construct has integrated into the genome.

VNTR markers: variable number of tandem repeat markers. Different individuals often contain specific-sized clusters of repeated DNA sequences. Such different-sized clusters can be assigned to individuals and specific chromosomes using a limited number of families.

Making transgenics

Currently five methods are used to make transgenic mice (Figure 9.5). Of these, microinjection, sperm-mediated transfer and retroviral insertion have been used to make transgenic domestic species (Palmiter and Brinster 1986; Gandolfi *et al.* 1989; Pursel *et al.* 1989; Evans and Moor, unpublished observations). For each method a considerable amount of infrastructure is required to provide sperm and eggs or embryos and their associated culture systems, donor animals and recipients as well as necessary surgical techniques. Only these three methods are discussed in detail here; concern about the safety of retroviral insertion means that it is not used routinely for transformation of mammals, although it is the main route to transgenesis in chickens and is also used for human gene therapy. Stem cell colonization does not generate germ-line transmission and is therefore not relevant to breeding stocks.

Microinjection

In most microinjection protocols, about 200–300 eggs are obtained from females induced to superovulate by injection of FSH over 2–4 days followed by prostaglandin to release the ovulated eggs. After IVF (detailed above) the DNA construct is microinjected into the larger, male pronucleus where, in as many as 20% of cases, it integrates into the genome (Figures 9.5 and 9.6). Injected zygotes are usually cultured *in vitro* for a short time and viable embryos are transferred in small batches (20–30 for the mouse, about 20 for the pig, 2–5 for the sheep, 2–10 for the cow) to suitably primed recipients of the appropriate stage of pregnancy (Biery *et al.* 1988; Simons *et al.* 1988; Pursel *et al.* 1989).

In domestic species about 10% of the embryos survive to term and are assayed for the presence of foreign DNA by biopsy of tail or ear tissue (Hammer *et al.* 1985). DNA is extracted from the biopsy material, hybridized with a radioactively labelled DNA probe for the transgene and positive animals detected by autoradiography. Expression of the integrated DNA (transgene) can then be detected either by analysis of RNA or by antibody detection of the transgene protein in tissues or in the circulation: overall, about 0.2–3% of injected eggs result in progeny that express the transgene. Generally, farm animals are at the lower end of the range. The advantages of microinjection are: (1) its relatively long history—10 years in the mouse and 5 years in domestic species; (2) the majority of positive progeny breed as true hemizygotes, i.e. 50% of the offspring are transgenic; (3) simple culture systems under well-established conditions. However, the effort and expense involved in generating transgenics by the microinjection method, with no guarantee of successful expression, has led to the search for simpler or more reliable systems.

Embryo stem cells

Embryo stem cells provide a good method for establishing and testing transgenes in the mouse (Figure 9.5). Their use in domestic species is undetermined. Embryo stem cells are derived from the early embryo at the blastocyst stage (see p. 438) and methods have been developed to allow the culture of mouse ES cells *in vitro*. Several groups are developing similar techniques to establish sheep and pig ES cell systems (Piedrahita *et al.* 1988; Evans *et al.* 1990; Notarianni *et al.* 1991; Notarianni and Evans 1992; Notarianni and Laurie 1992; Wilmut, unpublished observations). During this culture period, DNA can be introduced into the ES cells using simple, well-established techniques and, if a selectable marker is also introduced into the cells, those cells that have taken up the DNA can be selected and grown up as a pure population (Hooper *et al.* 1987; Kuehn

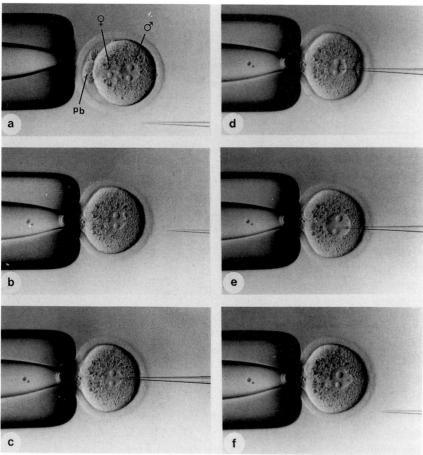

Figure 9.6 Microinjection of mouse zygote. (a) The zygote, held by suction to the pipette, contains a polar body (Pb) and larger, male (♂) and smaller, female (♀) pronuclei. (b) The injection pipette is aligned and (c) passes through the zona. (d) The pipette is 'jabbed' to ensure the plasma membrane is punctured and as the DNA solution is injected (e) the male pronucleus swells. (f) Finally the pipette is withdrawn ((a)–(f) from Monk, M. (ed.) (1987) *Mammalian development: a practical approach* by permission of the Oxford University Press).

et al. 1987). When cells from this pure, transgene-containing population are introduced into recipient blastocysts, they will differentiate and contribute to most or all of the tissues of the resulting organism. This chimeric organism will thus contain both transgenic and non-transgenic cells and, provided the transgenic ES cells have gone on to colonize the germ line, a proportion of their progeny will be homozygous transgenic individuals. The advantages of this system are thus: (1) a simpler manipulation procedure; (2) the availability of cultured cell systems; (3) an opportunity to assess gene integration and perhaps activity *in vitro*; and (4) the higher survival and transgenesis rates of manipulated animals. The main disadvantages are: (1) the chimeric nature of the transgenics with the possibility that the ES cells are not incorporated into the germ line; and (2) the difficulty of establishing and maintaining ES cells from domestic species.

Sperm-mediated transfer

Most recently, a dramatic report recapitulates an earlier discovery by Brackett *et al.* (1971) that promises to revolutionize transgenic biology. Brackett and colleagues investigated the uptake of SV40 viral DNA by rabbit sperm, and were able to show, by mixing sperm and DNA, that SV40 DNA was strongly associated with the sperm and could be passed into eggs after injection of the sperm *in utero*. This DNA was found to be still present at the 2-cell stage. Lavitrano and colleagues (1989) investigated the ability of mouse sperm to take up exogenous DNA (Figure 9.5). They incubated $1-2\times10^6$ mouse sperm/ml in a specially modified culture medium for 2–5 hours at 37 °C and then added DNA (final concentration of 0.4–2 µg/ml) for a further 30-minute incubation at 37 °C. This treated sperm was then used for IVF. Remarkably, they found that about 30% of the progeny contained the transgene. The results were complicated in that unusual arrangements of the transgene had occurred, and the transgene persisted in a non-integrated form. Furthermore, other groups have failed to reproduce these results (Brinster *et al.* 1989). Nevertheless, Lavitrano *et al.* (1989) reported that the transgene could be propagated to progeny and expression of the transgene was detected in several tissues. More recently, Gandolfi and colleagues (1989) have reported similar success in producing transgenic pigs. If this method can be routinely established, then the ability to produce transgenic animals will be within the reach of any laboratory capable of carrying out IVF.

Gene mapping

Where genetic traits have been identified, but no protein responsible for those traits has been identified, it is often difficult to identify where in the chromosome complement that gene is located, especially in domestic species when chromosome maps are of rather low resolution (Fries *et al.* 1989). Until recently, there was a large gap between the resolution of chromosome maps (about 10 000 kb) and the resolution of DNA analysis (1–100 kb). However, two techniques are helping to bridge this gap. First electrophoretic techniques capable of resolving DNA fragments in the range 100–5000 kb have been developed (Schwartz and Cantor 1984; Michiels *et al.* 1982). These electrophoretic methods are allied to the use of enzymes that cut the DNA only very rarely (about once every 200–500 kb) to generate fragments of a suitable size. In this way, DNA maps of regions of about 10 000 kb can be prepared.

Second, it has been recognized for a long time that much of the mammalian genome does not encode protein. Broadly speaking, DNA sequences are stable only when they are required for RNA or protein synthesis and, without such selective evolutionary pressure, the sequence is free to diverge. Such sequence divergence in non-coding DNA between individuals can affect the recognition sites of the restriction enzymes that cut DNA. Consequently, one individual may lack a site that is found in a second individual (Watkins 1988; Figure 9.7). This means that the two individuals produce restriction fragments of different lengths for the same region, so-called restriction fragment length polymorphisms (RFLPs). Such RFLPs can be assigned to specific chromosomes and if a genetic trait, say for wool production, has been localized to a specific chromosome also, then one can compare the inheritance of the trait with the inheritance of RFLPs along the chromosome to identify the RFLPs that map nearest to the trait. Together with long-range DNA mapping, these techniques can 'fill in' many of the gaps in the chromosome maps of domestic animals and many groups are currently engaged in mapping such genomes (Miller and Archibald 1993). The resolution of genome maps of domestic species is currently very poor. By identifying the regions of the genome to which specific traits map, it then becomes possible to map the gene more and more finely to allow its isolation. Among the genes of interest are those that confer disease resistance, alter the nature or frequency of reproductive behaviour or modify the composition or efficiency of meat, milk or wool production.

Exploiting transgenics

Ideally, the modular structure of genes should allow the synthesis of a chosen protein to be targeted to a specific tissue or at a specific time. At present, the range of regulatory sequences available is rather restricted, but several examples are worthy of consideration. In early work, the promoter most commonly used was the metallothionein promoter region

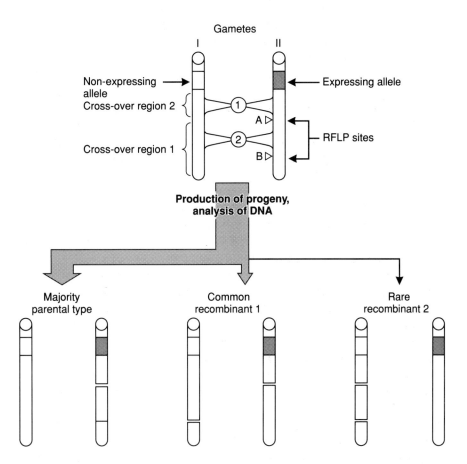

Figure 9.7 Mapping genes using DNA sequence divergence. In this example, the gene (or allele) is expressed by chromosomes of type II. These chromosomes also carry two restriction fragment length polymorphisms (RFLPs), one close to the allele (A) and one distal (B). When crossed to a chromosome from an individual carrying the non-expressing allele (type I), which does not carry RFLP sites A or B, three types of progeny may be produced. In the first, preponderant, case, the parental chromosomes are propagated and both RFLPs co-segregate with the expressing allele. Cross-overs or exchange between chromosomes at meiosis occur largely at random, the frequency depending on the distance between two markers. Hence cross-overs will occur most frequently between the distant RFLP, B, and the allele, as in recombinant 1. More rarely, cross-overs will occur between RFLP A and the allele, separating them as in recombinant 2. Thus, the RFLP that most frequently segregates with the expressing allele is the most closely linked. Mapping using VNTR sequences employs the same basic principles.

discussed above. Vize *et al.* (1988) used the human metallothionein IIA (hMT-IIA) promoter to drive a porcine GH gene and microinjected this construct into pig eggs. The aim of these experiments was to over-express the transgenic porcine GH gene in pigs to determine the effects of such expression. Of 423 injected embryos, 17 piglets were born; of these, six were transgenic and one expressed the GH transgene. This sow grew to market weight (90 kg) at 17 weeks, about 6 weeks before her littermates. However, several authors have reported severe pathologies, including liver and kidney disorder, arthritis and reproductive failure, in transgenic animals expressing high levels of GH (Pursel *et al.* 1989, 1990).

In order to avoid problems associated with poorly regulated expression, Polge and co-workers (1989) used a prolactin regulatory region to drive a GH gene in transgenic pigs. They were able to tightly regulate GH expression by inducing synthesis using sulpiride (which relieves the inhibition of prolactin by dopamine) or thyrotrophin releasing hormone, and this system promises to be useful in regulation.

An alternative to modulating the physiological system is to use the spare protein synthetic capacity of the organism to produce foreign proteins. Pursel and colleagues (1989) have investigated the expression of a series of DNA constructs in domestic species. They were able to obtain expression for a number of constructs, including those designed to over-express GH. Clearly, efficient expression of transgenes in domestic species can be obtained in these circumstances and, in many laboratories, the work of the next few years will be directed towards refining this expression.

Clark and colleagues have used transgenesis to synthesize foreign proteins in the milk of mice and sheep (Simons *et al.* 1987; Archibald *et al.* 1990; Wright *et al.* 1991). They first defined the regulatory regions of the sheep β-lactoglobulin gene by studying sheep β-lactoglobulin gene expression in transgenic mice. They then joined these regulatory sequences to the protein-coding regions for factor IX, a blood clotting factor required by some haemophiliacs. They chose this product because it is a scarce pharmaceutical compound that currently can be prepared only from human plasma and an alternative means of production would be invaluable. Although they obtained high levels of β-lactoglobulin in transgenic mice, the levels of factor IX synthesis in transgenic sheep were disappointingly low.

To address the problems of expression, a number of different gene constructs have been transferred into mice. Comparisons were made between genes with and without introns: it was found that the frequency of expression and the level of protein produced were greatest if all introns were present in the gene. Expression of α_1-antitrypsin in the sheep mammary gland was optimized using such methods. Several sheep expressing high levels of α_1-antitrypsin in their milk were produced (Wright *et al.*

1991). One ewe, called Tracy, synthesized 35 mg/ml of biologically active human protein in her milk. At current prices for α_1-antitrypsin, Tracy is a million-dollar sheep.

Paternity testing

We mentioned above that there is a considerable diversity between individuals in the sequences of non-coding DNA. Alec Jeffreys of Leicester University identified regions of the genome that are subject to especially high levels of sequence divergence, the so-called hypervariable sequences or VNTR markers (Jeffreys *et al.* 1986; Nakamura *et al.* 1987). The number and arrangement of such repeats varies between individuals and so when analysed on a gel the DNA of each individual produces a distinct pattern. The offspring will inherit half of their pattern of repeats from their mother and half from their father (Figure 9.8). This has been used in paternity testing in humans and can find the same application in testing parentage of domestic animals both in experimental and clinical situations. More recently, even more divergent (and therefore more informative) sequences have been described in human DNA. These are generated by variation in the number of short DNA sequences; the simplest of these so-called microsatellites is derived from tandem repeats of the sequence CT (Weber and May 1989). Using analysis of small blood samples, the DNA from the father, mother and progeny can be analysed to determine whether or not all the hypervariable bands in the progeny can be found in the two parents. If this is so, then there is only an exceedingly small probability that the tested putative parents are not the biological parents.

Prospects

New technologies in animal breeding are proceeding in two directions. In the first trend, attempts are being made to reduce the complexity of many procedures, to increase their efficiency, and to broaden their application. The second class of developments is toward the use of highly sophisticated techniques of transgenesis and nuclear or cellular manipulation.

The widespread use of AI is an example of a previously sophisticated technology taken to routine, practical use. It is likely that IVF will become similarly more widespread, especially if the *in vitro* development and maturation of oocytes obtained from abattoir material allows the maximum use of the female germ line. This technology has been established in

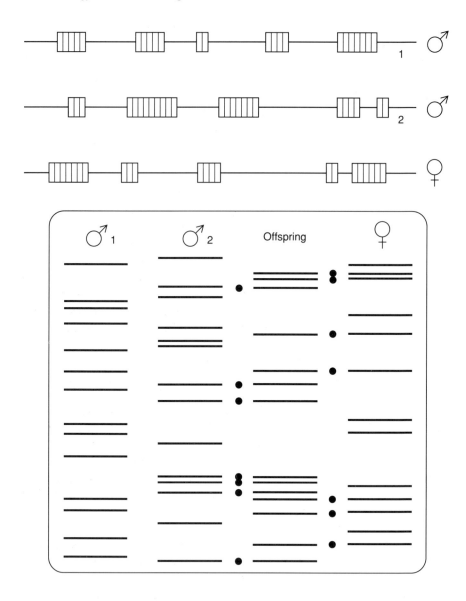

Figure 9.8 Paternity testing using minisatellite sequences. Minisatellites contain variable numbers of repeated units (open boxes) that are scattered throughout the genome (horizontal line). The locations and numbers of these are unique to the individual and when analysed on gels produce unique patterns of bands. Because half the offspring's chromosomes come from each parent, every DNA band in the offspring should be found in either the mother's or the father's pattern of bands. In this example it can be seen that the DNA from male number 2 satisfies this requirement.

most domestic species, at least in the laboratory. The techniques of parental testing using hypervariable DNA sequences are well established and should soon see commercial application if there is sufficient demand. This is likely in both livestock and in domestic pet pedigrees. Sexing embryos using PCR has been established using several DNA probes and is practical if widespread IVF is used. Similarly, if more laboratories can reproduce the experiments, producing transgenic animals by sperm-mediated transfer would be a technique available to any laboratory that can perform IVF.

This last example, however, emphasizes the need for basic work in order to generate DNA constructs suitable for transgenesis. In such a young field, it is not easy to predict the directions in which research will progress. However, some avenues seem to be especially favoured.

The alteration of growth and carcass composition in domestic species has met with mixed results. In the mouse, GH constructs resulted in pathological problems that were not so evident when growth hormone releasing factor (GRF) was used as the active protein; GRF is the hormone that stimulates GH expression and release. It may be that a more physiological response can be obtained by using a hormone one step further removed from the active events in promoting cell growth.

A second problem appears to be due to the continuous synthesis of GH in most transgenics; the natural hormone has a pulsatile release and attempts to tightly regulate GH release are likely to be more profitable (Clark *et al.* 1985). The prolactin promoter used by Polge and colleagues (1989) promises to be useful as its activity is negligible in the absence of inducers. An alternative is to use a promoter that is naturally induced in response to stimuli in the environment. In this category would be the cholecystokinin and gastrin genes, each of which is turned on in response to feeding. If these drive a GH gene, then one might expect to obtain GH synthesis in response to feeding and, if suitable signals could be found, to cause pulsatile release of GH into the circulation.

Control of reproductive behaviour is likely to be a further area of investigation. The hormonal regulation of ovulation is well established, resulting in many species in a seasonal breeding activity. The principal initiator of this pathway is the hormone melatonin, which stimulates output of gonadotrophin in response to day length. If the levels of melatonin or gonadotrophin could be altered in transgenic animals then the breeding cycle could be brought into a regulated system that is more suited to domestic conditions rather than the feral responses. It needs to be determined whether melatonin synthesis can be stimulated by elevated expression of the enzymes, such as hydroxyindole-*o*-methyltransferase. The hormonal regulation of ovulation involves complex interaction between oestrogen, FSH and luteinizing hormone (LH) and it seems unlikely that animals transgenic for these hormones will be especially useful unless either the system can be integrated or a single gene under transgenic control proves effective.

A more successful route may be to use the natural gene, present in the Booroola sheep, that causes them to release two eggs at ovulation producing twins more frequently than do most breeds of sheep (Piper *et al.* 1985). This gene is being actively sought using gene mapping techniques of the type outlined above. Transgenic biology should allow transfer of this gene into any suitable genetic background.

Several groups are attempting to transfer genes encoding cellulose-digesting enzymes to, in the first instance, mice in order to assess expression of cellulases in mice (Hazelwood and Gilbert 1989). The ultimate aim of such experiments is to take genes encoding cellulase enzymes of bacteria and to transfer them to pigs to improve the ability of these animals to digest cellulose and hemicellulose. The regulatory region used will be derived from an enzyme expressed in the pancreas, thus directing expression of the cellulase to the pancreas and resulting in its secretion from the pancreas into the small intestine. It is anticipated that such animals would obtain a greater energy yield from their feed if the cellulose content of their food was absorbed in the intestine.

Clearly, refinement of techniques designed to increase foreign protein production in either the milk or the bloodstream of transgenic animals would be of great value. Many human and animal proteins are used in therapy and are currently only available from human blood or cadavers or from slaughtered animals. The increased detection of slow virus diseases (such as scrapie in the sheep, bovine spongiform encephalopathy (BSE) in cattle and Creutzfeldt–Jakob disease in humans) has led to increasing concern about the safety of such scarce pharmaceutical proteins.

The technology of transgenesis would be revolutionized if the techniques of sperm transformation and development and maturation of oocytes *in vitro* (discussed below) were perfected for wide-scale use. If both transformed sperm and mature oocytes are available in essentially unlimited quantities then transgenesis becomes a far simpler and, potentially, much more widespread technique. It is likely then that the limiting step will become the isolation, characterization and reconstruction of suitable gene constructs and future emphasis will doubtless be on this aspect.

Finally, improvements in ES cell culture and DNA transfer have made it possible to modify endogenous genes. The site of DNA integration is usually random, but a variety of DNA constructs has been developed in order to increase the frequency with which homologous recombination occurs (Doetschmann *et al.* 1987; Thomas and Capecchi 1987; Mansour *et al.* 1988; Gossler *et al.* 1989; Zimmer and Grüss 1989). Homologous exchange between transgene and mammalian DNA is now efficient enough to use transgenes to: (1) repair a defective gene in valuable stock using a non-mutated transgene; (2) mutate to null function an undesirable or deleterious gene; or (3) alter the function or expression of an endogenous gene.

In some cases, unexpected side-effects have compromised the potential commercial value of transgenic experiments. As detailed an understanding as possible of physiological responses to transgene expression will always be an important prerequisite to the commercial exploitation of this technology. However, it does seem likely that transgenic techniques to alter growth or reproductive patterns will become well established, provided this increased sophistication in physiology and transgene design occurs. A similar increase in sophistication seems to be required to produce foreign proteins in the mammary gland of livestock species, where again basic work is directed towards determining sequences that affect protein processing and stability. Perhaps the use of transgenic animals to produce blood proteins, such as antibodies, in the bloodstream will be similarly affected by our imperfect understanding.

It seems that many biological and technical problems will need to be surmounted before the techniques of nuclear manipulation and stem cell or embryonic cell manipulation are routinely available for livestock species. Although many such techniques are well studied in the mouse, longer gestational phases make such studies more difficult in domestic species. However, recent improvement in the stability and totipotency of porcine ES cells is an example of a necessary technical advance.

Currently all mammalian nuclear transfer experiments are very laborious, error-prone and inefficient. These defects probably reflect the lack of understanding of developmental competence of nuclei, cytoplasmic competence and the influence of the cell cycle on successful reprogramming (Robl et al. 1986). Smith, L. C. et al. (1988) have shown that, in transfer of mouse pronuclei, synchrony of the cell cycle between donor and recipient embryos was about 30% more efficient than asynchronous transfers. By contrast, they found that both cytoplasts and karyoplasts from late in the cell cycle developed more frequently than those from early stages of the cell cycle. It is clear that refinement of the timing of nuclear transfers to optimize the compatibility between donor and recipient will greatly improve overall efficiency. Similarly, the data of Prather et al. (1987) showed that the competence of the oocyte recipients was affected by the age of the oocyte and a study of the ability of oocytes matured in vivo and in vitro for varying lengths of time will contribute to the maximization of the recipient's competence. The results of Cheong et al. (1993) detailed above further indicate that the early stages of the cell cycle provide the best material for further development.

A further unknown concerns the developmental ability of nuclei derived from blastocysts resulting from nuclear transfer. It seems probable that some nuclei will be capable of supporting normal development following serial transfer, but that the proportion of normal embryos will decline. As the rate of decrease will reflect the efficiency of each manipulative procedure and these are still being improved, it will be some time before an accurate estimate can be made of the ultimate potential yield of offspring from each donor embryo.

Fulka and Moor (1993) have recently described a chemical enucleation method for mouse embryos that avoids the classical manipulation normally used. If this method is suitable for domestic species, it will represent a further simplification of a complex technology.

Will such techniques find widespread use? It seems likely that it will be several years before the reliability of nuclear transfer techniques is high enough to justify its use. Currently the best success rates of nuclear transfer are well below 50% and each attempt costs many hundreds of pounds; by contrast, AI rates are over 70% and each costs only a few pounds. Nevertheless it has been estimated that a pure-bred dairy or beef cloned embryo could sell in the USA for over $100. Although such prices would not apply in Britain, it seems very likely that the technology will become financially viable in the near future.

Together, these technologies may drastically alter the efficiency and practice of livestock farming. It is important, therefore, that these applications are acceptable to the agricultural community as well as the wider public. Proposals for an open and informative registration scheme for the intended use of animals produced or modified by biotechnological processes are the most sensible way of ensuring that practical benefits, as well as any costs, are passed on to the producer and consumer. The benefits of such technologies could be very important and it must be ensured, therefore, that such technologies are implemented in a responsible fashion.

REFERENCES

Aanes W A (1988) Surgical management of foaling injuries. *Veterinary Clinics North America Equine Practice* 4(3): 417–39.

Abbitt B, Ball L, Kitto G P, Sitznan C G, Wilgenburg B, Raim L V et al. (1978) Effect of three methods of palpation for pregnancy diagnosis per rectum on embryonic and fetal attrition in cows. *Journal of the American Veterinary Medical Association* 173: 973–7.

Agrawala P L, Wagner V A, Geldermann H (1992) Sex determination and milk protein genotyping of preimplantation stage bovine embryos using multiplex PCR. *Theriogenology* 38: 969–78.

Agricultural Training Board (1989) *Artificial insemination of sheep.* TN 130.6, ATB, West Wickham, Kent, UK.

Aitken I D, Clarkson M J, Linklater K A (1990) Enzootic abortion of ewes. *Veterinary Record* 126: 136–8.

Akesson A, Henricson B (1972) Embryonic death in pigs caused by unbalanced karyotype. *Acta Veterinaria Scandinavica* 13: 151–60.

Alam M G S, Dobson H (1987) Pituitary responses to a challenge test of GnRH and oestradiol benzoate in post partum and regularly cyclic dairy cows. *Animal Reproduction Science* 14: 1–9.

Allen D (1990) *Planned beef production and marketing.* Blackwell, Oxford, pp 88–90.

Allen W R, Antczak D F, Wade J F (1989) Equine embryo transfer II. *Equine Veterinary Journal* 8

Alonso R A, Cantu J M (1982) A Robertsonian translocation in the domestic pig (Sus scrofa) 37, XX,– 13, 17, t rob(13; 17) *Annales de Genetique* 25: 50–2.

Amann R P (1989) Treatment of sperm to predetermine sex. *Theriogenology* 31: 49–60.

Anamthawat-Jonsson K, Long S E, Basrur P K, Adalsteinsson S (1992) Reciprocal translocation (13; 20) (q12; q22) in an Icelandic sheep. *Research in Veterinary Science* 52: 367–70.

Anderson S, Curran M K (1990) Selection and response within the nucleus of a sheep group-breeding scheme. *Animal Production* 51(3): 593–9.

Ansari H A, Jung H R, Heidiger R, Fries R, Konig H, Stranzinger G (1991) A balanced autosomal reciprocal translocation in an azoospermic bull. In *Proceedings 7th North American Colloquium on Domestic Animal Cytogenetics and Gene Mapping*, p 23.

Archibald A L, McClenaghan M, Hornsey V, Simon J P, Clark A J

(1990) High level expression of biologically active human α-1-antitrypsin in the milk of transgenic mice. *Proceedings of the National Academy of Sciences USA* **87**: 5178–82.

Armstrong D T, Pfitzner A P, Warnes G M, Ralph M M, Seamark R F (1983a) Endocrine responses of goats after induction of superovulation with PMSG and FSH. *Journal of Reproduction and Fertility* **67**: 395–401.

Armstrong D T, Pfitzner A P, Warnes G M, Seamark R F (1983b) Superovulation treatments and embryo transfer in Angora goats. *Journal of Reproduction and Fertility* **67**: 403–10.

Arthur G H, Noakes D E, Pearson H (1989) *Veterinary reproduction and obstetrics*, 6th edn. Bailliere Tindall, London, p 184.

Asbury A C (1984) Uterine defense mechanisms in the mare: the use of intrauterine plasma in the management of endometritis. *Theriogenology* **21**: 387–93.

Ashbrook P F (1982) Year-around breeding for uniform milk production. In *Proceedings of the Third International Conference on Goat Production and Disease, January 1982, Tucson, Arizona*, pp 153–4.

Atkins K D (1986) A genetic analysis of the components of lifetime productivity in Scottish Blackface Sheep. *Animal Production* **43**(3): 405–19.

Ayalon N (1978) A review of embryonic mortality in cattle. *Journal of Reproduction and Fertility* **54**: 483–93.

Bahri I, Bonneau M, Boscher J, Popescu C P (1984) Double heterozygote for reciprocal translocation in pigs. In *Proceedings of the 6th European Colloquium on Cytogenetics of Domestic Animals, Zurich*, pp 275–89.

Ball P J H, Lamming G E (1983) Diagnosis of ovarian acyclicity in lactating dairy cows and evaluation of treatment with GnRH or PRID. *British Veterinary Journal* **139**: 522–7.

Barnes F L, Robl J M, First N L (1987) Nuclear transplantation in mouse embryos: assessment of nuclear function.

Biology of Reproduction **36**: 1267–74.

Basrur P K, Gilman J P W (1964) Blood culture method for the study of bovine chromosomes. *Nature* **204**: 1335–7.

Becker W A (1984) *Manual of quantitative genetics*, 4th edn. Academic Enterprises, Washington.

Benmrad M, Stevenson J S (1980) Gonadotropin-releasing hormone and prostaglandin $F_{2\alpha}$ for postpartum dairy cows: Estrus, ovulation, and fertility traits. *Journal of Dairy Science* **69**: 800–11.

Berardino D Di, Iannuzzi L, Ferrara L, Matassino D (1979) A new case of Robertsonian translocation in cattle. *Journal of Heredity* **70**: 436–8.

Berland H M, Sharma A, Cribiu E P, Darre R, Boscher J, Popescu C P (1988) A new case of Robertsonian translocation in cattle. *Journal of Heredity* **79**: 33–6.

BEVA code of practice for veterinary surgeons in the UK and Ireland using artificial insemination for breeding equids.

Bichard M, David P J (1985) Effectiveness of genetic selection for prolificacy in pigs. *Journal of Reproduction and Fertility* Suppl. 33: 127–38.

Biery K A, Bondioli K R, De Mayo F J (1988) Gene transfer by pronuclear injection in the bovine. *Theriogenology* **29**: 224.

Blackmore D K (1960) Some observations on dystokia in the ewe. *Veterinary Record* **72**: 631–5.

Blockley M A de B, Wilkins J F (1984) Field application of the ram serving capacity test. In Lindsay D R, Pearce D T (eds) *Reproduction in sheep*. Cambridge University Press, Cambridge. pp 53–8.

Bloom S E, Goodpasture C (1976) An improved technique for selective silver staining of nucleolar organiser regions in human chromosomes. *Human Genetics* **34**: 199–206.

Boland M P, Crosby T F, Gordon I (1982) Induction of lambing: comparison of the effects of prostaglandin, oestradiol benzoate and dexamethasone. *Journal of Agricultural Science* **98**(2): 391–5.

Bongso A, Basrur P K (1976) Chromosome anomalies in Canadian Guernsey bulls. *Cornell Veterinarian* **66**: 476–89.

Bonneau M, Boscher J, Delate J J, Legault C, Popescu C P (1991) Deux nouvelles translocations reciproques impliquant le chromosome 6 chez le porc domestique. *Annales de Genetique* **34**: 65–9.

Borsberry S, Dobson H (1989) Periparturient diseases and their effect on reproductive performance in five dairy herds. *Veterinary Record* **124**: 217–19.

Bostedt H, Hirsch J, Rudloff P R, Sobiraj A (1984) Beta-blocker carazolol ('Suacron') influencing parturition in sows. In *Proceedings of the International Pig Veterinary Society*, p 278.

Boundy T (1985) *Care and examination of rams*, Vet 41. Unit for Veterinary Continuing Education, The Royal Veterinary College, University of London.

Boundy T (1992) Routine ram examination. *In Practice* **14**(5): 219–28.

Bouters R, Bonte P, Spincemaille J, Vandeplassche M (1974) Het chromosomenonderzoek bijde huisdieren 11 De afwijkingeninde geslachtschromosomen als oorzakelijke of begeleidnede factor van onvruchtbaarheid. *Vlams Diergeneeskungig Tijdschrift* **43**: 85–91.

Bowen J M (1987) Venereal diseases of stallions. In Robinson N E (ed) *Current therapy in equine medicine*. W B Saunders, Philadelphia, pp 567–71.

Bracher V, Allen W R (1992) Videoendoscopic evaluation of the mare's uterus I: Findings in normal fertile mares. *Equine Veterinary Journal* **24**: 274–8.

Bracher V, Neuschaefer A, Allen W R (1991) The effect of intra-uterine infusion of kerosene on the endometrium of mares. *Journal of Reproduction and Fertility* Suppl. 44, 706–7.

Bracher V, Mathais S, Allen W R (1992) Videoendoscopic evaluation of the mare's uterus II: Findings in subfertile mares. *Equine Veterinary Journal* **24**: 279–84.

Brackett B G, Baranska W, Sawicki W, Koprowski H (1971) Uptake of heterologous genome by mammalian spermatozoa and its transfer to ova through fertilization. *Proceedings of the National Academy of Sciences USA* **68**: 353–7.

Bradford G E, Hart R, Quirke J F, Land R B (1972) Genetic control of the duration of gestation in sheep. *Journal of Reproduction and Fertility* **30**: 459–63.

Bradley A, Evans M, Kaufman M H, Robertson E (1984) Formation of germ line chimaeras from embryo-derived teratocarcinoma cell lines. *Nature* **309**: 255–6.

Bretzlaff K N, Lock T F, Badertscher R (1985) Ultrasound detection of embryonic and fetal death in a dairy goat herd. *Abstracts from the Eighteenth Meeting Midwestern Section American Society of Animal Science, Chicago*, p 120.

Bretzlaff K N, Elmore R G, Nuti L C (1989) Use of an enzyme immunoassay to determine concentrations of progesterone in caprine plasma and milk. *Journal of the American Veterinary Medical Association* **194**(5): 664–8.

Brinsko S P, Varner D D (1992) Artificial insemination and preservation of semen. *Veterinary Clinics North America Equine Practice* **8**(1): 205–19.

Brinster R L, Sandgren E P, Behringer R R, Palmiter R D (1989) No simple solution for making transgenic mice. *Cell* **59**: 239–41.

Bruere A N (1969) Male sterility and an autosomal translocation in Romney sheep. *Cytogenetics* **8**: 209–18.

Bruere A N (1974) The segregation patterns and fertility of sheep heterozygous and homozygous for three different Robertsonian translocations. *Journal of Reproduction and Fertility* **41**: 453–64.

Bruere A N (1975) Further evidence of normal fertility and the formation of balanced gametes in sheep with one or more different Robertsonian translocations. *Journal of Reproduction and Fertility* 45: 323–31.

Bruere A N, Chapman H M (1973) Autosomal translocations in two exotic breeds of cattle in New Zealand. *Veterinary Record* 92: 615–18.

Bruere A N, Mills R A (1971) Observations on the incidence of Robertsonian translocations and associated testicular changes in a flock of New Zealand Romney sheep. *Cytogenetics* 10: 260–72.

Bruere A N, Chapman H M, Wyllie DR (1972) Chromosome polymorphism and its possible implications in the select Drysdale breed of sheep. *Cytogenetics* 11: 233–46.

Bruere A N, Evans E P, Burtenshaw MD, Brown B B (1978a) Centric fusion polymorphisms in Romney Marsh sheep of England. *Journal of Heredity* 69: 8–10.

Bruere A N, Blue M G, Jaine P M, Walker K S, Henderson L M, Chapman H M (1978b) Preliminary observations on the equine XO syndrome. *New Zealand Veterinary Journal* 26: 145–6.

Buckrell B C (1988) Applications of ultrasonography in reproduction in sheep and goats. *Theriogenology* 29(1): 71–84.

Cash R S G, Ousey J C, Rossdale P D (1985) Rapid strip test method to assist management of foaling mares. *Equine Veterinary Journal* 17: 61.

Caspersson T, Faber S, Foley G E, Knudynowski J, Modest EJ, Simonsson E et al. (1968) Chemical differentiation along metaphase chromosomes. *Experimental Cell Research* 49: 219–22.

Chemineau P (1983) Effect on oestrus and ovulation of exposing creole goats to the male at three times of the year. *Journal of Reproduction and Fertility* 67: 65–72.

Cheong H-T, Takahashi Y, Kanagawa H (1993) Birth of mice after transplantation of earch cell-cycle-stage embryonic nuclei into enucleated oocytes. *Biology of Reproduction* 48: 958–63.

Chew B P, Keller H F, Erb R E, Malven P V (1977) Periparturient concentrations of prolactin, progesterone and the estrogens in blood plasma of cows retaining and not retaining fetal membranes. *Journal of Animal Science* 44: 1055–60.

Christenson R K (1993) Ovulation rate and embryonic survival in Chinese Meishan and white crossbred pigs. *Journal of Animal Science* 71: 3060–6.

Church R B (1987) Embryo manipulation and gene transfer in domestic animals. *Trends in Biotechnology* 5: 13–19.

Clark K, Leman A D (1984) The effects of weaning age on subsequent litter size and farrowing rate in a large U.S. confinement unit. In *Proceedings of the International Pig Veterinary Society*, p 357.

Clark R G, Jansson J O, Isacsson O, Robinson I C A F (1985) Intravenous growth hormone: growth responses to patterned infusions in hypophysectomised rats. *Journal of Endocrinology* 104: 53–61.

Cole D J A (1990) Nutritional strategies to optimize reproduction in pigs. In Cole D J A, Foxcroft G R, Weir B J (eds) *Control of pig reproduction*. Journals of Reproduction and Fertility Ltd, Cambridge, pp 67–82.

Colenbrander B, Kemp B (1990) Factors influencing semen quality in pigs. In Cole D J A, Foxcroft G R, Weir B J (eds) *Control of pig reproduction*. Journals of Reproduction and Fertility Ltd, Cambridge, pp 105–15.

Colenbrander B, Feitsma H, Grooten H J (1993) Optimizing semen production for artificial insemination in swine. In Foxcroft G R, Hunter M G, Doberska C (eds) *Control of pig reproduction IV*. The Journals of Reproduction and Fertility Ltd, Cambridge, pp 207–15.

Conboy H S (1992) Training the novice stallion for artificial breeding. *Veteri-*

nary Clinics North America Equine Practice **8**(1): 101–11.

Coulter G H, Foote R H (1979) Bovine testicular measurements as indicators of reproductive performance and their relationship to productive tracts in cattle: a review. *Theriogenology* **11**: 297–311.

Coulter G H, Mapeltoft R J, Kobuz G C, Cates W F (1987) Scrotal circumference of two-year-old bulls of several beef breeds *Theriogenology* **27**: 485–91.

Cox J E, Redhead P, Dawson F (1986) Comparison of the measurement of plasma testosterone and plasma oestrogens for the diagnosis of cryptorchidism in the horse. *Equine Veterinary Journal* **18**(3): 179–82.

Cran D G (1992) Gender preselection in mammals In Lauria A, Gandolfi F (eds) *Embryonic manipulation and genetic engineering.* Portland Press, London, pp 125–34.

Cran D G, Johnson, L, Miller N G A, Cochrane D, Polge C (1993) Production of bovine calves following separation of X- and Y-chromosome-bearing sperm after IVF. *Veterinary Record* **132**: 40–1.

Cribiu E P, Matejka M, Darre R, Durand V, Berland H M, Bouvet A (1989) Identification of chromosomes involved in a Robertsonian translocation in cattle. *Genetics Selection Evolution* **21**: 555–60.

Darre R, Berland H M, Quiennec G (1974) Une nouvelle translocation Robertsonienne chez les bovins. *Annales de Genetique et de Selection Animale* **6**: 297–304.

Davies G, Heard T W, Jackson G H, Lund L J, Miller W M, Muirhead M R (1985) *Pig Health Recording, Production and Finance, A Producer's Guide.* The Pig Veterinary Society, Malmesbury, Wilts.

de Alba J, Kennedy BW (1985) Milk production in the Latin-American milking Criollo and its crosses with the Jersey. *Animal Production* **41**(2): 143–50.

Dobson H (1978) Radioimmunoassay of FSH in the plasma of post-partum dairy cows. *Journal of Reproduction and Fertility* **52**: 45–9.

Dobson H (1988) Softening and dilation of the uterine cervix. In Clark J R (ed) *Oxford Review in Reproductive Biology,* vol 10. Oxford University Press, Oxford, pp 491–514.

Dobson H, Alam M G S (1987) Preliminary investigations into the endocrine feedback system of subfertile cows: location of a common lesion (rate limiting step). *Journal of Endocrinology* **113**: 167–71.

Dobson H, Fitzpatrick R J (1976) Clinical application of the progesterone-in-milk test. *British Veterinary Journal* **132**: 538–42.

Dobson H, Cooper M J, Furr B J A (1975) Synchronization of oestrus with ICI 79,939 an analogue of PGF2 alpha and associated changes in plasma progesterone, oestradiol 17 beta and LH in heifers. *Journal of Reproduction and Fertility* **42**: 141–4.

Doetschmann T, Gregg R G, Maeda N, Hooper M L, Melton D W, Thomson S *et al.* (1987) Targetted correction of a mutant HPRT gene in mouse embryonic stem cells. *Nature* **1330**: 576–8.

Dusza L, Tilton J E (1990) Role of prolactin in the regulation of ovarian function in pigs. In Cole D J A, Foxcroft G R, Weir B J (eds) *Control of pig reproduction.* Journals of Reproduction and Fertility Ltd, Cambridge, pp 33–45.

Dutrillaux B (1973) Nouveau systeme de marquage chromosomique: les bandes T. *Chromosoma* **41**: 395–402.

Dutrillaux B, Lejeune J (1971) Sur une nouvelle technique d'analyse du caryotype humain. *Comptes Rendus de L'Academie de Science. Paris Series D* **272**: 2638–40.

Dutrillaux B, Laurent C, Couturier J, Lejeune J (1973) Coloration des chromosomes humains par l'acridine orange apres traitment par le 5-bromdeoxyuridine. *Comptes Rendus de L'Academie de Science (Paris)* **276**: 3179–81.

Eales A, Small J (1995) *Practical lambing and lamb care: a veterinary guide*, 2nd edn. Longman, London.

East N E (1983) Pregnancy toxaemia, abortions, and periparturient diseases. *Veterinary Clinics of North America: Large Animal Practice* **5**(3): 601–18.

Eiberg H (1974) New selective giemsa technique for human chromosomes, C_d staining. *Nature* **248**: 55.

Einarsson S, Rojkittikhun T (1993) Effects of nutrition on pregnant and lactating sows. In Foxcroft G R, Hunter M G, Doberska C (eds) *Control of pig reproduction IV*. The Journals of Reproduction and Fertility Ltd, Cambridge, pp 229–39.

Eldridge F E (1974) A dicentric Robertsonian translocation in a Dexter cow. *Journal of Heredity* **65**: 353–5.

Eldridge F E (1985) *Cytogenetics of livestock*. AVI Publishing Company Incorporated, Westport, Connecticut.

Eldridge F E, Blazak W K (1977) Chromosome analysis of fertile female heterosexual twins in cattle. *Journal of Dairy Science* **60**: 458–63.

Ellsworth S M, Paul R S, Bunch T D (1979) A 14/28 dicentric Robertsonian translocation in a Holstein cow. *Theriogenology* **11**: 165–71.

Elsen J M, Bodin L, Thimonier J (1991) (eds) *Major genes for reproduction in sheep*. Proceedings of the 2nd International Workshop, Toulouse, France, July 1990. Institute National de la Recherche Agronomique, Paris.

Evans G, Maxwell W M C (1987) *Salamon's artificial insemination of sheep and goats*. Butterworths, Sydney.

Evans H E, Sack W O (1973) Prenatal development of domestic and laboratory mammals: growth curves, external features and selected references. *Anatomy, Histology and Embryology* **2**: 11–45.

Evans M J, Notarianni E, Laurie S, Moor R M (1990) Derivation and preliminary characterization of pluripotent cell lines from porcine and bovine blastocysts. *Theriogenology* **33**: 125–8.

Falconer DS (1989) *Introduction to quantitative genetics*, 3rd edn. Longman, Harlow, pp 163–86.

Fechheimer N S, Herschler M S, Gilmore LO (1963) Sex chromosome mosaicism in unlike sexed cattle twins. In *Proceedings of the 11th International Conference on Genetics, The Hague*, vol 1, p 265.

Findlater R C F, Haresign W, Curnock R M, Beck N F G (1991) Evaluation of intrauterine insemination of sheep with frozen semen: effects of time of insemination and semen dose on conception rates. *Animal Production* **53**(1): 89–96.

Flint A P F, Ricketts A P (1979) Control of placental endocrine function; role of enzyme activation in the onset of labour. *Journal of Steroid Biochemistry* **11**: 493–500.

Flowers W L, Esbenade K L (1993) Optimizing management of natural and artificial matings in swine. In Foxcroft G R, Hunter M G, Doberska C (eds) *Control of pig reproduction IV*. The Journals of Reproduction and Fertility Ltd, Cambridge, pp 217–28.

Forbes J M (1967) Factors affecting the gestation length in sheep. *Journal of Agricultural Science* **68**: 191–4.

Ford C E and Clegg H M (1969) Reciprocal translocations. *British Medical Bulletin* **25**: 110–114.

Ford C E, Pollock D L, Gustavsson I (1980) Proceedings of the 1st International Conference for the Standardisation of Banded Karyotypes of Domestic Animals, Reading, 1976. *Hereditas* **92**: 145–62.

Ford S P, Youngs C R (1993) Early embryonic development in prolific Meishan pigs. In Foxcroft G R, Hunter M G, Doberska C (eds) *Control of pig reproduction IV*. The Journals of Reproduction and Fertility Ltd, Cambridge, pp 271–8.

Forster M, Willeke H, Richter L (1981) Eine autosomale, reziproke 1/16 translocation bei Deutschen Landrasse Schweinen. *Zuchthygiene* **16**: 54–7.

Foster D L, Yellon S M, Olster D H (1985) Internal and external determinants of the timing of puberty in the female. *Journal of Reproduction and Fertility* 75: 327–44.

French Anderson W (1992) Human gene therapy. *Science* 256: 808–15.

Fries R, Beckmann J S, Georges M, Soller M, Womack J (1989) The bovine gene map. *Animal Genetics* 20: 3–29.

Fulka J Jr, Moor R M (1993) Noninvasive chemical enucleation of mouse oocytes. *Molecular Reproduction and Development* 34: 427–30.

Gall C (1981) Goats in agriculture: distribution, importance and development. In Gall C (ed) *Goat production.* Academic Press, London, pp. 1–34.

Gandolfi F, Lavitrano M, Camaioni A, Spadafora C, Siracusa G, Lauria A (1989) The use of sperm-mediated gene transfer for the generation of transgenic pigs. *Journal of Reproduction and Fertility Abstract Series,* No. 4, p 10.

Gary F, Concordet D, Berland H M, Berthelot X, Darre R (1991) 1/29 Robertsonian translocation in Blonde d'Aquitaine bulls: frequency and effects on semen characteristic. *Genetics Selection Evolution* 23 (suppl. 1): 117s–19s.

Genus (1993) *Genus Dairy Bulls 1993.*

Genus (1994) *Dairy Directory 1994.*

Gibson J P (1987) The options and prospects for genetically altering milk composition in dairy cattle. *Animal Breeding Abstracts* 55: 231–43.

Gilbert R O, Marlow C H B (1992) A field study of patterns of unobserved foetal losses as determined by rectal palpation in foaling, barren and maiden Thoroughbred mares. *Equine Veterinary Journal* 24: 184–7.

Ginther O J (1986) *Ultrasonic imaging and reproductive events in the mare.* W. I. Equiservices, Cross Plains.

Ginther O J (1989) Twin embryos in the mare II: post fixation embryo reduction. *Equine Veterinary Journal* 21: 171–4.

Ginther O J (1989) Twin embryos in the mare I: from ovulation to fixation. *Equine Veterinary Journal* 21: 166–70.

Ginther O J (1990) Prolonged luteal activity in mares: a semantic quagmire. *Equine Veterinary Journal* 22: 152–6.

Giovanni A de, Succi G, Molteni L, Castiglioni M (1979) A new autosomal translocation in Grigia Alpina breed. *Abstracts of the 1st International Symposium on Research in Cytogenetics and Disease Resistance in Animals and Man.*

Giovanni A de, Popescu C P, Succi G, Molteni L (1980) Meiotic study of a new autosomal translocation in the Alpine Grey Cattle. In *Proceedings of the 4th European Colloquium on Cytogenetics of Domestic Animals, Uppsala,* pp 158–63.

Glahn-Luft B, Wassmuth R (1980) *Proceedings of the 31st Annual Meeting of the European Association of Animal Production.*

Gluzman Y, Schenk T (1983) *Enhancers and eukaryotic gene expression.* Cold Spring Harbor Laboratory, New York.

Goodman R L (1988) Neuroendocrine control of the ovine estrous cycle. In Knobil E, Neill J J (eds) *The physiology of reproduction.* Raven Press, New York, pp 1929–69.

Goodpasture C, Bloom S E (1975) Visualization of nucleolar organiser regions in mammalian chromosomes using silver staining. *Chromosoma* 53: 37–50.

Gordon I (1983) Control and manipulation of reproduction in sheep. In Gordon I (ed) *Controlled breeding in farm animals.* Pergamon Press, Oxford, pp 155–290.

Gordon I, Lu K H (1990) Production of embryos *in vitro* and its impact on livestock production. *Theriogenology* 33: 77–88.

Gossler A, Joyner A L, Rossant J, Sharnes W C (1989) Mouse embryonic stem cells and reporter constructs to detect developmentally regulated genes. *Science* 244: 463–5.

Grosveld F, van Assendelft G B, Greeves D R, Kollias G (1987) Position-independent, high-level expression of the human ß-globin gene in transgenic mice. *Cell* **51**: 975–85.

Gu Y, Haley C S, Thompson R (1989) Estimates of genetic and phenotypic parameters of growth and carcase traits from closed lines of pigs on restricted feeding. *Animal Production* **49**(3): 467–76.

Gunn R G (1968) A note on difficult birth in Scottish hill flocks. *Animal Production* **10**: 213–15.

Gurdon J B (1974) *The control of gene expression in animal development.* Clarendon Press, Oxford.

Gustavsson I (1979) Symposium: Cytogenetics of farm animals. Distribution and effects of the 1/29 Robertsonian translocation in cattle. *Journal of Dairy Science* **62**: 825–35.

Gustavsson I (1984) Reciprocal translocations in the pig (an interim report of a Swedish survey). In *Proceedings of the 6th European Colloquium on Cytogenetics of Domestic animals, Zurich*, pp 80–6.

Gustavsson I, Jonsson L (1991) Partial monosomy 14 and partial trisomy 15 in stillborn piglets produced by a boar carrying a rcp(14; 15) (q29; q24). In *Proceedings 7th North American Colloquium on Domestic Animal Cytogenetics and Gene Mapping*, p 1.

Gustavsson I, Rockborn G (1964) Chromosome abnormality in three cases of lymphatic leukaemia in cattle. *Nature* **203**: 990.

Gustavsson I, Settergren I (1984) Reciprocal translocation and transfer of centromeric heterochromatin in the domestic pig karyotype. *Hereditas* **100**: 1–5.

Gustavsson I, Settergren I, King W A (1982) Identification of three spontaneous reciprocal translocations in the domestic pig. In *Proceedings of the 5th European Colloquium on Cytogenetics of Domestic Animals, Milan*, pp 281–7.

Gustavsson I, Villagomez D A F, Alabay B, Ploen L (1989a) Reciprocal chromosome translocation, rcp(2p$^+$; 14q$^-$) in a boar demonstrating testicular hypoplasia, abnormal semen picture and decreased litter size. In *Proceedings of the 6th North American Colloquium on Cytogenetics of Domestic Animals, West LaFayette*, p 5.

Gustavsson I, Switonski M, Iannuzzi L, Ploen L, Larsson K (1989b) Banding studies and synaptonemal complex analysis of an X–autosome translocation in the pig. *Cytogenetics and Cell Genetics* **50**: 188–94.

Hageltorn M, Gustavsson I, Zech L (1973) The Q- and G- banding patterns of a t(11p$^+$; 15q$^-$) in the domestic pig. *Hereditas* **75**: 147–51.

Hageltorn M, Gustavsson I, Zech L (1976) Detailed analysis of a reciprocal translocation (13q$^-$; 14q$^+$) in the domestic pig by G- and Q- staining techniques. *Hereditas* **83**: 268–72.

Haibel G K (1988) Real-time ultrasonic fetal head measurement and gestational age in dairy goats. *Theriogenology* **30**(6): 1053–7.

Haley C S, Lee G J (1993) Genetic basis of prolificacy in Meishan pigs. In Foxcroft G R, Hunter M G, Doberska C (eds) *Control of pig reproduction IV.* The Journals of Reproduction and Fertility Ltd, Cambridge, pp 247–59.

Halnan C R (1985) Sex chromosome mosaicism and infertility in mares. *Veterinary Record* **116**: 542–3.

Hammer R E, Pursel V G, Rexroad C E Jr, Wall R J, Bolt D J, Ebert K *et al.* (1985) Production of transgenic rabbits, sheep and pigs by microinjection. *Nature* **315**: 680–3.

Hanada H, Muramatsu S, Abe T, Fukjshima T (1981) Robertsonian chromosome polymorphism found in a local herd of Japanese Black cattle. *Annales de Genetique et de Selection Animale* **13**: 205–11.

Handyside A, Hooper M L, Kaufman M A, Wilmut I (1987) Towards the isolation of embryonal stem cell lines from the sheep. *Roux's Archive of Developmental Biology* **196**: 185–90.

Hanrahan J P, Quirke J F (1985) Contribution of variation in ovulation rate and embryo survival to within breed variation in litter size. In Land R B and Robinson D W (eds) *Genetics of reproduction in sheep.* Butterworths, London, pp 193–201.

Hansen-Melander E, Melander Y (1970) Mosaicism for translocation heterozygosity in a malformed pig. *Hereditas* **64**: 199–202.

Haresign W (1990) Controlling reproduction in sheep. Proceedings of BSAP conference: New Developments in Sheep Production 1989, Malvern, UK.

Haresign W (1991) Breeding manipulation in sheep with melatonin. In *Sheep Veterinary Society Proceedings of Meetings 1989–90*, vol 14, pp 104–12.

Hartigan P J (1977) The role of non-specific uterine infection in the infertility of clinically normal repeat-breeder cows. *Veterinary Science Communications* **1**: 307–21.

Hartigan P J (1979) Some data on the length of gestation and on dystokia in primiparous cows in a Grade A Charollais herd. *Irish Vet. J.* **33**: 7–11.

Hartigan P J, Griffin J F T, Nunn W R (1974) Some observations on *Corynebacterium pyogenes* infection of the bovine uterus. *Theriogenology* **1**: 153–67.

Harvey M J A (1976) Veterinary cytogenetics. *Veterinary Record* **98**: 479–81.

Hasler J F, McCauley A D, Schermerhorn E C, Foote R H (1983) Superovulatory responses of Holstein cows. *Theriogenology* **19**: 83–100.

Hazelwood G P, Gilbert H J (1989) Genetic engineering and ruminant digestion. In *Bioscience in Animal Production. Royal Agricultural Society of England International Symposium,* pp 79–86. Stoneleigh, England.

Heap R B, Davis A J, Fleet I R, Goode J A, Hamon M, Nowak R A et al. (1988) Maternal recognition of pregnancy. In *Proceedings 11th International Congress on Animal Reproduction and A.I., Dublin,* vol 5, pp 55–60.

Hemsworth P H, Hansen C, Winfield C G (1989) The influence of mating conditions on the sexual behaviour of male and female pigs. *Applied Animal Behaviour Science* **23**: 207–14.

Henderson D (1985) Control of the breeding season in sheep and goats. *In Practice* **7**(4): 118–23.

Hindson J (1989) Examination of the sheep flock before tupping. *In Practice* **11**(4): 149–55.

Hindson J C, Winter A C (1990) *Outline of Clinical Diagnosis in Sheep,* Wright, London.

Hinrichs K (1992) Embryo transfer. In Robinson N E (ed) *Current therapy in equine medicine,* 3rd edn. W B Saunders, Philadelphia, pp 637–40.

Hinrichs K, Hunt P R (1990) Ultrasound as an aid to diagnosis of granulosa cell tumour in the mare. *Equine Veterinary Journal* **22**: 99–103.

Holdsworth R J, Heap R B, Booth J M, Hamon M (1982) A rapid direct RIA for the measurement of oestrone sulphate in the milk of dairy cows and its use in pregnancy diagnosis. *Journal of Endocrinology* **95**: 7–12.

Hook, EB (1977) Exclusion of chromosomal mosaicism: Tables of 90%, 95%, and 99% confidence limits and comments on use. *American Journal of Human Genetics* **29**: 94–7.

Hooper M, Hardy K, Handyside A, Hunter S, Monte M (1987) HPRT-deficient (Lesch–Nyhan) mouse embryos derived from germ line colonization by cultured cells. *Nature* **326**: 292–5.

Horzinek M C, den Boon J A, Snijder E J, Chirnside E D, de Vries A A F, Spaan W J M (1991) The virus of equine arteritis. In *Proceedings Equine Infectious Diseases VI,* pp 201–5.

Howarth S, Lucke V M, Pearson H (1991) Squamous cell carcinoma of the equine external genitalia: a review and assessment of penile amputation and urethrostomy as a surgical treatment. *Equine Vet. J.* **23**: 53–8.

Howlett S K, Barton S C, Surani M A (1987) Nuclear cytoplasmic interactions following nuclear transplantation in mouse embryos. *Development* **101**: 915–23.

Hughes J P, Trommershausen-Smith A (1977) Infertility in the horse associated with chromosomal abnormalities. *Australian Veterinary Journal* 53: 253–7.

Hughes J P, Kennedy P C, Benirschke K (1975) XO-gonadal dysgenesis in the mare (Report of two cases) *Equine Veterinary Journal* 7: 109–12.

Hurtgen J (1987) Stallion genital abnormalities. In Robinson N E (ed) *Current therapy in equine medicine*, 2nd edn. W B Saunders, Philadelphia, pp 558–62.

Hyman J M, Poulding R H (1972) In Warley G D (ed) *Animal tissue culture*. Butterworths, London. pp 147–165.

Iannuzzi I, Rangel-Figueiredo T, di Meo G P, Ferrara L (1991) A new centric fusion translocation in cattle. In *Proceedings 7th North American Colloquium on Domestic Animals Cytogenetics and Gene Mapping*, p 24.

ISCN (1978) An international system for human cytogenetic nomenclature, 1978. *Cytogenetics and Cell Genetics* 21: 309–404.

ISCNDA (1989) (1990) International system for cytogenetic nomenclature of domestic animals. *Cytogenetics and Cell Genetics* 53: 65–79.

Jackson P G G (1972) *Dystocia in the sow*. FRCVS Thesis.

Jainudeen M R, Hafez E S E (1987) Gestation, prenatal physiology and parturition. In Hafez E S E (ed) *Reproduction in farm animals*. Lea and Febiger, Philadelphia, pp 229–59.

Jeffcott L B, Rossdale P D, Freestone J, Frank C J, Towers-Clarke P F (1982) An assessment of wastage in Thoroughbred racing from conception to 4 years of age. *Equine Veterinary Journal* 14: 185–98.

Jeffreys A J, Wilson V, Thein S L (1986) Individual-specific 'fingerprints' of human DNA. *Nature* 316: 76–9.

Johnson L A (1992) Recent progress in preselection of swine for sex. *Pig News and Information* 13: 63N–65N.

Johnson L A, Flook J P, Hawk H W (1989) Sex preselection in rabbits: live births from X and Y sperm separated by DNA and cell sorting. *Biology of Reproduction* 41: 199–203.

Johnson R K, Zimmerman D R, Lamberson W R, Sasaki S (1985) Influencing prolificacy of sows by selection for physiological factors. *Journal of Reproduction and Fertility* Suppl. 33: 139–49.

Jost A, Vigier B, Prepin J, Perchellet J (1973) Studies on sex differentiation in mammals. *Recent Progress in Hormone Research* 29: 1–41.

Kaker M L, Murray R D, Dobson H (1984) Plasma hormone changes in cows during induced or spontaneous calvings and the early post partum period. *Veterinary Record* 115: 378–82.

Kastelic J P, Curran S, Pierson R A, Ginther O J (1988) Ultrasonic evaluation of the bovine conceptus. *Theriogenology* 29: 39–54.

Keeling B J, Crighton D B (1984) Reversibility of the effects of active immunization against LH-RH. In Crighton D B (ed) *Immunological aspects of reproduction in mammals*. Butterworths, London, pp 379–99.

Kenny R M (1978) Cyclic and pathologic changes in the mare endometrium as detected by biopsy with a note on early embryonic death. *Journal of the American Veterinary Medical Association* 172: 241.

Kenny R M (1983) *Manual for clinical fertility evaluation of the stallion*. Society for Theriogenology, Hasting, N E.

Kenny R M, Cummings M R (1990) Potential control of stallion penile shedding of *Pseudomonas aeruginosa* and *Klebsiella pneumoniae*. In *Proceedings Symposium Voortplanting Pard, Gent, Belgium*.

Kenny R M, Bergman R V, Cooper W L, Morse G W (1975) Minimal contamination techniques for breeding mares: techniques and preliminary findings. In *Proceedings 21st American Association Equine Practice*, p 327.

Kent M G, Shoffner R N, Buoen L, Weber A F (1986) XY sex reversal syndrome in the domestic horse. *Cytogenetics and Cell Genetics* 42: 8–18.

King W A, Gustavsson I, Popescu C P, Linares T (1981) Gametic products transmitted by rcp(13q$^-$; 14q$^+$) translocation heterozygous pigs and resulting embryonic loss. *Hereditas* 95: 239–46.

Kirkbride C A (1982) Diagnostic approach to abortions in cattle. *The Compendium on Continuing Veterinary Education* 4 (suppl.): 341–6.

Klug E (1987) Ejaculation failure. In Robinson N E (ed) *Current therapy in equine medicine*, 2nd edn. W B Saunders, Philadelphia, pp 562–3.

Kovacs A, Meszaros I, Sellyei M, Vass L (1973) Mosaic centric fusion in a Holstein Friesian bull. *Acta Biologica Academiae Scientiarum Hungaricae* 24: 215–20.

Kuehn M R, Bradley A, Robertson E J, Evans M J (1987) A potential animal model for Lesch–Nyhan syndrome through introduction of HPRT mutations into mice. *Nature* 326: 295–8.

Kuokkanen M-T, Makinen A (1987) A reciprocal translocation (7q$^-$; 12q$^+$) in the domestic pig. *Hereditas* 106: 147–9.

Kuokkanen M-T, Makinen A (1988) Reciprocal chromosome translocations, (1p$^-$; 11q$^+$) and (1p$^+$; 15q$^-$) in domestic pigs with reduced litter size. *Hereditas* 109: 69–73.

Land R B, Robinson D W (1985) *Genetics of reproduction in sheep.* Butterworths, London.

Land R B, Atkins K D, Roberts R C (1983) Genetic improvement of reproductive performance. In Haresign W (ed) *Sheep production.* Butterworths, London, pp 515–35.

Latt S A (1973) Micro-fluorometric detection of deoxyribonucleic acid replication in human metaphase chromosomes (33258 Hoechst/BrdU fluorescence). *Proceedings of the National Academy of Sciences USA* 70: 3395–9.

Lavitrano M, Camaioni A, Fazio V M, Dolci S, Farace M G, Spadafora C (1989) Sperm cells as vectors for introducing foreign DNA into eggs: genetic transformation of mice. *Cell* 57: 717–23.

Lawson J L, Forrest D W, Shelton M (1984) Reproductive response to suckling manipulation in Spanish does. *Theriogenology* 21(5): 747–55.

Lee G J, Land R B (1985) Testis size LH response to LH-RH as male criteria of female reproductive performance. In Land RB, Robinson DW (eds) *Genetics of reproduction in sheep.* Butterworths, London, pp 333–42.

Leonard M, Kirzenbann M, Cotinot C, Chené P, Heyman Y, Shunarka M G *et al.* (1987) Sexing bovine embryos using Y chromosome specific DNA probe. *Theriogenology* 27: 248.

Lewis W H E (1979) Performance testing—development and achievements. British Cattle Breeders Club, Winter Conference, Cambridge 1979. Digest no. 34.

Ley W B, Bowen J M, Sponenberg D P, Lessard P N (1989) Dimethyl sulfoxide intrauterine therapy in the mare: effects on endometrial histological features and biopsy classification. *Theriogenology* 29: 1091–8.

Locniskar F, Gustavsson I, Hageltorn M, Zech L (1976) Cytological origin and points of exchange of a reciprocal chromosome translocation (1p$^-$; 6q$^+$) in the domestic pig. *Hereditas* 83: 272–5.

Logue D N (1978) Chromosome banding studies in cattle. *Research in Veterinary Science* 25: 1–6.

Logue D N, Harvey M J A (1978) A 14/20 Robertsonian translocation in Swiss Simmental cattle. *Research in Veterinary Science* 25: 7–12.

Lojda L, Rubes J, Stavikova M, Harsanskova J (1976) Chromosomal findings in some reproductive disorders in bulls. In *Proceedings of 8th International Congress on Animal Reproduction and Artificial Insemination, Krakow* vol 1, p 158.

Long S E (1977) Cytogenetic examination of pre-implantation blastocysts of ewes mated to rams heterozygous for the Massey 1 (t_1) translocation. *Cytogenetics and Cell Genetics* **18**: 82–9.

Long S E (1978) Chiasma counts and non-disjunction frequencies in a normal ram and in rams carrying the Massey I (t_1) Robertsonian translocation. *Journal of Reproduction and Fertility* **53**: 353–6.

Long S E (1985) Centric fusion translocations in cattle: A review. *Veterinary Record* **116**: 516–18.

Long S E (1988) Chromosome anomalies and infertility in the mare. *Equine Veterinary Journal* **20**: 89–93.

Long S E (1993) Incidence of the rob. t(1; 29) centric fusion translocation in British White cattle in Britain. *Veterinary Record* **132**: 165–6.

Love R J, Evans G, Klupiec C (1993) Seasonal effects on fertility in gilts and sows. In Foxcroft G R, Hunter M G, Doberska C (eds) *Control of pig reproduction IV*. The Journals of Reproduction and Fertility Ltd, Cambridge, pp 191–206.

Lynch J J, Hinch G N, Adams D B (1992) *The behaviour of sheep*. CAB International, Wallingford, UK.

McCrea M R (1976) Parameters of breeding and production performance in a closed Clun flock over 13 years. In *Sheep Veterinary Society Proceedings of Meetings 1976–1978*. pp 76–83.

McDonnell S M (1992a) Ejaculation: Physiology and dysfunction. *Veterinary Clinics North America Equine Practice* **8**(1): 57–70.

McDonnell S M (1992b) Normal and abnormal sexual behaviour. *Veterinary Clinics North America Equine Practice* **8**(1): 71–91.

McDonnell S M, Love C C (1990) Manual stimulation collection of semen from stallions: training time, sexual behaviour and semen. *Theriogenology* **33**: 1201.

McFeely R A, Klunder L R, Goldman J B (1988) A Robertsonian translocation in a sow with reduced litter size. In *Proceedings of the 8th European Colloquium on Cytogenetics of Domestic Animals, Bristol*, pp 35–8.

McGladdery A J, Rossdale P D (1992) Ultrasound scanning of the mare for the early diagnosis of pregnancy. *Equine Veterinary Education* **4**(4): 198–203.

McGrath J, Salter D (1983) Nuclear transplantation in the mouse embryo by microsurgery and cell fusion. *Science* **220**: 1300–2.

McKelvey W A C, Robinson J J (1986) Embryo survival and growth in the ewe—recent studies on the effects of nutrition and novel techniques for the recovery and transfer of embryos. In *Annual report of studies in animal nutrition and allied sciences*, vol 41. The Rowett Research Institute, pp 9–25.

McKinnon A O, Squires E L (1988) Equine embryo transfer. *Veterinary Clinics North America Equine Practice* **4**: 305–33.

McLeod B J, Haresign W, Lamming G E (1982) Response of seasonally anoestrous ewes to small-dose multiple injections of GnRH with and without progesterone pretreatment. *Journal of Reproduction and Fertility* **65**: 223–30.

Macmillan K L (1978) Oestrus synchronisation with a prostaglandin analogue. III. Special aspects of synchronisation. *New Zealand Veterinary Journal* **26**: 104–8.

Macmillan K L (1988). Maximizing the use of AI in cattle. In *Proceedings of the XI International Congress on Animal Reproduction and Artificial Insemination*, vol 5, pp 265–75.

McQuirk B (1990) Operational aspects of a MOET nucleus dairy breeding scheme. In *Proceedings of the Fourth World Congress on Genetics applied to Livestock Production*, July 1990, Edinburgh, pp 259–62.

Madan K, Ford C E, Polge C (1978) A reciprocal translocation, t(6p$^+$; 14q$^-$) in the pig. *Journal of Reproduction and Fertility* **53**: 395–8.

Makinen A, Remes E (1986) Low fertility in pigs with rcp(4q$^+$;13q$^-$) translocation. *Hereditas* **104**: 223–9.

Makinen A, Kuokkanen M-T, Niini T, Pertola L (1987) A complex three-break point translocation in the domestic pig. *Acta Veterinaria Scandinavica* **28**: 189–96.

Mansour S L, Thomas K R, Capecchi M R (1988) Disruption of the proto-oncogene *int-2* in mouse embryo-derived stem cells: a general strategy for targeting mutations to non-selectable genes. *Nature* **336**: 348–52.

Marcum J B (1974) The freemartin syndrome. *Animal Breeding Abstracts* **42**: 227–42.

Marcum J B, Lasley J F, Day B N (1972) Variability of sex chromosome chimerism in cattle from heterosexual multiple births. *Cytogenetics* **11**: 388–99.

Marrable A W (1971) *The embryonic pig: a chronological account.* Sir Isaac Pitman and Sons Ltd, London

Martin G B, Oldham C M, Cognie Y, Pearce D T (1986) The physiological responses of anovulatory ewes to the introduction of rams—a review. *Livestock Production Science* **15**: 219–47.

Marx J L (1988) Cloning sheep and cattle embryos. *Science* **239**: 463–4.

Masuda H, Shioya Y, Fukjhara R (1980) Robertsonian translocation in Japanese Black cattle. *Japanese Journal of Zootechnical Science* **51**: 26–32.

Mayr B, Schleger W (1981) Cytogenetic survey in Austrian bulls and boars. *Zentralblatt fur Veterinarmedzin Reihe A* **28**: 70–5.

Mayr B, Themsessel H, Wockl F, Schleger W (1979) Reciprocal translocation, 60, XY, t(10; 11) (41; 14) in cattle. *Zeitschrift fur Tierzuchtung und Zuchtungsbiologie* **96**: 44–7.

Mayr B, Krutzler H, Auer H, Schleger W (1983) Reciprocal translocation 60, XY, t(8; 15) (21; 24) in cattle. *Journal of Reproduction and Fertility* **69**: 629–30.

Meat and Livestock Commission (1981) *Feeding the ewe.* MLC, Milton Keynes.

Meat and Livestock Commission (1982) *Sheep artificial insemination.* MLC, Milton Keynes.

Meat and Livestock Commission (1988) Beef breeding services. In *Beef year book.* Meat and Livestock Commission, pp 75–89.

Meat and Livestock Commission (1989) and (1991) *Sheep yearbook.* MLC, Milton Keynes.

Meat and Livestock Commission (1989) Sheep breeding. In *Sheep yearbook.* Meat and Livestock Commission, pp 69–80.

Meat and Livestock Commission (1990) Update on MLC-funded research projects. In *Sheep yearbook.* Meat and Livestock Commission, pp 67–8.

Meat and Livestock Commission (1992) *Sheep yearbook.* MLC, Milton Keynes.

Memon M A (1983) Male infertility. *Veterinary Clinics of North America: Large Animal Practice* **5**(3): 619–35.

Merck Veterinary Manual, 7th edn (1991) Merck & Co., Inc., Rahway, NJ, pp 1143–50.

Meredith M J (1977) Clinical examination of the ovaries and cervix of the sow. *Veterinary Record* **101**: 70–4.

Meredith M J (1981) Clinical techniques for the examination of infertile sows. *Pig Veterinary Society Proceedings* **8**: 49–53.

Meredith M J (1982) Mating injuries in gilts. In *Proceedings International Pig Veterinary Society, Mexico,* p 210.

Meredith M J (1983) A new approach to the assessment of reproductive performance of commercial pig herds. *Pig News and Information* **4**: 283–7.

Meredith M J (1989) Pregnancy diagnosis in higher performance pig herds—is it a waste of resources? *Pig News and Information* **10**: 477–80.

Meredith M J (1991) Non-specific bacterial infections of the genital tract in female pigs. *Pig Veterinary Journal* **27**: 110–21.

Meredith M J (1994) *Porcine reproductive and respiratory syndrome,* 7th edn, revised January 1994. Pig Disease Information Centre, Cambridge.

Meredith M J, Maddock S J (1995) Porcine reproductive ultrasonography. In Goddard P J (ed) *Veterinary ultrasonography*. CAB International, Wallingford, Oxfordshire.

Meyer K, Brotherstone S, Hill W G (1987) Inheritance of linear type traits in dairy cattle and correlations with milk production. *Animal Production* 44(1): 1–10.

Michiels F, Burmeister M, Lehrach H (1987) Derivation of clones close to met by preparative field inversion gel electrophoresis. *Science* 236: 1305–7.

Milk Marketing Board (1983) *Report of the Breeding and Production Organisation* 33: 50.

Milk Marketing Board (1986) *Report of the Breeding and Production Organisation* 36: 72–5.

Miller J R, Archibald A L (1993) 5′ and 3′ SINE-PCR allows genotyping of pig families without cloning and sequencing steps. *Mammalian Genome* 4: 234–46.

Ministry of Agriculture, Fisheries & Food (1986) *Nutrient allowances for cattle and sheep*. P2087, MAFF Publications, Alnwick.

Miyake Y-I, Kawata K, Ishikawa T, Umezu M (1977) Translocation heterozygosity in a malformed piglet and its normal littermates. *Teratology* 16: 163–6.

Monniaux D, Chupin D, Saumande J (1983) Superovulatory responses of cattle. *Theriogenology* 19: 55–82.

Morrell J M, Dresser D W (1989) Offspring from inseminations with mammalian sperm stained with Hoechst 33342, either with or without flow cytometry. *Mutation Research* 224: 177–83.

Morrison D G, Humes P E, Godke R A (1983) The use of dimenhydrinate in conjunction with dexamethasone for induction of parturition in dairy cattle. *Theriogenology* 19: 221–33.

Morrow D A, Roberts S J, McEntee K (1969) Post partum ovarian activity and involution of uterus and cervix. 1) Ovarian activity. *Cornell Veterinarian* 59: 173–90.

Muirhead M R (1986) Epidemiology and control of vaginal discharges in the sow after service. *Veterinary Record* 119: 233–5.

Mullan B P, Close W H, Cole D J A (1989) Predicting nutrient responses of the lactating sow. In Haresign W, Cole D J A (eds) *Recent advances in animal nutrition—1989*. Butterworth, London, pp 229–43.

Muller Z (1987) Practicalities of insemination of mares with deep-frozen semen. *Journal of Reproduction and Fertility* Suppl. 35: 121.

Mumford J A (1985) Preparing for equine arteritis. *Equine Veterinary Journal* 17: 6–11.

Nakamura Y, Leppert M, O'Connell P, Wolff T, Jolm T, Culver M et al. (1987) Variable number of tandem repeat (VNTR) markers for human gene mapping. *Science* 235: 1616–22.

Nanda A S, Ward W R, Dobson H (1988) A retrospective analysis of the efficacy of different hormone treatments of cystic ovarian disease in cattle. *Veterinary Record* 122: 155–8.

Naude R T, Hofmeyr H S (1981) Meat production. In Gall C (ed) *Goat production*. Academic Press, London, pp 285–307.

Newcomb R, Rowson L E A, Trounson A O (1976) The entry of superovulated eggs into the uterus. In Rowson L E A (ed) *Egg transfer in cattle*. Commission of the European Communities, Luxembourg, pp 1–15.

Nicholas F W (1987) *Veterinary genetics*. Oxford University Press, Oxford, p 387.

Nicholas F W, Smith C (1983) Increased rates of genetic change in dairy cattle by embryo transfer and splitting. *Animal Production* 36(3): 341–53.

Notarianni E, Evans M J (1992) Transgenesis and genetic engineering in domestic animals. In Murray J A H (ed) *Transgenesis: applications of gene transfer*. John Wiley & Sons, Chichester, pp 251–81.

Notarianni E, Laurie S (1992) Embryonic stem cells from domestic animals: establishment and potential applications. In Lauria A, Gandolfi F (eds) *Embryonic development and manipulation in animal production.* Portland Press, London, pp 175–82.

Notarianni E, Galli C, Moor R M, Evans M J (1991) Derivation of pluripotent, embryonic cell lines from pig and sheep. *Journal of Reproduction and Fertility* Suppl. 43: 255–360.

O'Farrell K J (1982) Effects of management factors on the reproductive performance of the postpartum dairy cow. *Current Topics in Veterinary Medicine and Animal Science* 20: 510–29.

O'Farrell K J (1985) Role of management in dairy herd fertility. *Irish Veterinary Journal* 29: 118–24.

Palmer E, Driancourt M A, Ortavant R (1982) Photoperiodic stimulation of the mare during winter anoestrus. *Journal of Reproduction and Fertility* Suppl. 32: 275–82.

Palmiter R D, Brinster R L (1986) Germ line transformation of mice. *Annual Review of Genetics* 20: 465–99.

Palmiter R D, Brinster M, Hammer R E, Trumbauer M E, Rosefeld M G, Birnberg N C *et al.* (1982) Dramatic growth of mice that develop from eggs microinjected with metallothionein–growth hormonal fusion genes. *Nature* 300: 611–15.

Papp M, Kovacs A (1978) Routine chromosomal examination of AI bulls in Hungary. *Annales de Genetique et de Selection Animale* 10: 593.

Papp M, Kovacs A (1980) 5/18 di-centric Robertsonian translocation in a Simmental bull. In *Proceedings of the 4th European Colloquium on Cytogenetics of Domestic Animals, Uppsala,* pp 51–4.

Pardue M L, Gall J G (1970) Chromosomal localisation of mouse satellite DNA. *Science* 168: 1356–8.

Parrat AC, Simm G (1987) Selection indices for terminal sires to improve lean meat production from sheep in the United Kingdom. *Animal Production* 45(1): 87–96.

Pascoe R R (1979) Observations on the length and angle of declination of the vulva and its relation to fertility in the mare. *Journal of Reproduction and Fertility* Suppl. 27: 229–305.

Paterson A M, Pearce G P (1990) Attainment of puberty in domestic gilts reared under long-day or short-day artificial light regimes. *Animal Reproduction Science* 23: 135–44.

Paterson A M, Martin G B, Foldes A, Maxwell C A, Pearce G P (1992) Concentrations of plasma melatonin and luteinizing hormone in domestic gilts under artificial long or short days. *Journal of Reproduction and Fertility* 94: 85–95.

Pearce P D, Ansari H A, Maher D W (1990) Two new centric fusions in domestic sheep. *Proceedings 9th European Colloquium on Cytogenetics of Domestic Animals, Toulouse, France, 7–13 July, 1990,* Abstract 26.

Pearson A M (1988) Managing the modern boar. *Pig Veterinary Society Proceedings* 21: 67–72.

Pepper R T, Dobson H (1987) Preliminary results of treatment and endocrinology of chronic endometritis in the dairy cow. *Veterinary Record* 120: 53–6.

Perry P, Wolff S (1974) New giemsa method for the differential staining of sister chromatids. *Nature* 251: 156–8.

Peura T, Aalto J, Hyttinen J M, Rainio V, Turunen M, Janne J (1991) Birth of calves developed from embryos of predetermined sex. *Acta Veterinaria Scandinavica* 32: 283–6.

Pickett B W, Voss J L, Squires E L, Aman (1981) *Maximising reproductive efficiency in the stallion.* Colorado State University Press.

Piedrahita J A, Anderson G B, Martin G R, BonDurant R H, Pashen R L (1988) Isolation of embryonic stem cell-line colonies from porcine embryos (abstract). *Theriogenology* 29: 286.

Pigplan Management Services (1994) *Quarterly Data Sheet 94/1.* Meat and Livestock Commission, Milton Keynes.

Piper L R, Bindon B M, Davis G H (1985) The single gene inheritance in the prolificacy of the Booroola Merino. In Land R B, Robinson D W (eds) *The genetics of reproduction in sheep.* Butterworths, London, pp 115–25.

Pirchner F (1985) Genetic structure of populations. In Chapman A B (ed) *General and quantitative genetics.* Elsevier, Amsterdam, pp 227–48.

Polge E J C, Barton S C, Surani M A H, Miller J R, Wagner T, Rottman F *et al.* (1989) Induced expression of a bovine growth hormone construct in transgenic pigs. In Heap, Prosser and Lamming (eds) *Biotechnology in growth regulation.* Butterworths, London, pp 189–99.

Pollock D L, Bowman J C (1974) A Robertsonian translocation in British Friesian cattle. *Journal of Reproduction and Fertility* 40: 423–32.

Pollott G E, Kilkenny J B (1976) A note on the use of condition scoring in commercial sheep flocks. *Animal Production* 23: 261–4.

Pope W F, Xie S, Broermann D M, Nephew K P (1990) Causes and consequences of early embryonic diversity in pigs. In Cole D J A, Foxcroft G R, Weir B J (eds) *Control of pig reproduction.* Journals of Reproduction and Fertility Ltd, Cambridge, pp 251–60.

Popescu C P (1977) A new type of Robertsonian translocation in cattle. *Journal of Heredity* 68: 139–42.

Popescu C P, Boscher J (1982) Cytogenetics of pre-implantation embryos produced by pigs heterozygous for the reciprocal translocation ($4q^+$; $14q^-$). *Cytogenetics and Cell Genetics* 34: 119–23.

Popescu C P, Boscher J (1986) A new reciprocal translocation in a hypoprolific boar. *Genetique Selection Evolution* 18: 123–30.

Popescu C P, Legault C (1979) Une nouvelle translocation reciproque t($4q^-$; $14q^-$) chez le porc domestique (*Sus scrofa domestica*). *Annales de Genetique et de Selection Animale* 11: 361–9.

Popescu C P, Boscher J, Tixier M (1983) Une nouvelle translocation reciproque t($7q^-$; $15q^+$) chez un verrat 'hypoprolifique'. *Genetique Selection Evolution* 15: 479–88.

Popescu C P, Bonneau M, Tixier M, Bahri I, Boscher J (1984) Reciprocal translocations in pigs. Their detection and consequences on animal performance and economic losses. *Journal of Heredity* 75: 448–52.

Pouret E J M (1982) Surgical technique for the correction of pneumo- and urovagina. *Equine Veterinary Journal* 14: 249–50.

Power M M (1986) XY sex reversal in a mare. *Equine Veterinary Journal* 18: 233–6.

Prather R S, First N L (1989) Nuclear transfer in mammalian embryos. *International Reviews of Cytology* (in press).

Prather R S, Barnes F L, Sims M M, Robl J M, Eyestone W H, First N L (1987) Nuclear transplantation in the bovine embryo: assessment of donor nuclei and recipient oocyte. *Biology of Reproduction* 37: 859–66.

Pursel V G, Pinkert C A, Miller K F, Bolt D J, Campbell R G, Palmiter R D *et al.* (1989) Genetic engineering of livestock. *Science* 244: 1281–8.

Pursel V G, Hammer R E, Bolt R E, Palmiter R D, Brinster R L (1990) Integration, expression and germ-line transmission of growth-related genes in pigs. *Journal of Reproduction and Fertility* Suppl. 41: 173–82.

Radostits O M, Blood D C (1985) *Herd health.* W B Saunders, Philadelphia.

Rahe C H, Owens R E, Fleeger J C, Newton H J, Harms P G (1980) Pattern of plasma luteinizing hormone in the cystic cow: dependence upon the period of cycle. *Endocrinology* 107: 498–503.

Ral G, Andersson K, Sundgren P E (1978) Crossbreeding effects in practical pig production. EAAP Meeting, Stockholm, June 1978.

Rantanen N W, Kincaid B (1988) Ultrasound guided foetal cardiac puncture: A method of twin reduction in the mare. In *Proceedings 34th Annual Convention Association Equine Practitioners*, pp 173–80.

Ricketts S W (1989) The barren mare: Diagnosis, prognosis, prophylaxis and treatment for genital abnormality. Part 1&2. *In Practice* 11: 119–25 and 156–64.

Ricketts S W, Alonso S (1991) Assessment of the breeding prognosis of mares using paired endometrial biopsy techniques. *Equine Veterinary Journal* 23: 185–8.

Ricketts S W, Alonso S (1991) The effect of age and parity on the development of equine chronic endometrial disease. *Equine Veterinary Journal* 23: 189–92.

Ricketts S W, Young A, Medici E B (1993) Uterine and clitoral cultures. In *Equine reproduction*. Lea and Febiger, Philadelphia, pp 234–45.

Ricordeau G (1981) Genetics: breeding plans. In Gall C (ed) *Goat production*. Academic Press, London, pp 111–69.

Roberts S J (1986) *Veterinary obstetrics and genital diseases (theriogenology)*. David and Charles, North Pomfret, Vermont.

Roberts S J (1986) *Veterinary obstetrics and genital diseases*. Published by the author, Woodstock, Vermont, p 21.

Robertson E J (1987) *Teratocarcinomas and embryonic stem cells: a practical approach*. IRL Press, Oxford.

Robl J M, Gilligan B, Critser E S, First N L (1986) Nuclear transplantation in mouse embryos: assessment of recipient cell stages. *Biology of Reproduction* 34: 733–9.

Robl J M, Prather R, Barnes F, Eyestone W, Northey D, Gilligan B *et al.* (1987) Nuclear transplantation in bovine embryos. *Journal of Animal Science* 64: 642–7.

Roche J F, Ireland J J (1984) Manipulation of ovulation in cattle. In *Proceedings of 10th International Congress on Animal Reproduction and A.I.*, vol 4, IV-9–IV-17.

Roldan E R S, Meroni M S, Lauzewitsch I V (1984) Two abnormal chromosomes found in one cell line of a mosaic cow with low fertility. *Genetique Selection Evolution* 16: 136–42.

Russel A J F (1985) Nutrition of the pregnant ewe. *In Practice* 7(1): 23–8.

Sasser R G, Ruder C A, Ivani K A, Butler J E, Hamilton W C (1986) Detection of pregnancy by RIA of a novel pregnancy specific protein in serum of cows and a profile of serum concentrations during gestation. *Biology of Reproduction* 35: 936–42.

Scaramuzzi R J, Campbell B K, Cognie Y, Downing J A (1987) Applications of immunological techniques to enhance reproductive performance in the ewe. In Fayez M M, Owen J B (eds) *New techniques in sheep production*. Butterworths, London, pp 47–56.

Schanbacher B D, Ford J J (1976) Seasonal profiles of plasma luteinizing hormone, testosterone and estradiol in the ram. *Endocrinology* 99: 752–7.

Schepper G C de, Aalbers J G, te Brake J H A (1982) Double reciprocal translocation heterozygosity in a bull. *Veterinary Record* 110: 197–9.

Schwartz D C, Cantor C R (1984) Separation of yeast chromosome-size DNAs by pulsed field gel electrophoresis. *Cell* 37: 67–75.

Schwerin M, Golisch D, Ritter E (1986) A Robertsonian translocation in swine. *Genetique Selection Evolution* 18: 367–74.

Scott H M, Ferguson J A, Pastrana R, Madani M O K, Williams H L (1983) A study of infertility in Scottish Blackface sheep in Colombia, South America. *British Veterinary Journal* 139: 349–54.

Seabright M (1972a) The use of proteolytic enzymes for the mapping of structural rearrangements in the chromosomes of man. *Chromosoma* 36: 204–10.

Seabright M (1972b) Human chromosome banding. *Lancet* i: 967.

Sharp A J, Wachtel S S, Benirschke K (1980) H-Y antigen in a fertile XY female horse. *Journal of Reproduction and Fertility* 58: 157–60.

References

Shelton M (1986) Abortion in Angora goats. In Morrow D A (ed) *Current therapy in theriogenology 2.* W B Saunders, Philadelphia, pp 610–12.

Shelton M, Groff J L (1984) Reproductive efficiency in Angora goats. Texas Agricultural Experiment Station Bulletin 1485.

Shelton M, Stewart J (1973) Partitioning losses in reproductive efficiency in Angora goats. Texas Agricultural Experiment Station Bulletin PR-3187.

Silver M (1987) Successful induction of labour in sheep. *Veterinary Record* **120**: 299–300.

Simm G, Smith C, Prescott J H D (1986) Selection indices to improve the efficiency of lean meat production in cattle. *Animal Production* **42**(2): 183–93.

Simons J P, Land R B (1987) Transgenic livestock. *Journal of Reproduction and Fertility* Suppl. 34: 237–50.

Simons J P, McClenaghan M, Clark A J (1987) Alteration of the quality of milk by expression of a sheep ß-lactoglobulin gene in transgenic mice. *Nature* **328**: 530–2.

Simons J P, Wilmut I, Clark A J, Archibald A L, Bishop J O, Lathe R (1988) Gene transfer into sheep. *Biotechnology* **6**: 179–83.

Simpson D J (1987) Venereal diseases of mares. In Robinson N E (ed) *Current therapy in equine medicine*, 2nd edn. W B Saunders, Philadelphia.

Sirad M A, Parrish J J, Ware C B, Leibfried-Rutledge M L, First N L (1988) The culture of bovine embryos to obtain developmentally competent embryos. *Biology of Reproduction* **39**: 546–52.

Smith A G, Heath J K, Donaldson D D, Wong G G, Moreau J, Stahl M *et al.* (1988) Inhibition of pluripotential embryonic stem cell differentiation by purified polypeptides. *Nature* **336**: 668–90.

Smith C, King J W B (1962) Genetic parameters of British Large White bacon pigs. *Animal Production* **4**(1): 128–43.

Smith C, Ross G J S (1965) Genetic parameters of British Landrace bacon pigs. *Animal Production* **7**(3): 291–301.

Smith G S, Van Camp S D, Basrur P K (1977) A fertile female co-twin to a male calf. *Canadian Veterinary Journal* **18**: 287–9.

Smith J F (1985) Protein, energy and ovulation rate. In Land R B, Robinson D W (eds) *Genetics of reproduction in sheep.* Butterworths, London.

Smith K C (1991) Mating patterns and reproductive wastage. In *Sheep Veterinary Society Proceedings of Meetings 1991*, vol **15**, pp 103–8.

Smith K C (1995) Diagnostic aids in reproductively abnormal ewes. In: *Sheep Veterinary Society Proceedings of Meetings 1993–94*, **18**, 175–9.

Smith L C, Wilmut I (1989) Influence of nuclear and cytoplasmic activity on the development *in vivo* of sheep embryos after nuclear transplantation. *Biology of Reproduction* **40**: 1027–35.

Smith L C, Wilmut I (1990) Factors affecting the viability of nuclear transplanted embryos. *Theriogenology* **33**: 153–62.

Smith L C, Wilmut I, Hunter R H F (1988) Influence of cell cycle stage at nuclear transplantation on the development *in vitro* of mouse embryos. *Journal of Reproduction and Fertility* **84**: 619–24.

Smith M C (1986) Causes and diagnosis of abortion in goats. In Morrow D A (ed) *Current therapy in theriogenology 2.* W B Saunders, Philadelphia.

Smith M C, Sherman D M (1994) Reproductive system. In: *Goat Medicine*, Lea & Febiger, Philadelphia.

Spence J, Aitchinson G (1986) Clinical aspects of dental disease in sheep. *In Practice* **8**(4): 128–35.

Squires E L (1993) Embryo transfer. In *Equine reproduction.* Lea and Febiger, Philadelphia, pp 357–67.

Stashak T S, Vandeplassche M (1993) *Cesarean section in equine reproduction.* Lea and Febiger, Philadelphia, pp 437–43.

Stranzinger G F, Forster M (1976) Autosomal translocations in German

Simmental and German brown cattle. *Experientia* **32**: 24–7.

Succi G, de Giovanni Macchi A M, Molteni L (1982) Preliminary observations on the influence of 25/27 translocation on fertility and milk production of grey alpine cows. In *Proceedings of the 5th European Colloquium on Cytogenetics of Domestic Animals, Milan*, pp 142–7.

Sumner A T (1972) A simple technique for demonstrating centromeric heterochromatin. *Experimental Cell Research* **75**: 304–6.

Surani M A H, Barton S C, Norris M L (1984) Development of reconstituted mouse eggs suggests imprinting of the genome during gametogenesis. *Nature* **308**: 548–50.

Symons A M, Arendt J, Poulton A L, English J (1988) The induction of ovulation with melatonin. In *Proceedings 11th International Congress on Animal Reproduction and A.I., Dublin*, vol 5, pp 155–9.

Tarkowski A K, Balakier H (1980) Nucleo-cytoplasmic interactions in cell hybrids between mouse oocytes, blastomeres and somatic cells. *Journal of Embryology and Experimental Morphology* **55**: 319–30.

Tarocco C, Franchi F, Croci G (1987) A new reciprocal translocation involving chromosomes 1/14 in boar. *Genetique Selection Evolution* **19**: 381–6.

Taylor D J (1989) *Pig diseases*, 5th edn. Published by the author, Glasgow.

Thatcher W W, Hansen P J, Bazer F W (1988) Role of the conceptus in the establishment of pregnancy. In *Proceedings of 11th International Congress on Animal Reproduction and A.I., Dublin*, vol 5, pp 45–54.

Thomas K R, Capecchi M R (1987) Site-directed mutagenesis by gene targeting in mouse embryo-derived stem cells. *Cell* **51**: 503–12.

Thoroughbred Breeders Association (1992) *A code of practice for the control of Equine Viral Arteritis (E.V.A.), Contagious Equine Metritis (C.E.M.) and other equine venereal diseases for 1992 covering season in France, Germany, Ireland, Italy and the U.K. U.K. code for Equine Herpes Virus 1 infections.*

Tielgy A H, Fathalla M, Omar M A, Al-Dahash S (1982) The clinical and morphological characteristics of the uterus of the goat during the period of involution. *Canadian Veterinary Journal* **23**: 138–40.

Tjio J H, Whang J (1962) Chromosome preparations of bone marrow cells without prior *in vitro* culture or *in vivo* colchicine administration. *Stain Technology* **37**: 17–21.

Trower C J (1991) The induction of parturition in ewes as an aid to flock management. In *Sheep Veterinary Society Proceedings of Meetings 1991*, vol 15, pp 109–12.

Tschudi P, Zahner B, Kupfer U, Stampfli G (1977) Chromosomenuntersuchungen an schweizerischen Rinderrassen. *Schweizer Archiv fur Tierheilkunde, Switzerland* **119**: 329–36.

Tzocheva K (1990) A new reciprocal chromosome translocation ($1p^-$; $11p^+$) in a boar karyotype. In *Proceedings of the 9th European Colloquium on Cytogenetics of Domestic Animals, Toulouse, France, July 7–13*, Abstract 29.

Umberger S H, Lewis G S (1992) Melengestrol acetate (MGA) for estrous synchronization and induction of estrus in spring-breeding ewes. *Sheep Research Journal* **8**(2): 59–62.

Van Brunt J (1988) Molecular farming: transgenic animals as bioreactors. *Biotechnology* **6**: 1149–54.

Van Camp S C (1988) Endometrial biopsy of the mare: A review and update. *Veterinary Clinics North America Equine Practice* **4**(2): 229–46.

Vandeplassche M (1980) Obstetrician's view of the physiology of equine parturition and dystocia. *Equine Veterinary Journal* **12**: 45.

Van Rensburg S W J, de Vos W H (1962) Ovulatory failure in bovines. *Onderstepoort Journal of Veterinary Research* **29**: 55–79.

Varley M A, Foxcroft G R (1990) Endocrinology of the lactating and weaned sow. In Cole D J A, Foxcroft

G R, Weir B J (eds) *Control of pig reproduction*. Journals of Reproduction and Fertility Ltd, Cambridge, pp 47–61.

Villagomez D A F, Gustavsson I, Ploen L (1991a) Synaptonemal complex analysis of reciprocal chromosome translocations in the domestic pig. *Genetics Selection Evolution* 23 (suppl. 1): 217s–21s.

Villagomez D A F, Switonski M, Singh B, Fisher K R S, Gustavsson I, Basrur P K (1991b) Synaptonemal complex analysis of an X–autosome translocation carrier in the domestic pig. *Genetics Selection Evolution* 23 (suppl. 1): 222s–5s.

Vize P D, Michalska A E, Ashman R, Lloyd B, Stone B A, Quinn P et al. (1988) Introduction of a porcine growth hormone fusion gene into transgenic pigs promotes growth. *Journal of Cell Science* 90: 295–300.

Walkland C (1992) Durocs add quality, but at a price. *Pig Farming* 40(3): 19–20.

Wall R J, Pursel V G, Hammer R E, Brinster R L (1985) Development of porcine ova that were centrifuged to permit visualization of pronuclei and nuclei. *Biology of Reproduction* 32: 645–51.

Wassarman P M, Bleil J D, Cascio J D, La Marca M J, Letourneau G E, Mrozak S C et al. (1981) Programming of gene expression during mammalian oogenesis. In Jagiello G, Vogel H J (eds) *Bioregulators of reproduction*. Academic Press, New York, pp 119–50.

Watkins P C (1988) Restriction fragment length polymorphism (RFLP): applications in human chromosomal mapping and genetic disorder research. *Biotechniques* 6: 310–18.

Watson E D (1988) Uterine defence mechanisms in mares resistant and susceptible to persistent endometritis: A review. *Equine Veterinary Journal* 20: 397–400.

Webb R, Lamming G E, Haynes N B, Hafs H D, Manns J G (1977) Response of cyclic and postpartum suckled cows to injections of synthetic LH-RH. *Journal of Reproduction and Fertility* 50: 203–10.

Weber J A, Woods G L (1992) Transrectal ultrasonography for the evaluation of stallion accessory sex glands. *Veterinary Clinics North America Equine Practice* 8(1): 183–90.

Webster G M and Haresign W (1981) A note on the use of Dexamethasone to induce parturition in the ewe. *Animal Production* 32: 341–44.

White R A S, Allen W R (1985) Use of ultrasound echography for the differential diagnosis of a granulosa cell tumour in a mare. *Equine Veterinary Journal* 17: 401–2.

Whittemore C (1993) *The science and practice of pig production*. Longman, Harlow.

Whitwell K E (1980) Investigations into foetal and neonatal losses in the horse. *Veterinary Clinics North America* 2: 313.

Willadsen S M (1986) Nuclear transplantation in sheep embryos. *Nature* 320: 63–5.

Williams H Ll (1977) Environmental control of oestrus with particular attention to alterations of daylength. In *Proceedings 28th Annual Meeting of the European Association of Animal Production, Brussels*. M-SG/5.04, pp 1–6.

Williams H Ll (1984) The effects of the physical and social environments on reproduction in adult sheep and goats. In *Proceedings of the 10th International Congress on Animal Reproduction and Artificial Insemination, Illinois, USA*, vol IV, pp 31–8.

Williams H Ll (1994a) Facilities for handling intensively managed sheep. In Grandier T (ed) *Livestock handling and transport*. CAB International, Wallingford, UK, pp 159–78.

Williams H Ll (1994b) Sheep and melatonin. In Raw M E, Parkinson T J (eds) *The Veterinary Annual*, vol 34, pp 58–70.

Williams H Ll, Hanif M (1990) The use of melatonin in the preparation of rams for out-of-season breeding. In *Sheep Veterinary Society Proceedings of Meetings 1989–90*, vol 14, pp 113–16.

Williams H Ll, Ward S J (1988) Melatonin and light treatment of ewes for autumn lambing. *Reproduction, Nutrition, Development* **28**: 79–85.

Wilmut I (1986) Cryopreservation of mammalian eggs and embryo. In Gwatkin R B L (ed) *Manipulation of mammalian development.* Plenum Press, New York, pp 217–47.

Wilmut I (1987) Embryo transfer. In Fayez I, Marai M, Owen J B (eds.) *New techniques in sheep production.* Butterworths, London, pp 79–89.

Wilmut I, Smith L C (1988) Biotechnology and the bovine embryo: at present and in the future. In *Proceedings of the 4th Congress of the European Embryo Transfer Association.* European Embryo Transfer Association, Lyon, France, pp 19–31.

Wilmut I, Ashworth C J, Sales D I (1985) The influence of embryo stage and maternal hormone profiles on embryo survival in farm animals. *Theriogenology* **23**: 107–20.

Wilmut I, Sales D I, Ainsworth C J (1986) Maternal and embryonic factors associated with prenatal loss in mammals. *Journal of Reproduction and Fertility* **76**: 851–64.

Wilsmore A J (1986) Birth injury in a flock of Poll Dorset ewes. *British Veterinary Journal* **142**: 233–7.

Wilsmore A J (1989) Birth injury and perinatal loss in lambs. *In Practice* **11**(6): 239–43.

Wilson T D (1990) Identification of the 1/29 Robertsonian translocation chromosome in British Friesian cattle. *Veterinary Record* **126**: 37–9.

Wingfield Digby N J (1978) The technique and clinical application of endometrial cytology in mares. *Equine Veterinary Journal* **10**: 167–70.

Wingfield Digby N J, Ricketts S W (1982) A method for clitoral sinusectomy. *In Practice* **4**: 145.

Winqvist G (1954) Morphology of the blood and the haemopoietic organs in cattle under normal and some experimental conditions. *Acta Anatomica* Suppl. 21: 1–22.

Wright G, Carver A, Cotton D, Reeves D, Scott A, Simons P et al. (1991) High level expression of active human alpha-1-antitrypsin in the milk of transgenic sheep. *Bio/Technology* **9**: 830–4.

Xu K P, Greve T, Smith S, Hyttel P (1986) Chronological changes of bovine follicular oocyte maturation *in vitro. Acta Veterinaria Scandinavica* 27: 505–19.

Yang H, Solinas S, Jung H R, Bolt R, Fries R, Stranzinger G (1991) *Proceedings of 7th North American Colloquium on Domestic Animal Cytogenetics and Gene Mapping, (Philadelphia, PA, July 8–11),* p 6.

Young I M, Anderson D B (1986) First service conception rate in dairy cows treated with dinoprost tromethamine early post partum. *Veterinary Record* **118**: 212–13.

Zang J, Ricketts S W, Tanner S J (1990) Antisperm antibodies in the semen of a stallion following testicular trauma. *Equine Veterinary Journal* **22**: 138–41.

Zimmer A, Grüss P (1989) Production of chimaeric mice containing embryonic stem (ES) cells carrying a homeobox Hox 1.1 allele mutated by homologous recombination. *Nature* **338**: 150–5.

INDEX

Index

Index

Index